Vitreoretinal Surgery

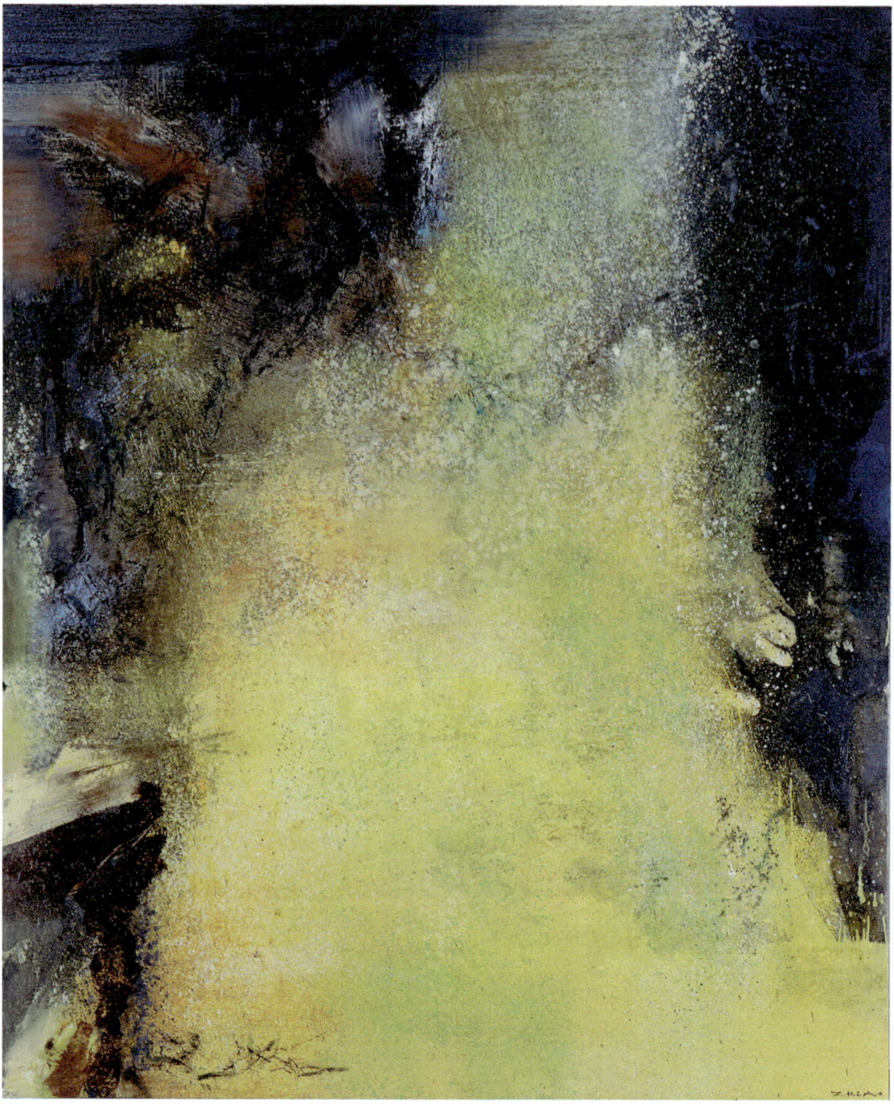

An oil painting by Zao Wou-Ki embodies the harmonious coexistence of tranquility and passion, as well as the boundless vitality born from their fusion. For us as vitreoretinal surgeons, these same qualities are essential to our craft.

ZAO Wou-Ki (1920–2013)
25.04.88, 1988
Oil on canvas, 200 × 162 cm
Private collection

Zhaotian Zhang • Ulrich Spandau

Vitreoretinal Surgery

Underlying Logic and Basic Skill

Springer

Zhaotian Zhang
Zhongshan Ophthalmic Center
Sun Yat-Sen University
Guangzhou, China

Ulrich Spandau
Ophthalmology
University of Uppsala
Uppsala, Uppsala Län, Sweden

ISBN 978-3-032-25270-8 ISBN 978-3-032-25271-5 (eBook)
https://doi.org/10.1007/978-3-032-25271-5

This Springer imprint is published by the registered company Springer Nature Switzerland AG
The registered company address is: Gewerbestrasse 11, 6330 Cham, Switzerland

This book is dedicated to my mentor, Professor Shaochong Zhang, with thanks for his kindness and motivation; to my idols, the painter Zao Wou-Ki and the architect I.M. Pei, for their inspiration in bridging East and West; to my dear friends Ulrich Spandau and Geoffrey Emerson for their great encouragement; to every colleague at Zhongshan Ophthalmic Center for their constant support; and to my family, for their unfading love.

—Zhaotian Zhang, MD, FASRS

Foreword 1

It is a pleasure to introduce this textbook of retinal surgery techniques for my friends and colleagues, Zhaotian Zhang and Ulrich Spandau.

This book offers introspective guidance for aspiring retina surgeons as they embark on and mature in their careers, emphasizing continuous learning, resilience, and composure. Retina surgery is a field that blends profound reward with frequent challenge and periodic failure.

Learning and mastering vitreoretinal surgery requires both solid theoretical knowledge and extensive practical training. There is no substitute for surgical experience and great mentors. Surgeons must cultivate deep understanding, humility, and patience—prioritizing careful judgment over speed.

The learning curve of a retinal surgeon is steep. Even steps that seem simple at first can hide complexity and risk. An open-minded and pragmatic attitude is essential in surgery, so that we may adapt to new techniques in an ever-changing field. Nevertheless, surgical situations are not always predictable. Sometimes a surgeon can surmount a tricky situation by remembering an old technique, or a case they saw or heard of from a predecessor.

Vitreoretinal surgery remains a growing and demanding field. The authors encourage approaching it with optimism, respect, and a commitment to technical excellence as well as compassion for patients. As an aspiring surgeon myself, I appreciate this philosophy and take it to heart. I am also grateful to have this insightful and comprehensive text at my side for moments when I need a suggestion or even a quick review of the basics. Thank you and bravo, Zhaotian and Ulrich.

Minneapolis, MN, USA — Geoffrey G. Emerson, MD, PhD

Foreword 2

In the intricate microcosm of the eye, vitreoretinal surgery represents one of medicine's most profound intersections of art and science. It is a discipline in constant flux, where technological innovation and refined clinical wisdom converge to restore not just sight, but hope for millions. This book, a collaborative endeavor between leading experts from Uppsala University Hospital and the Zhongshan Ophthalmic Center (ZOC), is conceived in this very spirit of dynamic evolution.

It is a natural extension of the Bright-X—a cultural and strategic philosophy I have distilled to guide our mission at ZOC. The name Bright-X encapsulates a dual commitment: intellectually, it stands for Borrow & Build, Road & Reach, Intelligence & Integration, Global & Governance, Health & Happy, Technology & Talent, and Cross & Unknown. Politically, it resonates with a broader vision: Belt & Road Initiative: Great Health Together. It is our belief that by illuminating the path for global ophthalmology, we can advance the health of nations along the Belt and Road and beyond, fostering a world where shared knowledge leads to shared well-being.

As the largest public ophthalmic hospital in China, the sole ophthalmic specialty hospital administered by China's National Health Commission, and the World Health Organization Collaborating Center for Eye Care and Vision in China, ZOC has long been recognized as a leader in ophthalmic care. In November 2024, we took another historic step forward with the official inauguration of the International Ophthalmology Medical Center, a landmark initiative designed to serve as a global platform for cutting-edge research, talent cultivation, and cross-border collaboration in eye health.

Our commitment to research excellence is reflected in our sustained global impact. According to the Nature Index annual rankings, ZOC has ranked first in the world among all ophthalmic institutions for three consecutive years since 2023. This unprecedented achievement in both Health Sciences and Biological Sciences underscores our dedication to advancing the frontiers of ophthalmic science and translating discovery into clinical impact on a global scale.

Beyond our research and clinical achievements, ZOC takes pride in its role as a bridge connecting ophthalmic communities across continents. As the headquarters of the Asia-Pacific Academy of Ophthalmology and the President Office of the Afro-Asian Council of Ophthalmology, we have long served as a convening force for dialogue and collaboration among eye care professionals across Asia, Africa, Europe, and the Americas.

The foundation of this work is rooted in Borrow & Build. It respectfully borrows from the foundational knowledge laid by pioneers while building upon it with the rich, collective clinical experience of both Chinese and European masters. By weaving together the vast surgical volumes seen at ZOC with the refined techniques of Uppsala, we have built a guide that transcends any single institution's perspective.

This book, therefore, paves a new Road & Reach. It charts a clear educational pathway for surgeons at every level, from the novice grasping the underlying logic of vitrectomy to the seasoned expert navigating complex pathologies. Our reach extends from our operating rooms in Guangzhou and Uppsala to the global community, embodying the "Road" in our philosophy—connecting colleagues and patients across continents in a shared pursuit of excellence.

This endeavor is powered by Intelligence & Integration. The book integrates core physical principles with cutting-edge surgical methodologies. But more than that, it reflects a deep integration of minds—combining European rigor with Asian innovation to foster the clinical intelligence that defines wise, adaptable surgeons.

As a World Health Organization Collaborating Center and the headquarters of leading international ophthalmic societies, ZOC bears a profound responsibility in the realm of Global & Governance. This book is a tangible expression of our commitment to global eye health governance. By sharing knowledge and setting educational benchmarks, we actively contribute to the "Great Health Together" vision, fostering the cross-border collaboration essential to addressing the universal challenge of blindness.

Ultimately, our goal is Health & Happy. Every principle detailed, every technique analyzed, is in service of this singular outcome: restoring healthy vision and, with it, the happiness and quality of life for patients worldwide.

This achievement would not be possible without our most valuable asset: our people. It underscores the critical importance of Technology & Talent. While we embrace technological advancement, we firmly believe it is most powerful when wielded by talented, well-trained hands—the very hands this book seeks to cultivate.

Finally, this project is a venture into the Cross & Unknown. It is a cross-cultural partnership that enriches us all. By venturing into the unknown territories of complex diseases together, we model the very collaboration that will unlock the future of medicine.

Published with Springer Nature, this book marks a significant milestone in ZOC's journey as a global leader in ophthalmology. It is our hope that *Vitreoretinal Surgery: Underlying Logic and Basic Skill* serves not as an endpoint, but as a catalyst for future discoveries. At ZOC, we stand ready to deepen these global partnerships, to share Chinese wisdom and Asian solutions, and to continue our shared journey toward a world where no one is needlessly blind.

Director, Zhongshan Ophthalmic Center (ZOC) Hao-tian Lin, MD
President, Zhongshan Ophthalmic Center Hospital
Sun Yat-sen University
Guangzhou, China

Preface

Vitreoretinal surgery demands a high level of both manual precision and mental clarity. It's a field where miracles can be created to bring light and hope to darkness and desperation. For retina surgeons, mastering vitreoretinal surgery requires a long learning process, a steep learning curve, and the ability to shoulder immense responsibility. Yet, it is also a field filled with obstacles and challenges, while bringing a unique sense of professional accomplishment.

Over the past century, vitreoretinal surgery has undergone tremendous development. What was once regarded as an inaccessible and uncertain territory has gradually become a mature surgical discipline due to the refined instruments, improved visualization systems, and increasingly sophisticated surgical concepts. Many pioneers devoted their lives to exploring this field, despite the conditions being far less favorable than we enjoy today. Their perseverance transformed the treatment of retinal diseases from an uncertain attempt into a reliable and effective surgical practice.

Despite the achievements up till now, vitreoretinal surgery remains the Benben stone of the pyramid of ophthalmology. The eye is a delicate and complex organ, offering the narrow confines of the vitreous cavity and unstable intraocular environments for retinal surgeons to repair the fragile tissues. Each case is quite unique, and the surgeon is required to make decisions before, during, and after surgery. In such circumstances, technique alone is inadequate.

Many young surgeons begin their training by memorizing surgical steps. They learn how to set up the machine, where to place the trocars, how to perform fluid–air exchange, and how to apply laser photocoagulation. These steps are necessary but not sufficient. When facing unexpected situations—an undetected retinal break, a sudden hemorrhage, or an unstable intraocular pressure—repetition of standard procedures will not get you out of the trap. At that moment, only a clear understanding of the underlying logic can guide the surgeon forward.

The essence of vitreoretinal surgery is not a sequence of movements, but a way of thinking. Each surgical maneuver is a response to the physical, anatomical, and pathological conditions inside the eye. The behavior of fluids, the elasticity of tissues, and the interaction between instruments and intraocular structures all follow certain principles. If these principles are understood, the surgery becomes logical and coherent. If ignored, even the skillful hands may encounter unnecessary difficulties.

During years of clinical practice and teaching, we have observed that many trainees struggle not because of their lack of diligence, but because of their lack of understanding of the underlying principles. They could perform well in routine cases, but may get stuck when conditions deviate from the expected pattern.

This book, coauthored by two experienced retina surgeons from China and Europe, is born from a conviction that the advancement of surgical care thrives on the synthesis of diverse experiences, philosophies, and techniques. It represents a deliberate effort to bridge geographical and methodological perspectives, bringing together the rich, evolving narrative of vitreoretinal surgery in China with the established and innovative practices from Europe.

We hope to present vitreoretinal surgery as an integrated discipline, in which theory and practice are inseparable. Each chapter attempts to answer not only the question of how a procedure is performed, but also why it should be performed. By understanding the reasoning behind each step, the reader may develop the ability to adapt to different situations and to make sound surgical decisions.

Another important intention of this book is to promote the exchange of surgical experience across different regions. Vitreoretinal surgery has developed along diverse paths due to variations in training systems, different clinical environments and technological resources, which have led to different surgical philosophies and techniques. These differences should not be considered as contradictions, but as valuable sources of knowledge.

This book brings together experiences from both China and Europe. By presenting these perspectives side by side, we hope to provide readers with a broader understanding of vitreoretinal surgery. Exchanging clinical experiences is particularly important in the current epoch, when scientific communication is no longer limited by geography. The progress of medicine depends on openness, collaboration, and the willingness to learn from one another.

The first part of this book focuses on the conceptual foundations and practical principles of vitreoretinal surgery. It begins with the historical development and the contributions of major pioneers. It then introduces the physical principles that govern intraocular surgery, the evolution and characteristics of tamponade agents, and essential aspects of preoperative evaluation. Subsequent chapters discuss common surgical conditions, including retinal detachment, proliferative diabetic retinopathy, epiretinal membrane, macular hole, and proliferative vitreoretinopathy. Special attention is given to challenging situations and pediatric cases, where careful judgment is especially important.

Recognizing the growing importance of digital communication, a chapter is also devoted to the editing and sharing of surgical videos. Currently, surgical videos have become an essential medium for education and academic communication in ophthalmology. Learning how to present surgical work clearly and responsibly is of great importance during a surgeon's professional development.

The second part of the book presents vitreoretinal techniques and experiences from Europe. These chapters illustrate different approaches to both routine and complex surgeries, offering readers alternative perspectives and practical insights. By comparing different strategies, surgeons may better understand the strengths and limitations of each approach and make adaptations based on their own clinical environments.

This book is the brainchild of close collaboration among colleagues from different countries. Such cooperation reflects the spirit of modern medicine, where knowledge is shared across borders for the benefit of patients worldwide. We are deeply grateful to all contributors who generously shared their experience and wisdom.

We also acknowledge the mentors who guided us at the beginning of our surgical careers. Their patience, strictness, and encouragement shaped our professional attitudes and surgical habits. Above all, we thank all our patients. Each surgical improvement, every new technique, and every lesson learned in the operating room ultimately come from the trust they place in us.

Vitreoretinal surgery is a lifelong journey. It requires not only technical skill, but also perseverance, humility, and continuous learning. Techniques will change, instruments will improve, and concepts will evolve. But the fundamental principles—respect for tissue, careful observation, rational decision-making, and responsibility toward patients—will remain eternal.

If this book helps young surgeons understand these principles more clearly, approach surgery with greater confidence, and avoid unnecessary mistakes, its purpose will have been achieved.

Vitreoretinal surgery will continue to advance, and future generations will undoubtedly surpass what has been accomplished today. We hope this book will serve as a small step along this path, contributing to the shared goal of preserving and restoring vision.

Finally, we would like to express our gratitude to Yuntong Li, Wenjia Yan, Yangming Xu, Baizhou Chen, and Shudi Mao for their great help in organizing the book.

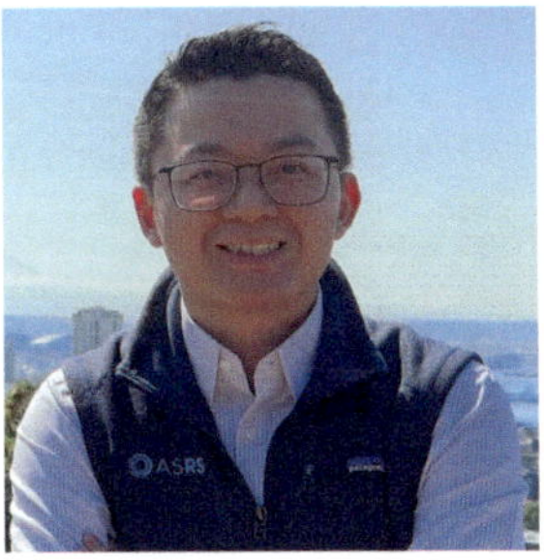

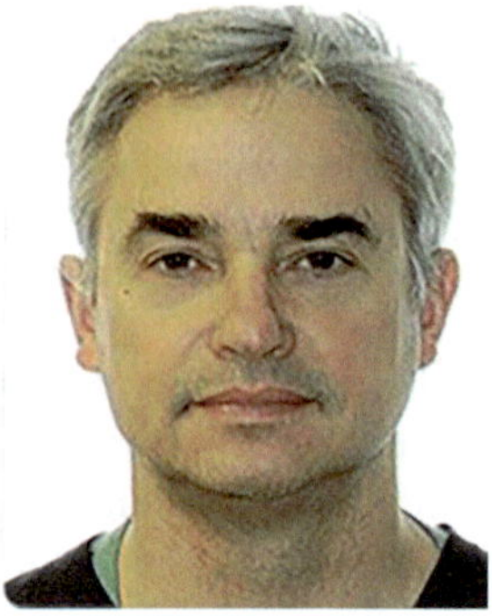

Guangzhou, China Zhaotian Zhang
Uppsala, Uppsala Län, Sweden Ulrich Spandau

Competing Interests

The authors have no competing interests to declare that are relevant to the content of this manuscript.

Contents

Part I Basics of Vitreoretinal Surgery

1 A Brief History of the Development of Vitreoretinal Surgery 3
1.1 The Evolution of Treatment Eras for Rhegmatogenous Retinal Detachment 3
1.1.1 Pre-Jules Gonin Era 3
1.1.2 Post-Jules Gonin Era 5
1.2 The Evolution of Retinopexy Methods 6
1.3 The Development of Scleral Buckling 6
1.4 The Development of Modern Vitrectomy 8
1.5 The Continuous Improvement of Vitreoretinal Surgery 9
1.6 Summary 11

2 Physical Principles Underlying Vitreoretinal Surgery 13
2.1 Bernoulli's Principle 13
2.2 Hydrostatic Pressure in Fluids 15
2.3 Poiseuille Equation 16
2.4 Surface Tension and Interfacial Tension 17
2.4.1 Surface Tension 17
2.4.2 Interfacial Tension 18
2.4.3 The Manifestation of Surface/Interfacial Tension in Intraocular Tamponade Agents 18
2.4.4 The Relationship Between Interfacial Tension and Retinal Reattachment 19
2.5 Boyle's Law 20
2.6 Fick's Diffusion Law 22
2.7 Other Physical Principles 23
2.8 Summary 23

3 Intraocular Tamponade Agents 25
3.1 The Evolution of Intraocular Tamponade Agents 25
3.2 Common Physical Properties of Intraocular Tamponade Agents 26
3.2.1 Density 26
3.2.2 Buoyancy 26
3.2.3 Interfacial Tension 27
3.2.4 Viscosity 28

3.3 Gases 29
3.3.1 Function and Metabolism of Gases 29
3.3.2 Pneumatic Retinopexy 29
3.3.3 Other Indications for Gas Tamponade 32
3.3.4 Gas Injection Techniques 32
3.3.5 Precautions when Preparing for and Performing Intravitreal Gas Injection 33
3.3.6 Precautions After Intravitreal Gas Injection 34
3.4 Silicone Oil 39
3.4.1 Physical and Chemical Properties 39
3.4.2 Silicone Oil Usage Rate 39
3.4.3 Effects and Indications of Silicone Oil Tamponade 40
3.4.4 Techniques of Silicone Oil Injection 41
3.4.5 Complications and Management of Silicone Oil 43
3.5 Heavy Liquid 53
3.5.1 Physical and Chemical Properties 53
3.5.2 Indications and Usage of Heavy Liquid 54
3.5.3 Indications and Effects of Heavy Liquid 55
3.5.4 Injection and Drainage of Heavy Liquid 58
3.6 Summary 61

Part II Vitrectomy in China

4 Preoperative Preparation and Anesthesia 65
4.1 Doctor-Patient Interaction 65
4.2 Preparation of the Surgeon 66
4.3 Choice of Anesthesia 69
4.3.1 Local Anesthesia 70
4.3.2 General Anesthesia 74
4.4 Summary 74

5 Basic Steps and Techniques of Vitrectomy 75
5.1 Common Terms and Instruments 75
5.1.1 Instrument Diameter 75
5.1.2 Trocar-Cannula System 75
5.1.3 Vitrectomy Machine 77
5.2 Basic Steps 77
5.2.1 Selection of PPV 77
5.2.2 Basic Objectives of PPV 78
5.2.3 Basic Operation of PPV 78
5.3 Practical Skills and Detailed Illustration 83
5.3.1 Creation of Scleral Incision 83
5.3.2 Safety of the Perfusion Line 87
5.3.3 Posterior Vitreous Detachment (PVD) 88
5.3.4 Safe Removal of Sufficient Vitreous 95
5.3.5 Common Mistakes in Light Pipe Operation 96

5.3.6 How to Perform Scleral Indentation Well 97
5.3.7 Understanding the Safe Operation of Intraocular Instruments from a Geometric Perspective 98
5.4 Summary 99

6 Surgical Intervention of Rhegmatogenous Retinal Detachment: Part 1 (Scleral Buckling) 101
6.1 Current Status of Scleral Buckling 101
6.2 Indications for Scleral Buckling 102
6.2.1 Pathological Mechanism of Rhegmatogenous Retinal Detachment 103
6.2.2 Functions of Scleral Buckling 105
6.2.3 Indications for Scleral Buckling 105
6.2.4 Relative Contraindications for Scleral Buckling 110
6.3 Preoperative Break Localization for Scleral Buckling 110
6.3.1 Emphasize the Application of Three-Mirror Lens Examination 110
6.3.2 Lincoff's Rules 111
6.4 Basic Steps and Precautions of Scleral Buckling 113
6.4.1 Understand Different Philosophies of Scleral Buckling 113
6.4.2 Basic Steps of Scleral Buckling 113
6.5 Different Operations in Scleral Buckling 122
6.5.1 Break Localization and Sealing Under Indirect Ophthalmoscope and Microscopes 122
6.5.2 Subretinal Fluid Drainage 123
6.5.3 Scleral Encircling 126
6.5.4 Modified Methods in Scleral Buckling 127
6.5.5 Modified Suturing Technique to Produce Temporary Scleral Buckling Effect for Noncomplex Rhegmatogenous Retinal Detachment 128
6.6 Postoperative Complications and Management of Scleral Buckling . . 130
6.6.1 Persistent Subretinal Fluid 130
6.6.2 Recurrent Retinal Detachment 131
6.6.3 Elevated Intraocular Pressure 131
6.6.4 Anterior Segment Ischemia 132
6.6.5 Explant Displacement and Extrusion 133
6.6.6 Extraocular Muscle Dysfunction 133
6.6.7 Refractive Changes 133
6.6.8 Common Issues of Retinal Detachment 134
6.7 Summary 134

7 Surgical Intervention of Rhegmatogenous Retinal Detachment: Part 2 (Pars Plana Vitrectomy) 135
7.1 Patient Selection for Vitrectomy 135
7.2 Why You Should Be Familiar with the Underlying Logic of Parameters Settings on Vitrectomy Machine 136

7.3 Fundamental Steps and Key Precautions . . . 137
7.3.1 Cutting Central Vitreous . . . 137
7.3.2 Confirming or Creating Posterior Vitreous Detachment . . . 138
7.3.3 Relieving Traction on Primary Retinal Breaks . . . 138
7.3.4 Examination of the Peripheral Retina (Generally Performed Simultaneously with Step 5) . . . 139
7.3.5 Removing Peripheral Vitreous . . . 139
7.3.6 Reattaching the Retina . . . 140
7.3.7 Sealing Retinal Breaks . . . 140
7.3.8 Intraocular Tamponade Agents . . . 142
7.3.9 Adjusting Intraocular Pressure . . . 143
7.3.10 Closing Scleral Incisions and Advising the Patient to Maintain a Face-Down Position . . . 143
7.4 Details of Air/Fluid Exchange . . . 143
7.4.1 Advantages and Disadvantages . . . 143
7.4.2 Key Points and Difficulties . . . 144
7.4.3 Application of Flute Needle . . . 145
7.4.4 Cooperation of Patient's Head Position and Eye Position . . . 147
7.5 Systematic Approach to Prevent Inadvertent Perfusion in Eyes with Extensive Choroidal Detachment, Suprachoroidal Fluid, and Hypotony During Pars Plana Vitrectomy . . . 148
7.6 Etiology and Surgical Treatment of Giant Retinal Tear . . . 151
7.6.1 Pathological Basis . . . 151
7.6.2 Surgical Principles . . . 151
7.6.3 Surgical Strategies . . . 153
7.7 Surgical Treatment of Retinal Detachment Secondary to or Concomitant with Macular Hole . . . 155
7.8 How to Modify the Surgical Approach When Primary Break(s) Cannot Be Found . . . 158
7.9 Additional Steps to Ensure Possibly Higher Long-Term Reattachment Rate . . . 159
7.9.1 360° Laser Encircling . . . 159
7.9.2 Scleral Buckling . . . 159
7.10 Surgical Complications and the Management . . . 161
7.11 Summary . . . 161

8 Surgical Management of Diabetic Retinopathy . . . 163
8.1 Underlying Logic for Surgeons to Better Understand Surgical Techniques . . . 163
8.1.1 Retinal Proliferative Changes . . . 164
8.1.2 Vitreous Status . . . 165
8.2 How to Better Analyze Dilemmas when Surgical Intervention Is the Only Option . . . 166
8.2.1 Significant Discrepancy Between Preoperative and Intraoperative Findings . . . 167
8.2.2 A Fine Line Between Treatment and Harm . . . 167

8.2.3 Coordination of Interventional Strategies 167
8.3 When to Use Anti-VEGF. 168
8.4 Surgical Treatment of Vitreous Hemorrhage 170
8.4.1 Diagnostic Evaluation and Etiology of Vitreous Hemorrhage 170
8.4.2 Timing of Surgery for Vitreous Hemorrhage. 171
8.4.3 Surgical Techniques and Intraoperative Precautions 172
8.4.4 Management of Postoperative Recurrent Hemorrhage 176
8.5 Techniques for Relieving Vitreoretinal Traction 177
8.5.1 Segmentation Technique 178
8.5.2 Delamination Technique 178
8.5.3 En Bloc Technique. 180
8.6 Vital Dyes and Intraocular Tamponade Agents 180
8.6.1 Staining Agents 180
8.6.2 Tamponades 182
8.7 How to Get Rid of Intraoperative Dilemmas. 184
8.7.1 Corneal Edema. 184
8.7.2 Lens Opacity 184
8.7.3 Pupillary Constriction 184
8.7.4 Iatrogenic Retinal Tears. 185
8.7.5 Intraoperative Bleeding 185
8.8 Postoperative Complications and the Management. 187
8.8.1 Elevated Intraocular Pressure. 187
8.8.2 Uveal Reaction and Inflammation 187
8.8.3 Lens Opacity 188
8.8.4 Iris Neovascularization and Secondary Glaucoma 188
8.8.5 Anterior Hyaloidal Fibrovascular Proliferation. 188
8.8.6 Intraocular Fibrin Syndrome 189
8.8.7 Vitreous Hemorrhage. 189
8.9 Summary 191

9 Surgical Management of Epiretinal Membrane 193
9.1 Clinical Characteristics 193
9.1.1 Classification and Etiology of ERM 193
9.1.2 Staging of Idiopathic Epiretinal Membrane. 194
9.2 Etiology of Epiretinal Membrane 195
9.2.1 Cellular Components of ERM 196
9.3 Evaluation and Differential Diagnosis. 197
9.4 Surgical Timing and Prognostic Factors 198
9.4.1 Surgical Timing 198
9.4.2 Prognostic Factors 200
9.5 Standard Surgical Steps 201
9.6 Use of Vital Dyes 202
9.6.1 Triamcinolone Acetonide (TA) 202
9.6.2 Indocyanine Green (ICG) 203
9.6.3 Brilliant Blue G (BBG) 204

9.7 Underlying Logic and Practical Skills of Membrane Peeling 204
9.7.1 Preparation 204
9.7.2 Flap Initiation Methods 207
9.7.3 Expanding the Flap 209
9.7.4 Deciding Whether to Peel the ILM 209
9.8 Complications 209
9.8.1 Intraoperative Complications 209
9.8.2 Postoperative Complications 210
9.9 Summary 211

10 Surgical Intervention of the Macular Hole 213
10.1 How Macular Hole Became a Curable Disease: Lessons for Surgeons 213
10.2 Classification and Staging of MH 215
10.2.1 Classification 215
10.2.2 Staging of Idiopathic Macular Hole (IMH) 215
10.3 Etiology of Macular Hole 217
10.4 Routine Surgical Procedures 218
10.5 Use of Dyes 219
10.5.1 Commonly Used Dyes 219
10.5.2 Modified Approaches to ILM Staining 220
10.6 Underlying Logic and Practical Skills of Internal Limiting Membrane Peeling 222
10.6.1 Challenges for Novice Surgeons 222
10.6.2 Flap Initiation Techniques 224
10.6.3 Extending the ILM Flap 225
10.6.4 ILM Flap Techniques 228
10.7 Complications 228
10.8 Summary 229

11 Prevention and Management of Proliferative Vitreoretinopathy 231
11.1 Etiology 231
11.1.1 Cell Composition of Proliferative Vitreoretinopathy 231
11.1.2 Regulation of Cell Proliferation and Migration 232
11.1.3 Extracellular Matrix Remodeling 233
11.1.4 Susceptibility Genes 233
11.2 Clinical Classification and Staging of PVR 233
11.2.1 Clinical Manifestations 233
11.2.2 Grading 237
11.3 Risk Factors of Occurrence and Development of PVR 237
11.4 Surgical Strategies for Improving Long-Term Outcomes in Severe PVR 240
11.4.1 Identification and Release of Preretinal Proliferation 240
11.4.2 Retinotomy and Retinectomy 242
11.4.3 Radial Retinotomy 245
11.4.4 Scleral Encircling and Buckling 245
11.5 Summary 246

12 Vitreoretinal Surgery in Children and Adolescents 247
12.1 General Characteristics and Unique Challenges 247
12.2 Surgical Management of ROP 250
12.2.1 Overview of the Third Edition of ROP Classification 250
12.2.2 Anti-VEGF Intraocular Injection 253
12.2.3 Retinal Laser Photocoagulation 255
12.2.4 Vitreoretinal Surgery 256
12.3 Rhegmatogenous Retinal Detachment Secondary to FEVR 258
12.3.1 Overview 258
12.3.2 Clinical Staging of FEVR 259
12.3.3 FEVR and RRD 259
12.3.4 Principles of Surgical Management 260
12.4 Retinal Detachment Secondary to Stickler Syndrome 261
12.4.1 Typology of Stickler Syndrome 262
12.4.2 Clinical Features of Stickler Syndrome 262
12.5 Summary 264

13 Editing and Presentation of Surgical Videos 265
13.1 Unique Characteristics of Vitreoretinal Surgical Videos 265
13.2 Core Elements of Surgical Videos 266
13.3 Basic Parameters of Surgical Videos 267
13.4 How to Adjust Your Camera and Microscope 269
13.5 Choosing the Right Editing Software for Efficiency and Quality 270
13.6 Fundamental Steps and Matters Needing Attention 272
13.7 Protection of Patient Privacy and Intellectual Property 278
13.8 Showcase Your Art Works 278
13.9 Summary 279

Part III Vitrectomy in Europe

14 General Introduction to Vitreoretinal Surgery in Europe 283
14.1 Education of Vitreoretinal (VR) Surgery 283
14.2 Easy and Difficult Vitrectomy 283
14.3 Cataract Surgery and Vitrectomy 284

15 Combined Phaco/Vitrectomy 287
15.1 The Surgery 288
15.2 Main Surgical Steps 289
15.3 The Surgery Step-by-Step 289
15.3.1 25G/27G Three-Port System with Chandelier Light 289
15.3.2 Phacoemulsification 289
15.3.3 Core Vitrectomy and Posterior Vitreous Detachment 292
15.3.4 Mark the Breaks with Endodiathermy 292
15.3.5 Injection of PFCL to Posterior Edge of Break and Drainage of Subretinal Fluid 293
15.3.6 Vitrectomy of the Tear Flap and the Peripheral Vitreous 293

15.3.7 PFCL Injection Up to Ora Serrata ... 294
15.3.8 Laser Therapy of Breaks ... 295
15.3.9 Trimming of Vitreous Base (Shaving) ... 296
15.3.10 Fluid Against Air Exchange ... 298
15.3.11 Drainage of Subretinal Fluid ... 298
15.3.12 Complete Laser Coagulation ... 301
15.3.13 Tamponade ... 301
15.3.14 Removal of the Trocar Cannulas ... 303
15.3.15 FAQ ... 307

16 Encircling Band, Vitrectomy, Retinotomy, and C_3F_8 (Stockholm Technique) ... 309
16.1 Surgery ... 311
16.2 Main Surgical Steps ... 311
16.3 Every Step in Detail ... 311
16.4 FAQ ... 313

17 Easy Diabetic Retinopathy ... 315
17.1 Introduction ... 315
17.2 Combined Phacoemulsification and Anti-VEGF Treatment ... 316
17.3 Vitrectomy ... 318
17.3.1 The Surgery Step-by-Step ... 319
17.3.2 Complications ... 321
17.4 FAQ ... 321

Part IV Difficult Vitrectomy in Europe

18 Usage of a Chandelier Light ... 325
18.1 Insertion of Chandelier Light ... 326

19 Vitrectomy for Difficult Retinal Detachment (PVR) ... 329
19.1 Introduction ... 329
19.2 Instruments for PVR Detachment ... 330
19.3 The Surgery Step-by-Step ... 330
19.4 Every Surgical Step in Detail ... 331
19.4.1 Encircling Band (cerclage) ... 331
19.4.2 Phacoemulsification and IOL Implantation ... 331
19.4.3 Pars Plana Vitrectomy ... 331
19.4.4 Vitreous Staining with Triamcinolone ... 333
19.4.5 Vitreous Base Shaving ... 333
19.4.6 Membrane Dissection ... 333
19.4.7 Removal of Epiretinal Membranes ... 334
19.4.8 Removal of Subretinal Proliferations ... 337
19.4.9 Retinotomy ... 337
19.4.10 Instillation of PFCL ... 338
19.4.11 Laser Photocoagulation ... 339
19.4.12 Prepare the Anterior Chamber ... 340
19.4.13 Tamponade ... 340

20 Difficult Proliferative Diabetic Retinopathy 347
20.1 Introduction 347
20.2 General Introduction 349
20.3 The Surgery Step-by-Step 351
20.3.1 Three-Port Trocar System with Chandelier Illumination 351
20.3.2 Posterior Hyaloid Rhexis 351
20.3.3 Removal of Tractional Membranes 354
20.3.4 Instruments for the Removal of Proliferations 354
20.3.5 Hemostasis 359
20.3.6 Removal of Attached Posterior Hyaloid in the Periphery 362
20.3.7 Panretinal Photocoagulation (PRP) Under BSS 364
20.3.8 Fluid Against Air Exchange 364
20.3.9 Intravitreal Avastin 365
20.3.10 Internal Postoperative Tamponade 365
20.3.11 Removal of Trocars 367
20.4 Complications 368
20.5 FAQ 368

Bibliography 371

Abbreviations

AC	Anterior Chamber
AGEs	Advanced Glycation End Products
AL	Axial Length
AMD	Age-related Macular Degeneration
BBG	Brilliant Blue G
BIOM	Binocular Indirect Ophthalmomicroscope
BSS	Balanced Saline Solution
C_2F_6	Perfluoroethane
C_3F_8	Perfluoropropane
CME	Cystoid Macular Edema
cpm	Cuts Per Minute
CSF	Colony-Stimulating Factor
D	Diopter
DOF	Depth of Field
ECG	Electrocardiogram
ECM	Extracellular Matrix
EGF	Epidermal Growth Factor
EMT	Epithelial–Mesenchymal Transition
ERM	Epiretinal Membrane
FA	Fluorescein Angiography
FDA	Food and Drug Administration
FEVR	Familial Exudative Vitreoretinopathy
fps	Frames Per Second
G	Gauge
GRT	Giant Retinal Tear
H.264/AVC	Advanced Video Coding
H.265/HEVC	High Efficiency Video Coding
ICG	Indocyanine Green
ICROP	International Classification of Retinopathy of Prematurity
IGF	Insulin-like Growth Factor
ILM	Internal Limiting Membrane
IMH	Idiopathic Macular Hole
IOP	Intraocular Pressure
IOL	Intraocular Lens

kbps	Kilobits per Second
KPs	Keratic Precipitates
LIO	Laser Indirect Ophthalmoscopy
MCP-1	Monocyte Chemoattractant Protein-1
MH	Macular Hole
MH-RD	Macular Hole Retinal Detachment
N_2O	Nitrous Oxide
NCT	Non-contact Tonometry
NRD	Non-rhegmatogenous Retinal Detachment
OCT	Optical Coherence Tomography
PAT	Preferences and Trends Survey (ASRS)
PCO	Posterior Capsule Opacification
PCV	Polypoidal Choroidal Vasculopathy
PD	Optic Disc Diameter
PDGF	Platelet-Derived Growth Factor
PDR	Proliferative Diabetic Retinopathy
PFCL	Perfluorocarbon Liquid
PFD	Perfluorodecalin
PFO	Perfluoro-octane
PFOB	Perfluorooctyl Bromide
PFTB	Perfluorotributylamine
PDMS	Polydimethylsiloxane
PPV	Pars Plana Vitrectomy
PRP	Panretinal Photocoagulation
PVD	Posterior Vitreous Detachment
PVR	Proliferative Vitreoretinopathy
RD	Retinal Detachment
ROP	Retinopathy of Prematurity
RPE	Retinal Pigment Epithelium
RRD	Rhegmatogenous Retinal Detachment
SF6	Sulfur Hexafluoride
TA	Triamcinolone Acetonide
TB	Trypan Blue
TGF-β	Transforming Growth Factor-Beta
TRD	Tractional Retinal Detachment
UBM	Ultrasound Biomicroscopy
VA	Visual Acuity
VEGF	Vascular Endothelial Growth Factor
VH	Vitreous Hemorrhage
VMT	Vitreomacular Traction
VR	Vitreoretinal

Part I

Basics of Vitreoretinal Surgery

A Brief History of the Development of Vitreoretinal Surgery

1

The history of vitreoretinal surgery is marked by exceptional pioneers who combined surgical talent with rigorous scientific inquiry. Leveraging rapid technological progress, they tirelessly refined their craft and expanded the horizons of what was thought possible. Their legacy has enabled today's surgeons to overcome the once-insurmountable obstacles of the fundus. Through their persistence, the dream of 'seeing' has become a clinical reality. We now revisit these individuals and events with profound reverence.

1.1 The Evolution of Treatment Eras for Rhegmatogenous Retinal Detachment

1.1.1 Pre-Jules Gonin Era

Beginning in 1805, scholars such as Ware, Wardrop, and Panizza published reports on retinal detachment, a sight-threatening disease. However, because the ophthalmoscope had not yet been invented, diagnosis could only be inferred from clinical symptoms. Not until the mid-nineteenth century, following the invention of the direct ophthalmoscope, did the diagnosis of retinal detachment become intuitive and reliable (Fig. 1.1). Even so, treatment of the disease remained in its infancy.

In 1805, Ware made the first attempt to treat retinal detachment by puncturing the sclera with a scalpel to drain subretinal fluid. Then, in 1863, Albrecht von Graefe (1828–1870) of Germany modified this approach: he intentionally created retinal breaks to allow subretinal fluid to escape into the vitreous cavity.

Von Graefe lost both parents by the age of 12. His father had been a renowned professor of ophthalmology at the University of Berlin. As an adult, von Graefe resolved to follow in his father's footsteps. He not only possessed superb medical skills but also insisted on providing free medical services to low-income patients. In 1854 and 1857, he founded, respectively, the ophthalmology journal *Albrecht von Graefes Archiv für Ophthalmologie* (now known as *Graefe's Archive for Clinical*

Z. Zhang, U. Spandau, *Vitreoretinal Surgery*,
https://doi.org/10.1007/978-3-032-25271-5_1

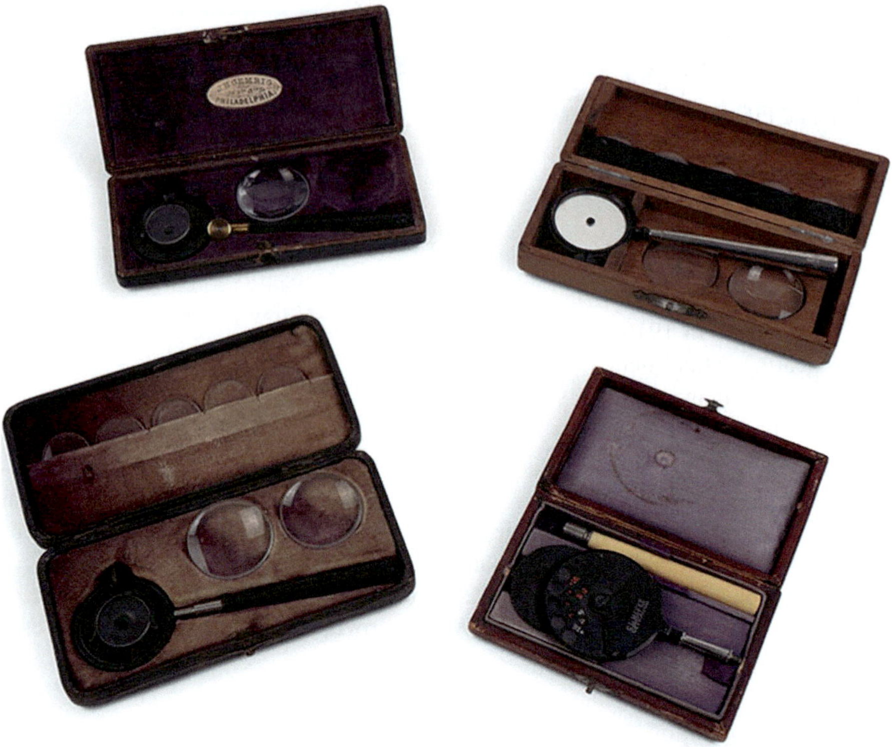

Fig. 1.1 Direct ophthalmoscope without a built-in light source commonly used in the early twentieth century. (Photo courtesy of the American Society of Retina Specialists History of Retina)

and Experimental Ophthalmology) and the *German Ophthalmological Society*. For his numerous foundational contributions to ophthalmology in the nineteenth century, he is remembered as the "father of modern ophthalmology."

In 1883, Grossman pioneered the subconjunctival injection of hypertonic saline to create an osmotic and hydrostatic gradient across the sclera, thereby promoting transscleral drainage of subretinal fluid. Other historical approaches sought to increase intraocular pressure as a treatment for retinal detachment. For instance, in 1925, Carbone advocated injecting vitreous and gelatin into the anterior chamber. Some surgeons injected rabbit vitreous, protein solutions, or filtered air into the vitreous cavity to raise intraocular pressure and reattach the retina. Still others went so far as to attempt suturing the retina to the ocular wall.

Despite these numerous efforts, the success rate of retinal detachment surgery remained extremely low. The community, once highly enthusiastic, gradually sank into despair. In 1904, retinal detachment was even declared an incurable disease at an international conference in Paris. This was by no means a rash conclusion: data from 1912 indicated that the reported success rate of retinal detachment among ophthalmologists in the United States was a mere 0.1%—a figure that cast the field into deep despair.

1.1.2 Post-Jules Gonin Era

The emergence of a gifted figure completely reversed this situation. That epoch-making ophthalmologist was Jules Gonin. Born into a culturally devoted family in Lausanne, Switzerland, Gonin displayed exceptional linguistic talent from an early age, mastering French, German, Latin, Greek, English, and Spanish. At 18, he entered the University of Lausanne to study medicine, and in 1896, he launched his distinguished career as an ophthalmologist.

Gonin's major contribution was his proposal that retinal breaks are the primary cause of retinal detachment, and therefore the key to successful surgery lies in sealing these breaks. In 1919, he designed a set of surgical instruments (Fig. 1.2) and began treating retinal detachment by cauterizing the sclera beneath the identified breaks, achieving increasingly satisfactory outcomes. Precise localization of all retinal breaks prior to surgery remains a core step of this technique.

Like most new theories and methods, Gonin's ideas and surgical techniques were not widely accepted by his peers at first. The community remained committed to the mainstream approach of directly draining subretinal fluid surgically. Nevertheless, Gonin held firm to his judgment and continued to carry out effective clinical practices. It was not until the International Congress of Ophthalmology in Amsterdam

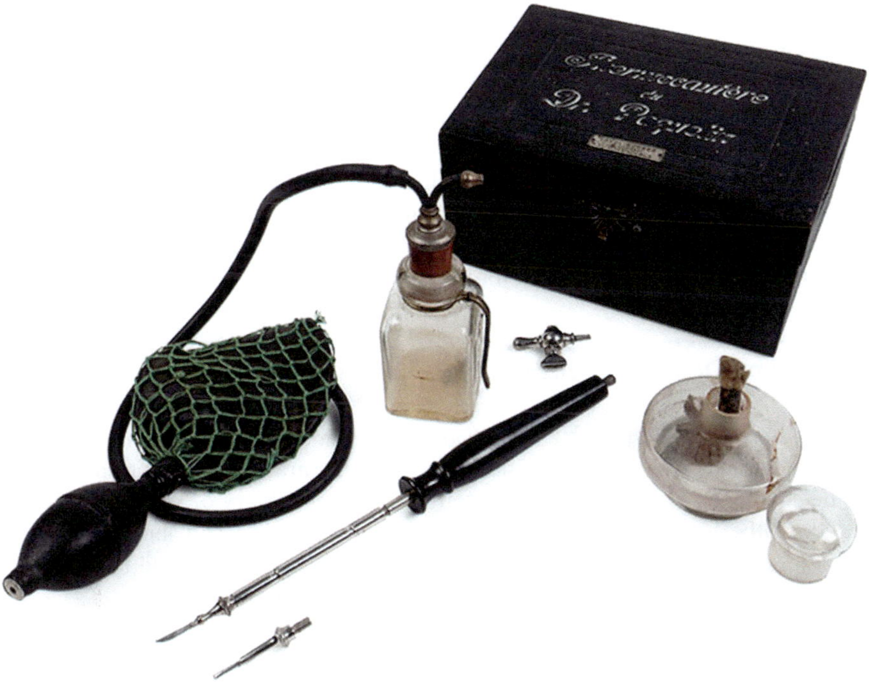

Fig. 1.2 Surgical instruments for retinal detachment designed by Jules Gonin. (Photo courtesy of the American Society of Retina Specialists History of Retina)

in 1929 that Jules Gonin presented objective, authentic case data to prove the validity of his theory and surgical technique to the world. From that point on, the treatment of retinal detachment entered the "Gonin Era," with anatomical success rates exceeding 50%—a truly inspiring achievement!

Jules Gonin passed away in May 1935. He was a philanthropist of noble medical ethics, donating most of his property during his lifetime to the blind who had lost the ability to work. According to subsequently declassified documents, he regrettably missed receiving the Nobel Prize by a single vote in the final years of his life.

1.2 The Evolution of Retinopexy Methods

The prerequisite for a successful retinal detachment surgery is sealing the primary break. This requires physical methods to create a tight adhesion between the retina and choroid, thereby sealing the break. The transscleral cauterization method proposed by Jules Gonin was widely used before the 1960s.

In 1931, Guist used potassium hydroxide to cauterize the choroid beneath retinal breaks to fix the detached retina. Meanwhile, Imre, von Szily, and Helmut Machemer (Robert Machemer's father) used electric current to scar the choroid and retina around the breaks. In 1954, Dellaporta performed thermocoagulation of retinal breaks for the first time. Although these methods achieved relatively high success rates, they were associated with significant iatrogenic damage, and related complications were frequently reported.

Meyer-Schwickerath observed that some individuals developed retinal and choroidal scars shortly after viewing a solar eclipse without adequate eye protection. Inspired by this phenomenon, he first proposed the technique of retinal photocoagulation in 1949, earning him the title of "father of retinal photocoagulation." In 1963, Campbell reported the first use of laser for retinal photocoagulation in human eyes. Since then, laser photocoagulation has gradually replaced earlier methods and remains the mainstream approach for retinopexy to this day.

1.3 The Development of Scleral Buckling

The development of scleral buckling was inspired by von Graefe's theory of retinal detachment, which hypothesized that an increase in intraocular volume caused retinal detachment. In 1903, Mueller performed the first surgery of scleral shortening to reduce the intraocular volume. Later, Blascovics introduced lamellar sclerectomy: after suturing the lamellar sclera, a surgical ridge was formed to indent the retinal break—this was also the prototype of modern scleral buckling.

In 1949, Ernst Custodis (1898–1990), a leading figure in scleral buckling from Düsseldorf, Germany, performed the first modern scleral buckling. Unlike the current technique, he used scleral thermocoagulation and polyvinyl. In 1956, Custodis reported that the success rate in 515 patients reached an impressive 83.3%—a new "world record" and attracted a worldwide attention.

Custodis argued that subretinal fluid drainage was unnecessary during scleral buckling; as long as the retinal break was properly indented, the subretinal fluid would be absorbed spontaneously.

Meanwhile, Charles Schepens (1912–2006) began performing scleral buckling in 1951. Born in Belgium, Schepens is regarded as one of the ten greatest ophthalmologists of the twentieth century. He majored in mathematics as an undergraduate and served in the Belgian Air Force. After Belgium was occupied, he moved to France and secretly joined an anti-fascist organization. He successfully saved many innocent lives and transmitted intelligence through mine tunnels. Although he was arrested multiple times, he was fortunate enough to escape each time. Later, he moved to England to avoid pursuit and began his career in ophthalmology. In 1947, he immigrated to the United States and established the world's first retinal treatment and research center. Drawing on his background in both mathematics and ophthalmology, he successfully developed the prototype of the world's first modern binocular indirect ophthalmoscopes. In 1956, Schepens used a polyethylene tube for scleral buckling for the first time.

Unlike Custodis, Schepens advocated draining subretinal fluid to ensure a better anatomical success rate of scleral buckling.

Another key figure in scleral buckling was Harvey Lincoff (1920–2017) from New York, United States. In 1955, he briefly observed Schepens' scleral buckling in Boston, United States, and was deeply impressed by the precision and efficiency of Schepens' surgical technique.

In 1958, Lincoff was sent to Bonn, Germany, to evaluate and learn the retinal photocoagulation technique invented by Meyer-Schwickerath. Following the advice of Edward Norton (1922–1994), he traveled to another city (Düsseldorf) to observe Custodis' scleral buckling. That year, Norton had just left Cornell University in New York to serve as the chief of Ophthalmology at the University of Miami School of Medicine. In 1962, he founded the Bascom Palmer Eye Institute, which soon became a cradle for many new ophthalmic technologies and theories.

At Custodis' clinic, Lincoff used his own indirect ophthalmoscopes to examine the patients after surgery. He found that even without subretinal fluid drainage, the retina of most patients remained well-attached on the first day after surgery. From then on, he began to advocate Custodis' concept and actively promoted it. Interestingly, at a conference later, Lincoff was invited to share this surgical approach; Schepens was also present at the conference and commented: "Not draining subretinal fluid is all right for New York doctors because New York doctors never sleep."

Lincoff made three additional contributions to scleral buckling: (1) improving the materials for scleral buckling; (2) introducing cryotherapy to get retinopexy (in 1963); and (3) proposing Lincoff's Law for identifying primary retinal break (in 1971). These contributions significantly improved the overall effectiveness of scleral buckling. Inspired by dermatologists' use of cryotherapy for skin lesions, Lincoff formally introduced cryotherapy into scleral buckling in 1963, which significantly reduced the incidence of complications caused by thermocoagulation.

To this day, scleral buckling remains divided into two schools: the Custodis-Lincoff School and the Schepens School. Both have their adherents and detractors worldwide. The ongoing debate over the necessity and safety of subretinal fluid drainage continues to be a fascinating topic in the field of vitreoretinal surgery.

1.4 The Development of Modern Vitrectomy

The essence of modern vitrectomy is captured in three letters: PPV (pars plana vitrectomy). The advent of PPV has opened broad horizons for the treatment of vitreoretinal diseases. Even before the PPV era, ophthalmologists had attempted to treat retinal detachment through vitrectomy. In the nineteenth century, pioneers such as von Graefe and Deutschmann introduced the concept of vitrectomy. However, due to the limitations of theories and instruments at that time, vitrectomy failed to arouse widespread interest for a long time. In 1915, von Hippel reported the first successful treatment of a patient with tractional retinal detachment by shaving the vitreous. In 1962, Kasner first proposed the open-sky vitrectomy. For certain vitreoretinal diseases (e.g., vitreous hemorrhage secondary to diabetic retinopathy), treatment could only be performed via opensky vitrectomy, which was highly invasive. As a result, most patients chose to abandon the treatment.

Ultimately, the introduction of PPV completely revolutionized the diagnosis and treatment of vitreoretinal diseases.

The founder of modern PPV was Robert Machemer (1933–2009) of Germany. Like von Graefe, he was a "second-generation ophthalmologist"—the son of an ophthalmologist. Unfortunately, he lost his father in childhood. His devoted mother worked tirelessly to raise him and his two brothers, ensuring that all three received a good higher education. To fund his university studies, Machemer once worked in an iron mine. In the 1960s, he went to the Bascom Palmer Eye Institute in the United States for further training. With his exceptional talent, he met Edward Norton—his career mentor—who soon offered him a formal position. Having endured hardships in his youth, Machemer deeply cherished this hard-won opportunity. At Bascom Palmer, he fully realized his potential and made significant contributions to vitreoretinal surgery within just a few years.

After numerous animal eye experiments, Machemer concluded that vitrectomy via the pars plana was the most ideal approach. He also pioneered continuous perfusion of the vitreous cavity to prevent ocular collapse. The harder one works, the luckier one gets: on April 20, 1970, Machemer performed the world's first closed PPV surgery. The patient had vitreous hemorrhage, and no significant complications occurred during or after the procedure. Postoperatively, the patient's visual acuity recovered well.

Over the following decade, the vitrectomy system underwent continuous optimization. The indications for PPV gradually expanded beyond its initial indication of vitreous hemorrhage. In 1975, Connor O'Malley modified Machemer's vitrectomy system, developing the "standard three-port" PPV configuration that remains in use today. Advances in surgical microscopy also played a key role in promoting the development and widespread adoption of PPV. In 1974, Parel invented a surgical microscope featuring a foot pedal controller and X-Y axis adjustment, which greatly facilitated vitreoretinal surgery.

Steve Charles of Memphis, Tennessee, invented the flute needle for draining subretinal fluid. Drawing on his background in electrical and mechanical engineering, he also made significant contributions to the advancement of vitrectomy machines. Furthermore, the development and application of various intraocular instruments—including intraocular scissors, intraocular forceps, intraocular laser photocoagulation probes, and chandelier lighting systems—have greatly enhanced the safety and efficiency of PPV.

Since 2002, vitreoretinal surgery has entered the minimally invasive era, with systems evolving through 25G, 23G, 25G+, and now 27G. A growing number of retina surgeons have adopted minimally invasive vitrectomy systems to replace the traditional 20G approach. Meanwhile, the role of scleral buckling has faced increasing challenges. Balancing innovation and tradition to find the most suitable treatment strategy for each patient is a question that our generation of ophthalmologists must reflect on more deeply.

1.5 The Continuous Improvement of Vitreoretinal Surgery

The rapid development and widespread adoption of vitrectomy also owe much to the pioneering contributions of other ophthalmologists. In 1962, Cibis reported the first use of silicone oil tamponade for retinal detachment. However, because PPV had not yet been invented, silicone oil could only be injected directly into the vitreous cavity without prior vitrectomy, leading to suboptimal results. With the advent of PPV, silicone oil quickly gained favor among retina surgeons. In 1978, Haut reported the first successful treatment of complex retinal detachment using PPV combined with silicone oil tamponade. In 1983, Hueneke first employed gas-fluid exchange for retinal reattachment. In 1984, Parike reported the first use of a combined approach—"PPV + intraocular laser photocoagulation + retinectomy + intraocular gas tamponade"—for the treatment of proliferative vitreoretinopathy (PVR).

The application of perfluorocarbon liquids (PFCLs) has also played an important role in advancing vitreoretinal surgery. Heavy liquid was initially developed as a blood substitute but later gained significant attention in vitreoretinal surgery. Before the introduction of heavy liquid, the surgical treatment of giant retinal tear presented enormous challenges. Some surgeons, including Machemer, went so far as to secure the patient to the operating table and tilt them into a prone position, cleverly using the buoyancy of gas to reattach the retina. While this was a major advancement at the time, it posed significant difficulties for both patients and surgeons.

A key figure in the popularization and application of heavy liquid is Stanley Chang, a Chinese-American ophthalmologist. Born in Shanghai, he emigrated to the United States with his parents at the age of two and later became an outstanding retina surgeon. In 1987, he began advocating for the intraocular use of heavy liquid and demonstrated its safety and efficacy through human and animal experiments.

The introduction of heavy liquids greatly facilitated retinal flattening, particularly during surgery for giant retinal tears, laser photocoagulation, and retinal reattachment. Another major contribution of Stanley Chang was the invention and promotion of the wide-field fundus imaging system. He also trained numerous ophthalmologists from around the world, including many from mainland China. In a recent interview, his advice to the new generation of retina specialists was: "Keep an open mind and don't forget to ask how you can improve what you are doing. Always focus on providing your best effort for your patient, who has immense trust in you."

Before the advent of PPV, idiopathic macular holes—like vitreous hemorrhage—were basically untreatable. In 1991, Kelly reported the first successful case of treating macular holes with PPV. Although the technique was met with numerous doubts from his peers, a series of subsequent clinical studies soon convinced everyone that macular holes could close spontaneously after surgical intervention. Taking macular hole surgery as a catalyst, the requirements for delicate operation in vitreoretinal surgery have been elevated to a new level. Claus Eckardt from Frankfurt, Germany, proved the importance of internal limiting membrane (ILM) peeling in the postoperative closure of macular hole with a series of clinical studies. He also further improved intraocular forceps, enabling ILM peeling to be faster and safer. Another important contribution of his was the application and promotion of the 23G vitrectomy system.

Norton, Lincoff, and Stanley Chang have also made great contributions to the use of intraocular gas. Multicenter clinical studies confirmed that inert gas exhibited nearly equal therapy effect with silicone oil. However, since the densities of both gas and silicone oil are lower than that of water, patients must maintain a face-down position for a period after surgery. This inevitably causes significant inconvenience to patients and results in poor sealing effects for those with inferior retinal break. Based on this, researchers have never given up searching for more ideal intraocular tamponade agents. In 2002, David Wong from Hong Kong, China, first introduced "heavy silicone oil" (density: $1.06\ g/cm^3$) in vitreoretinal surgery, and achieved satisfactory outcomes. This has provided another option for certain patients. We have reason to believe that more intraocular tamponade agents will be applied in the near future.

The introduction of anti-vascular endothelial growth factor (anti-VEGF)in vitreoretinal disorders is another important milestone in the history of vitreoretinal surgery. In the 1990s, animal studies confirmed that intravitreal injection of anti-VEGF could effectively inhibit iris neovascularization without causing obvious inflammatory reactions.

In the early 2000s, anti-VEGF drugs demonstrated good efficacy in several multicenter clinical trials. Some results were published in high-impact journals (e.g., *The New England Journal of Medicine*). In 2004, Macugen became the first anti-VEGF drug approved by the US Food and Drug Administration (FDA) for intravitreal injection for age-related macular degeneration (AMD). In 2006, Lucentis was also approved for the treatment of AMD. These pioneering researches not only saved the vision in countless AMD patients but also opened a new era in the treatment of proliferative diabetic retinopathy.

1.6 Summary

"If I have seen further, it is by standing on the shoulders of giants." Vitreoretinal surgery stands as a testament to the remarkable 200-year evolution of modern medicine. The historical trajectory of this field reveals that its progress is not merely a matter of linear time, but the result of several synergistic catalysts: (1) the courage of pioneering ophthalmologists who, undeterred by failure, transformed "incurable" conditions into treatable ones through relentless experimentation and clinical bravery; (2) a profound and versatile academic grounding that bridges basic science and clinical practice, allowing for the flexible application of knowledge across diverse fields; (3) the rapid advancement of high-precision engineering and digital technology, which has provided the sophisticated material infrastructure necessary for microscopic intraocular maneuvers; (4) extensive collaboration and the exchange of ideas among clinicians, interdisciplinary scientists, and the pharmaceutical industry. This collective ecosystem ensures the rapid refinement, validation, and global dissemination of transformative theories and surgical techniques.

Looking ahead, the future of vitreoretinal surgery lies in the transition from "microscopic precision" to "biological restoration." We are entering an era where robotic-assisted platforms will transcend the physical limits of human tremors, and artificial intelligence will provide real-time intraoperative guidance, transforming surgery from an art of experience into a data-driven science. Beyond mechanical refinement, the next frontier will be defined by the integration of gene therapy, stem cell transplantation, and bioengineered tissues. We are no longer just repairing the "architecture" of the eye; we are beginning to restore its "vitality".

Physical Principles Underlying Vitreoretinal Surgery

2

The continuous innovation of concepts and technologies in vitreoretinal surgery has led to a variety of surgical approaches, which have greatly benefited patients with vitreoretinal diseases. Today, the anatomical recovery and visual prognosis associated with different surgical methods have become a hot topic in vitreoretinal surgery. However, beginners often find it difficult to deeply understand the physical problems related to vitreoretinal surgery and may occasionally apply physical concepts incorrectly. Learning relevant physics knowledge enables retina surgeons to move beyond a perceptual, experience-based understanding and master vitreoretinal surgery at a more fundamental level—an ability that is particularly crucial for beginners. This chapter will briefly describe several major physical issues closely related to vitreoretinal surgery.

2.1 Bernoulli's Principle

In 1726, Daniel Bernoulli proposed Bernoulli's principle, which is essentially a statement of the conservation of mechanical energy in fluid flow. Important real-life examples of Bernoulli's principle include the design of airplane wings and the curved trajectory of a ball in sports—such as David Beckham's signature curved free kick.

Bernoulli's equation is:

$$p + \frac{1}{2}\rho v^2 + \rho g h = C.$$

- p: pressure at a point in the fluid
- v: velocity of the fluid at that point
- ρ: density of the fluid
- g: acceleration due to gravity

Z. Zhang, U. Spandau, *Vitreoretinal Surgery*,
https://doi.org/10.1007/978-3-032-25271-5_2

- *h*: height of the point
- *C*: constant

In the above formula, the variables related to vitreoretinal surgery are *p* and *v*, which are reflected in vitreoretinal surgery in the following two aspects:

1. Venturi pump in vitrectomy machine: When compressed air passes through a constricted section of a tube (the Venturi throat), its velocity increases, leading to a corresponding drop in static pressure. This creates a powerful and constant vacuum that is utilized for aspiration during vitrectomy (Fig. 2.1a).
2. Scleral buckling: A scleral ridge is formed to bulge inward and indent on the retinal break. This increases the velocity of vitreous humor flowing through the break. According to Bernoulli's principle, the increased flow velocity reduces fluid pressure around the break, helping to draw the break edges toward the ocular wall. The subretinal fluid is then absorbed by the retinal pigment epithelium, leading to anatomical reattachment of the detached retina.

   According to Bernoulli's principle, accurate localization and secure closure of the retinal break are the foundations for successful scleral buckling. This principle explains why some scleral buckling procedures achieve excellent anatomical outcomes without subretinal fluid drainage—or despite incomplete drainage. The increased flow velocity across the break reduces local fluid pressure, allowing the subretinal fluid to be absorbed by the retinal pigment epithelium over time, with the retina becoming fully reattached one to several days after surgery (Fig. 2.1b).

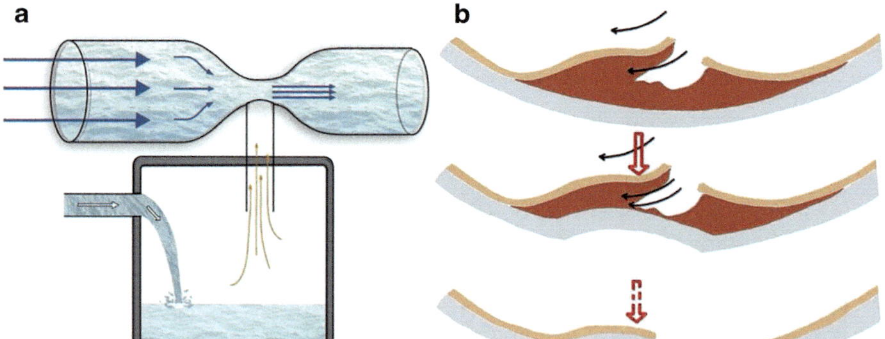

Fig. 2.1 Bernoulli's principle in vitreoretinal surgery. (**a**) Schematic diagram of a Venturi pump; (**b**) schematic diagram of scleral buckling

2.2 Hydrostatic Pressure in Fluids

The calculation of the hydrostatic pressure in fluids is a basic concept in physics, and it is also closely related to vitreoretinal surgery, mainly the estimation of liquid perfusion pressure.

New-generation vitrectomy machines feature integrated perfusion systems that use pressurized gas to drive the perfusion fluid, allowing for precise, real-time control of intraocular pressure. Nevertheless, the traditional gravity-fed (hanging bottle) method is still employed in certain clinical settings. In such cases, the hydrostatic pressure formula remains a reliable tool to estimate the perfusion pressure delivered to the eye based on the height of the infusion source.

The formula for hydrostatic pressure in fluids is:

$$P = \rho g h$$

- P: hydrostatic pressure in fluids
- ρ: liquid density
- g: gravitational acceleration
- h: height of fluid column

The above formulas are closely related to P and h. P generally represents the hydrostatic pressure exerted at the level of the eye, and h generally represents the vertical height of the perfusion liquid above the level of the eye (Fig. 2.2a).

First of all, we must know the densities of water (H_2O) and mercury (Hg), ρ (H_2O) = 1 g/cm^3, ρ (Hg) = 13.6 g/cm^3. At the same height, it is simply understood that the pressure exerted by water is 1/13.6 that of mercury.

During surgery, if we expect the intraocular perfusion pressure to be 30 mmHg, then in theory, we must hang the perfusion bottle at a height of 30 mm × 13.6 = 408 mm (40.8 cm) above the eyeball. Through simple conversion, the relationship between

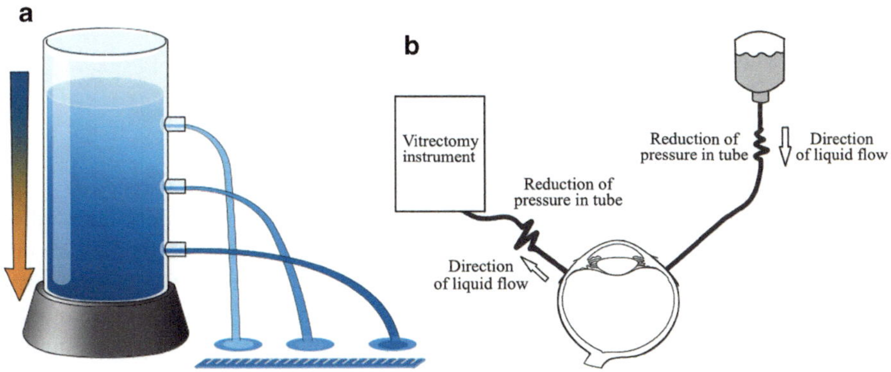

Fig. 2.2 Schematic diagram of the generation of hydrostatic pressure in fluid and its attenuation during surgery. (**a**) Pressure difference inside the liquid; (**b**) the attenuation effect of the tubes on pressure during vitrectomy surgery

perfusion bottle height, and the hydrostatic pressure can be simply calculated as: perfusion pressure (mmHg) = 0.74 × perfusion bottle height (cm).

But in reality, regardless of whether the perfusion pressure is generated by a hanging bottle or by a vitrectomy machine, we must take into account the negative impact of another force – the flow resistance within the tubes (Fig. 2.2b). When the perfusion fluid flows through the tube, the friction from the tube wall reduces the pressure. Therefore, when performing vitreoretinal surgery, the height of the perfusion bottle should be set higher than the theoretical value. At the same time, the surgeon should also avoid curling or folding the perfusion tube to avoid unpredictable reductions of pressure and accidental hypotony during surgery.

In addition to the friction of the tube itself, we must also pay attention to the reduction of perfusion pressure by the intravitreal tissue around the tip of the infusion cannula. Especially when using a 25G or 27G infusion cannula, is, the small perfusion fluid is sometimes difficult to overcome the blockage of the peripheral vitreous, leading to a decrease in intraocular pressure. Stable maintenance of intraocular pressure during vitrectomy requires the surgeon to "look ahead and behind" and promptly troubleshoot potential attenuation factors when hypotony occurs.

2.3 Poiseuille Equation

The Poiseuille equation primarily relates to the efficiency of silicone oil injection and drainage. Silicone oil we usually use is generally divided into two viscosities: 1,000 centistokes (cSt) and 5,000 cSt. From the Poiseuille equation, it can be seen that, using the same silicone oil injection and removal methods, the higher the silicone oil viscosity, the longer the surgical time.

The Poiseuille equation is:

$$Q = \pi r^4 \times \Delta p / \left(8\eta L\right).$$

- Q: volume flow rate
- r: radius of the tube
- Δp: pressure difference between the two ends of the tube
- η: viscosity coefficient of the liquid
- L: length of the tube

All variables in this equation are closely related to vitreoretinal surgery.

Before minimally invasive vitrectomy system (MIVS) was widely adopted in China, silicone oil drainage was typically performed by the surgeon using a 10-mL syringe connected to an intravenous indwelling needle. The needle was inserted into the vitreous cavity through a 20-gauge scleral incision, and the surgeon manually retracted the plunger to create negative pressure (Δp), thereby actively draining the silicone oil.

In addition to the well-known disadvantages of 20-gauge vitrectomy, the method described above also suffers from low efficiency due to the long length (L) of the indwelling needle. According to the Poiseuille equation, flow rate is inversely proportional to tube length ($Q \propto 1/L$). Therefore, increasing the needle length reduces the efficiency of silicone oil drainage, potentially offsetting any advantage conferred by the larger tube diameter.

In recent years, with the widespread development of minimally invasive vitrectomy, the pneumatic device built into the vitrectomy machine has freed the surgeon's hands, making silicone oil injection more convenient and quicker. Some commonly used vitrectomy machines can deliver silicone oil injection pressures up to 80 psi.

According to the Poiseuille equation, increasing the pressure difference across the tube can offset the reduced flow caused by a smaller instrument diameter, thereby maintaining the efficiency of silicone oil injection and removal. If a surgeon wishes to use MIVS to remove silicone oil, there are only two aspects that can be modified to overcome the disadvantage of a smaller tube diameter: increase the vacuum or decrease the length of the tube.

The author (Zhang) has proposed a machine-independent method to have silicone oil removal using a 10-mL syringe connected with a plastic tube. This technique is commonly used in China, which has two obvious advantages: (1) The vacuum by retracting the plunger can easily reach and exceed 650 mmHg; (2) The short plastic tube is easy to form a closed system including the vitreous cavity and the syringe, which is also easily available and low in cost. For details, please refer to the following chapter.

2.4 Surface Tension and Interfacial Tension

Understanding the concepts of surface tension and interfacial tension will help surgeons flexibly use various intraocular tamponade agents in vitreoretinal surgery, thereby achieving better retinal surgical outcomes.

2.4.1 Surface Tension

Surface tension is generated by the cohesive forces between liquid molecules. While a molecule within the bulk of a liquid is pulled equally in all directions by its neighbors, a molecule at the surface experiences a net inward force. This imbalance causes the surface layer to behave like a taut, elastic film that naturally contracts to minimize its surface area. Since a sphere provides the smallest surface area for a given volume, droplets—such as dew on a leaf—strive to maintain a spherical shape under the action of surface tension (Fig. 2.3a, b).

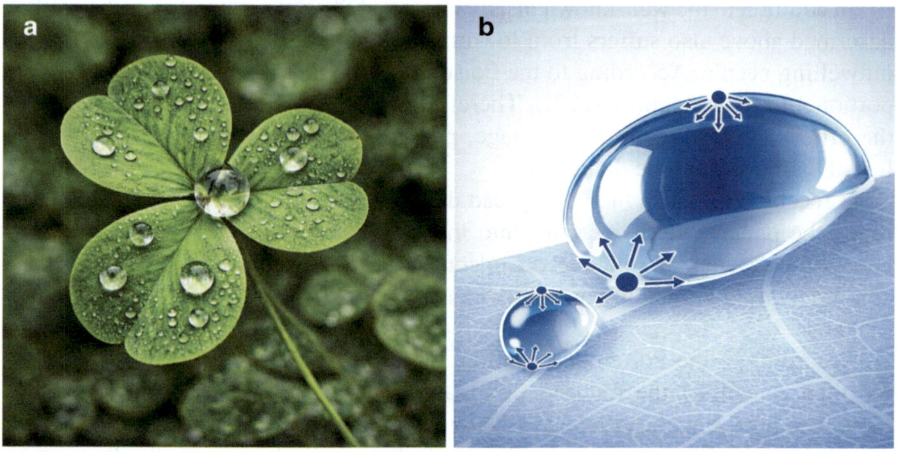

Fig. 2.3 Examples of surface tension. (**a**) The shape of dew drops on leaves is maintained by surface tension. (**b**) The principle of liquid surface tension

2.4.2 Interfacial Tension

Interfacial tension refers to the energy exists at the boundary between two immiscible phases. When a liquid contacts another immiscible liquid (such as silicone oil and water), the force is described as liquid-liquid interfacial tension. When it contacts a solid surface (such as the retina or an intraocular lens), it is solid-liquid interfacial tension. While surface tension (liquid-gas) and interfacial tension share the same physical nature, they should be distinguished in clinical logic. Relying solely on the concept of surface tension can be misleading; a deeper understanding of interfacial tension is essential to grasp how different intraocular tamponade agents interact with each other and with the ocular tissues.

2.4.3 The Manifestation of Surface/Interfacial Tension in Intraocular Tamponade Agents

In vitreoretinal surgery, balanced saline solution (BSS) is commonly used for intravitreal perfusion. BSS has a pH of approximately 7.4–7.5 and an osmotic pressure of about 300 mOsm/L, with physical properties essentially similar to those of water. After vitrectomy, the fluid remaining in the vitreous cavity also resembles water in its physical properties. When other intraocular tamponades—such as perfluorocarbon liquid, gas, or silicone oil—are introduced during surgery, these substances are immiscible with water. Therefore, it is the interfacial tension between these agents and water that must be considered, rather than their individual surface tension. This is a fundamental physical concept that requires clear understanding.

The connotation of the main physical parameters is interpreted as follows:

1. The viscosity indicates the difficulty of injection and removal of the tamponade agents.
2. The difference in refractive index between water and tamponade agents allows the surgeon to clearly identify their interface during surgery (such as heavy liquid with BSS). This difference also alters the refractive power of the operated eye postoperatively, depending on the tamponade agent used.
3. By exploiting the density difference between the tamponade agents (gas, silicone oil, or perfluorocarbon liquid) and the perfusion fluid (water-based), the surgeon can reposition the agent within the vitreous cavity by changing the patient's head position. This gravitational movement helps adequately tamponade the retinal break, improving anatomical recovery.
4. Surface tension allows a gas tamponade agent to remain as a single cohesive bubble within the fluid-filled vitreous cavity, resisting breakup into smaller bubbles. For liquid agents (e.g., silicone oil), resistance to dispersion (emulsification) depends more on viscosity and interfacial tension than on surface tension alone.
5. The interfacial tension between an intraocular tamponade agent (e.g., silicone oil or gas) and water determines the agent's ability to stably occupy a specific area of the retina, such as a macular hole or retinal break. This ability manifests in two ways: (1) During eye movements, the interfacial tension protects the retina from scouring and shear forces generated by the intravitreal fluid, preventing the edge of the retinal break from being lifted. This creates a stable, quiet environment for anatomical recovery. (2) The agent occupies the area around the retinal break, blocking intravitreal fluid from re-entering the subretinal space through the break. This provides sufficient time and space for complete absorption of the subretinal fluid and for the maturation of laser photocoagulation or cryoretinopexy scars.

2.4.4 The Relationship Between Interfacial Tension and Retinal Reattachment

From the above, the interfacial tension between the tamponade agent (gas or silicone oil) and water is a key factor in promoting retinal reattachment by creating a stable barrier and preventing fluid flow. However, surface tension itself should not be understood as a "force" that actively pushes the retina back.

During vitrectomy, air/fluid exchange is commonly performed to flatten the retina, with intraocular pressure transiently reaching 30–50 mmHg. However, if the retina has not been fully loosened—meaning traction from the vitreous base, epiretinal membranes, or proliferative vitreoretinopathy (PVR) bands has not been completely relieved—the short-term retinal reattachment observed after air/fluid exchange can be deceptive. The high-pressure gas bubble mechanically pushes the retina against the RPE, creating an illusion of reattachment. Once the intraocular pressure drops, the residual traction reasserts itself, the retina re-detaches, and the surgery ultimately fails.

The densities of gas and silicone oil are lower than that of water. When these agents fill the vitreous cavity, the retina at the uppermost surface of the agent experiences a buoyant force. However, the pressure generated by this buoyancy is extremely small and clinically negligible. Therefore, buoyancy from intraocular tamponade agents should not be confused with the "force" that actively drives retinal reattachment.

Similarly, during vitrectomy, perfluorocarbon liquid (PFCL) is injected to flatten the retina. Because PFCL has a density approximately twice that of water, the retina at the posterior pole is temporarily flattened by the gravitational force of the heavy liquid. However, if residual traction (from epiretinal membranes, vitreous base, or proliferative vitreoretinopathy) is not completely removed, the tension on the retina may overcome the interfacial tension between PFCL and the intravitreal fluid. This can cause the interface to break, allowing heavy liquid droplets to enter the subretinal space. The result is subretinal PFCL retention and/or failure of retinal reattachment.

Unlike gas, silicone oil is not gradually metabolized within the vitreous cavity. It can occupy most of the vitreous cavity for a relatively long period, acting as a long-term tamponade agent that mechanically holds the retina against the ocular wall. However, if various unfavorable factors (such as residual proliferative vitreoretinopathy membranes, incomplete vitreous base shaving, missed retinal breaks, or residual hemorrhage) are not completely removed during surgery, the probability of postoperative PVR increases. Silicone oil may temporarily mask these persistent tractional or inflammatory forces. Once the oil is removed, the retina is likely to detach again because the underlying pathology was never truly resolved.

In summary, the fundamental principle of retinal detachment surgery is to eliminate all sources of traction. This requires adequate vitrectomy, meticulous peeling of proliferative membranes and tractional bands, and, when necessary, addressing intrinsic retinal tension through relaxing retinotomy or retinectomy. Only after the retina has achieved maximum mobility—becoming soft, flat, and freely conformable to the ocular wall—can the chosen intraocular tamponade agent (gas, silicone oil, or perfluorocarbon liquid) perform its intended supportive role. Tamponade agents facilitate reattachment but cannot compensate for unresolved traction. Success depends on traction relief first; tamponade second.

2.5 Boyle's Law

Boyle's law was proposed by Irish chemist Robert Boyle in 1662 based on experimental results. It is also one of the earliest quantitative gas laws. Its core content is that under constant temperature and quantity, the volume of an ideal gas is inversely proportional to the pressure.

The formula of Boyle's law is:

$$\text{Pressure}_1 \times \text{Volume}_1 = \text{Pressure}_2 \times \text{Volume}_2.$$

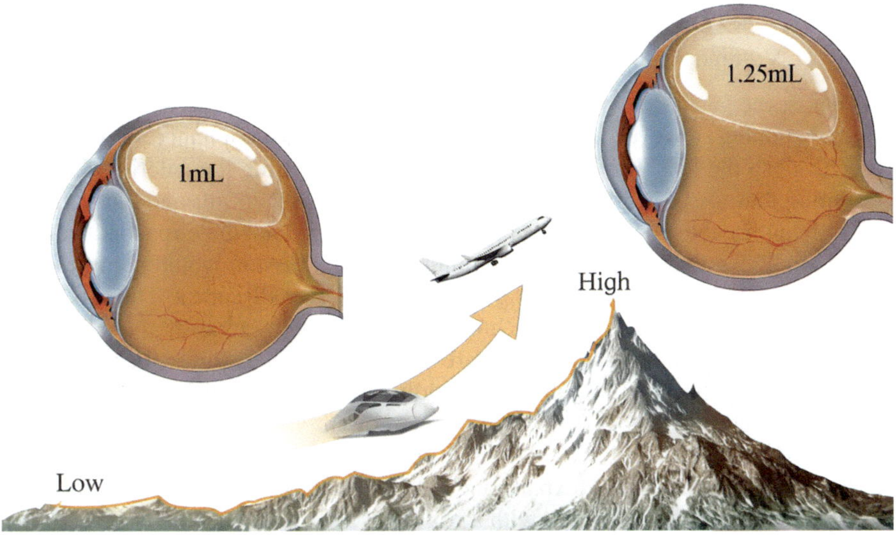

Fig. 2.4 Demonstration of volume expansion of intraocular gas when the patient moves from low altitude to high altitude under the state of intraocular gas tamponading

After vitreoretinal surgery, patients with intraocular gas tamponade must avoid sudden changes in atmospheric pressure, as these can cause abrupt intraocular pressure elevation due to gas expansion (Boyle's law). This is a critical component of postoperative education for both medical staff and patients. In countries with complex and variable terrain, and given the increasing convenience of modern transportation, patients may travel long distances within hours of discharge—often passing through significant altitude changes between the surgical center and their home. Such altitude-related atmospheric pressure changes act directly on the intraocular gas bubble, causing rapid IOP spikes that can lead to unnecessary and irreversible visual damage. Therefore, altitude restrictions must be clearly communicated, tailored to the gas type, and enforced until the gas bubble is sufficiently absorbed (Fig. 2.4).

For example, consider a patient who undergoes vitrectomy with intraocular gas tamponade at the Zhongshan Ophthalmic Center in Guangzhou, where the altitude is 10 m and the corresponding atmospheric pressure is 760 mmHg. The patient's postoperative intraocular pressure (IOP) is measured at 16 mmHg. Thus, the absolute pressure inside the vitreous cavity is: $\text{Pressure}_1 = 760 + 16 = 776$ mmHg. If the patient takes a high-speed rail journey back to Kunming immediately after discharge, the local altitude of Kunming is 1,891 m, with a corresponding atmospheric pressure of approximately 606 mmHg. Ignoring other factors (such as gas absorption or ocular compliance), the absolute pressure of the intraocular gas when the patient arrives in Kunming would be:

$$\text{Pressure}_2 = 606 + 16 = 622\,\text{mmHg}.$$

From the above formula, we can know:

$$\text{Volume}_2 / \text{Volume}_1 = \text{Pressure}_1 / \text{Pressure}_2 = 776 / 622 = 1.25.$$

That is, the gas in the vitreous cavity has a tendency to expand to 1.25 times its original volume. However, because the eyeball has limited compliance, the expanded gas will push the lens–iris diaphragm forward, compressing the anterior chamber. Assuming that the patient's anterior chamber volume is 0.25 mL and that 1 mL of gas remains in the eye upon discharge from Guangzhou, the expanded volume would be 1.25 mL upon arrival in Kunming. This expansion would compress the anterior chamber, potentially causing it to narrow or even disappear. The loss of the anterior chamber obstructs aqueous humor outflow, leading to a sharp rise in intraocular pressure. Such elevated IOP may result in central retinal artery occlusion and damage to the retinal neuroepithelium. Additionally, the lens may be pushed forward and develop significant opacification (cataract).

Similarly, if the patient takes a flight, the cabin pressure decreases during ascent, causing the intraocular gas to expand and leading to a sudden increase in intraocular pressure. Conversely, if a patient with a gas-filled eye rapidly descends from a high altitude to a low altitude, the gas volume will shrink, resulting in a sharp drop in intraocular pressure. Both scenarios may trigger a series of adverse clinical consequences.

2.6 Fick's Diffusion Law

Fick's law of diffusion states that when a gas diffuses through a thin layer of tissue, the volume of gas diffusing per unit time is directly proportional to the partial pressure difference of the gas across the tissue, directly proportional to the surface area available for diffusion, inversely proportional to the thickness of the tissue layer, and directly proportional to the diffusion coefficient of the gas.

In vitreoretinal surgery, Fick's diffusion law is mainly reflected in the expansion and absorption of inert gases.

Inert gases generally exhibit slower elimination kinetics from the vitreous cavity, reflecting differences in their molecular diffusion behavior and solubility characteristics. This is one of the reasons why an inert gas injected into the vitreous cavity must often be diluted with filtered air—and why the absorption time of the gas mixture is prolonged.

After surgery, patients with intraocular gas tamponade should avoid general anesthesia using nitrous oxide. Nitrous oxide rapidly diffuses into the intraocular gas bubble, causing acute gas expansion and a sharp rise in IOP, which may lead to rapid and severe vision loss. Case reports describing such complications have been published. Therefore, this issue requires careful attention from both surgeons and anesthesiologists.

Table 2.1 Physical problems in vitreoretinal surgery and their manifestations in surgery

Physical principles	Surgery related	Underlying logic
Bancroft rule	Emulsification of silicone oil	The protein in the eye acts as an emulsifier for silicone oil emulsification, and the mechanical movement of the eyeball also accelerates the emulsification of silicone oil droplets
Joule--Thomson effect	Scleral cryotherapy	The temperature of the eye wall drops, causing protein denaturation and resulting in retinal adhesion scars
Reynolds number	Silicone oil emulsification and inferior retina redetachment	Sufficient silicone oil tamponading reduces the Reynolds number of the liquid below the silicone oil, thereby reducing the scouring of the silicone oil and the retina by the liquid

2.7 Other Physical Principles

In addition to the above, there are still many physical problems (Table 2.1) in vitreoretinal surgery that we need to understand. Due to space limitations, the following table summarizes several other physical principles for reference.

2.8 Summary

"Judge the beauty of heaven and earth, and analyze the principles of all things." In closing this chapter, we return to this timeless wisdom, which reminds us that the mastery of any craft begins with a deep understanding of the laws that govern its existence. While the study of physics can often feel like a detached or even mundane academic exercise, its true brilliance is revealed the moment we connect it to the tangible challenges we face at the bedside and on the surgical table.

For the novice retina surgeon, physics is not merely a prerequisite subject; it is the very language of our daily practice. Our professional lives are inextricably linked to the physical world. Every diagnostic insight gained through the optical precision of the slit lamp and indirect ophthalmoscopy, and every therapeutic maneuver performed during vitrectomy or laser photocoagulation, is a direct application of profound physical theories. The instruments we hold are not just pieces of equipment—they are the culmination of centuries of engineering designed to manipulate light, fluid, and energy within the delicate architecture of the eye.

By contextualizing these concepts within specific clinical scenarios, we transform abstract formulas into intuitive surgical wisdom. As we move forward, let this chapter serve as the foundation for your technical growth. In the following chapters, we will continue to bridge the gap between theory and practice, exploring detailed physical problems through the lens of real-world surgery to ensure that your clinical journey is guided by both skill and scientific insight.

Intraocular Tamponade Agents

3

Intraocular tamponade refers to the technique of placing a series of substances into the vitreous cavity during vitreoretinal surgery to maintain intraocular pressure and to promote anatomical and functional recovery of the intraocular tissues. Based on their application scenario, intraocular tamponade agents are classified into two types: intraoperative and postoperative.

3.1 The Evolution of Intraocular Tamponade Agents

In 1911, Ohm first reported a successful case of retinal detachment treated by draining subretinal fluid and injecting filtered air into the eye; the report was published in the long-established ophthalmology journal *Albrecht von Graefes Archiv für Ophthalmologie*. In 1938, Rosengren of Gothenburg, Sweden, described in *Acta Ophthalmologica* the treatment of retinal detachment by injecting air into the vitreous cavity and introduced the term "tamponade" to refer to an intraocular tamponade agent. In 1962, Cibis from the University of Washington School of Medicine reported in the leading ophthalmology journal *Archives of Ophthalmology* (now *JAMA Ophthalmology*) their attempt to treat a severe case of retinal detachment with silicone oil, meticulously recording both the potential benefits and complications of silicone oil tamponade. Although the outcome was not satisfactory, the surgeons—embodying innovation and pioneering spirit—conducted rigorous scientific research and identified a new intraocular tamponade agent that was transparent and chemically stable.

The word "tamponade" (/ˌtæm.pəˈneɪd/) is derived from French and originally means "plugging" or "stuffing." In cardiology, the term appears in the well-known condition cardiac tamponade, where it describes compression and obstruction of normal tissue by external pressure. In vitreoretinal surgery, however, the term should not be understood literally as "plugging" or "stuffing."

Since the 1970s, with the advent and refinement of PPV technology, intraocular tamponade agents have become widely used in vitreoretinal surgery. Today, it

Z. Zhang, U. Spandau, *Vitreoretinal Surgery*,
https://doi.org/10.1007/978-3-032-25271-5_3

remains the preferred approach for many complex conditions. Beginners must familiarize themselves with the physical and chemical properties of various intraocular tamponade agents and fully understand their potential advantages and drawbacks. Such knowledge will enable them to make optimal intraoperative decisions and to prevent or promptly manage associated complications—whether intraoperative or postoperative.

3.2 Common Physical Properties of Intraocular Tamponade Agents

The neuroepithelium of the retina is composed of approximately 99% water. From a physical standpoint, it can be regarded as equivalent to water. Due to surface tension, a closely apposed yet immiscible curved interface forms between an intraocular tamponade agent and the retinal surface. This interface serves as a barrier, preventing fluid from entering from the vitreous cavity and thus providing optimal conditions for the closure of retinal breaks.

Understanding the role of intraocular tamponade agents within the vitreous cavity requires familiarity with four key physical properties: density, buoyancy, interfacial tension, and viscosity.

3.2.1 Density

Density is a measure of mass per unit volume, defined as the mass of an object divided by its volume. It is an intrinsic property of a substance, determined solely by the material's composition and independent of its mass or volume. Because aqueous humor, vitreous, and the retina are composed primarily of water, their densities are all approximately 1 g/cm^3. This value serves as the reference standard for classifying intraocular tamponade agents as either "light" or "heavy." For example, perfluorocarbon liquid (PFCL) is commonly referred to as a heavy liquid because its density exceeds 1 g/cm^3 (Fig. 3.1).

3.2.2 Buoyancy

Buoyancy is the vertically upward force exerted on an object immersed in a fluid (liquid or gas), acting opposite to gravity. The principle of buoyancy was discovered by Archimedes in 245 BCE. Unless otherwise specified, buoyancy generally refers to the upward force on an object submerged in a liquid.

In vitreoretinal surgery, we take advantage of the fact that silicone oil and gases have a lower density than water. Within the vitreous cavity, these agents experience an upward buoyant force from the intraocular fluid. When this upward force exceeds gravity, they rise to maximize contact with the superior retina. Because gases are much less dense than silicone oil, an equal volume of gas experiences a

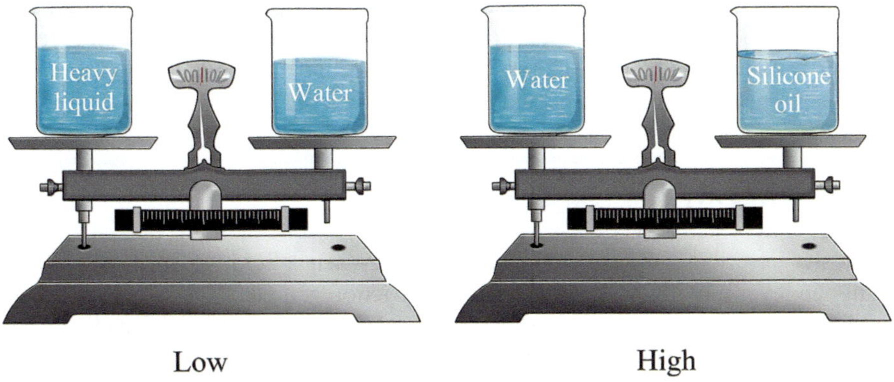

Fig. 3.1 Density comparison of heavy liquid, silicone oil, and water

Fig. 3.2 Buoyancy enables the intraocular gas bubble to ascend and tamponade the retinal break

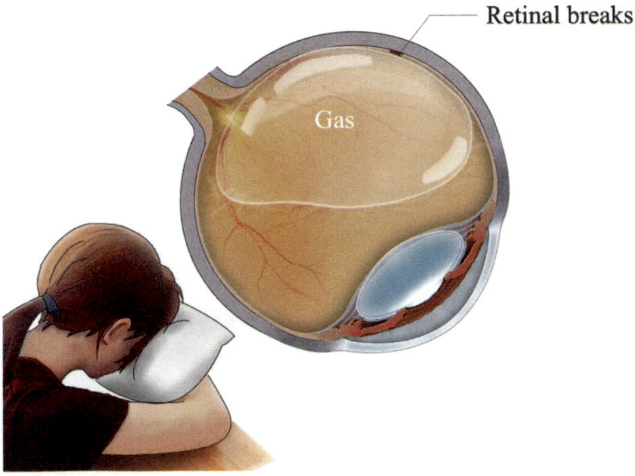

considerably greater upward force. Both gases and silicone oil exert their maximal buoyant effect at the highest point they reach within the eye. This principle partly explains why patients with intraocular gas or silicone oil tamponade must maintain a face-down position, and why retinal detachments caused by superior breaks generally have a higher surgical success rate (Fig. 3.2).

3.2.3 Interfacial Tension

Interfacial tension refers to the attractive molecular forces at the boundary between two immiscible fluids. At a gas-liquid interface, this force is specifically called surface tension, with the standard unit of mN/m. A substance with higher interfacial tension is better able to maintain a large cohesive bubble and resist breakup by external forces. When considering the interface with intraocular fluid and the retina, silicone oil, heavy liquids, and gas exhibit distinct differences (Fig. 3.3). Gas has a higher interfacial tension than both heavy liquid and silicone oil, which gives it greater resistance to fragmentation from subtle ocular movements. This property enables more effective coverage and tamponade of retinal breaks.

3.2.4 Viscosity

Viscosity describes a fluid's resistance to flow. When a fluid (gas or liquid) flows with one layer moving past another, internal friction generates resistance. In the SI system, the unit of kinematic viscosity is the stoke (St), defined as square meters per second (m^2/s). In practice, the centistoke (cSt) is commonly used, where 1 cSt = 1 mm^2/s. The lower the viscosity, the less energy is required to break a large bubble into small droplets. Among all intraocular tamponade agents, silicone oil has the highest viscosity. This is the fundamental physical reason why injecting and removing silicone oil are considerably more challenging than doing so with balanced salt solution or heavy liquids.

The key physical properties of commonly used intraocular tamponade agents are summarized in Table 3.1.

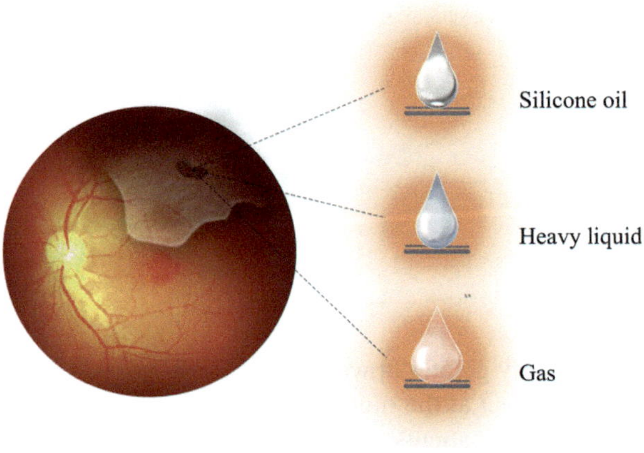

Fig. 3.3 Understanding the sealing effect of different intraocular tamponade agents on retinal breaks from the perspective of interfacial tension

Table 3.1 Physical properties of commonly used intraocular tamponade agents

Physical property	Water	Heavy liquid (C10F18)	Gas (air)	Silicone oil
Viscosity/cSt	1	2.7	15.7	1000/5000
Molecular weight	18	462	29	25,000/50,000
Refractive index	1.336	1.313	1.003	1.4
Density/($g \cdot cm^{-3}$)	1.0	1.8~2.0	0.001	0.97
Surface tension/($mN \cdot m^{-1}$)	73	19.0	70	21.3
Interfacial tension with water/($mN \cdot m^{-1}$)	–	57.8	70	40

3.3 Gases

3.3.1 Function and Metabolism of Gases

(1) Effect of Gases on the Retina

Based on their retention duration within the eye, gases used in vitreoretinal surgery are classified as either filtered air or inert gases. Both are colorless and odorless, and both are eventually absorbed and eliminated by the body. Compared with silicone oil and heavy liquids, gases have the highest interfacial tension against water. This property allows them to form an effective barrier that maximally isolates intravitreal humor from the subretinal space across retinal breaks. Consequently, this provides adequate space and time for break closure and retinal reattachment.

(2) Metabolism of Intraocular Gases

Before using gases for intraocular tamponading, it is essential to understand their pharmacokinetics within the eye, which is governed by Fick's law of diffusion. This law states that when two different gases are separated by a semipermeable membrane, each gas diffuses across the membrane until its partial pressure equilibrates on both sides. Differences in diffusion rates can lead to accumulation of the slower-diffusing gas on one side of the membrane, resulting in a volume imbalance.

Consider the vitreous cavity filled with C_3F_8 (molecular weight 188) while nitrogen (N_2, molecular weight 28) is present in the bloodstream. Because of its larger molecular weight, C_3F_8 diffuses through the ocular walls into the circulation much more slowly than nitrogen diffuses into the vitreous cavity. This difference in diffusion rates results in a net increase in intraocular gas volume (Fig. 3.4). If an excessively high concentration of inert gas is introduced into the eye, nitrogen from the blood may diffuse into the vitreous cavity too rapidly and in excessive amounts, causing a sharp rise in intraocular pressure. Therefore, the concentration of inert gases used must be strictly controlled.

Filtered air does not present an expansion problem because there is no significant nitrogen concentration gradient across the ocular wall. As a result, the volume of filtered air begins to decrease immediately after it is introduced into the vitreous cavity. The properties of various gases commonly used in vitreoretinal surgery are summarized in Table 3.2.

3.3.2 Pneumatic Retinopexy

(1) Principle and Application

Among all intraocular tamponade agents, gas exhibits the highest interfacial tension with water while its own weight is negligible, making gas particularly advantageous for sealing superior retinal breaks. Moreover, when combined with appropriate postoperative positioning, gas can effectively seal macular holes (using face-down positioning), as well as temporal and nasal breaks.

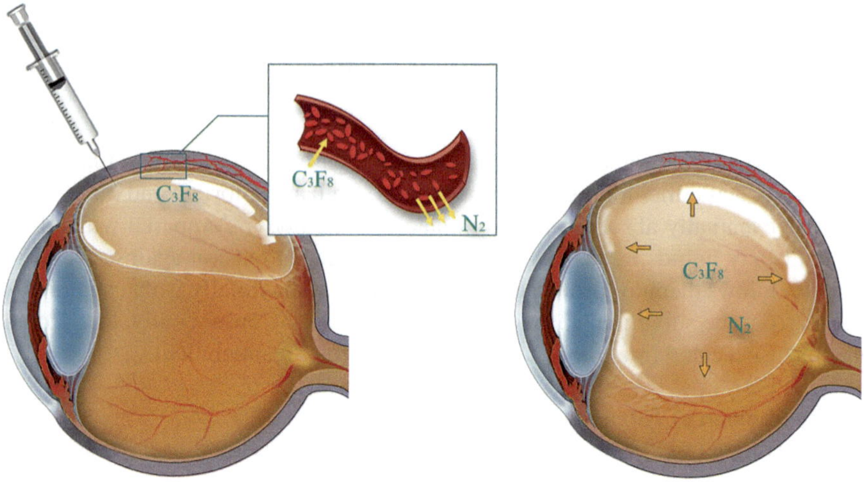

Fig. 3.4 According to Fick's law of diffusion, the volume of inert gas within the vitreous cavity undergoes dynamic changes. Because these gases remain in the vitreous cavity for a prolonged period, they are referred to as inert gases or long-acting gases

Table 3.2 Physical properties of commonly used gases and their pharmacokinetics in the vitreous cavity

Gas type	Molecular weight	Time to maximal expansion (h)	Retention in the eye (day)	Nonexpansile concentration (%)	Maximal ratio of expansion
Air	29	–	5~7	–	–
SF6	146	24~48	7~14	20	2
C2F6	138	36~60	28~35	16	3.3
C3F8	188	72~96	42~56	12	4

(2) Patient Selection

Pneumatic retinopexy was initially used to treat uncomplicated RRD, typically when the break(s) were located within the superior eight clock hours (i.e., the 8:00 to 4:00 o'clock positions). In our clinical practice, however, this procedure is rarely considered as the first-line treatment. Therefore, our limited experience restricts us from elaborating on its technical details.

Here, we focus on a randomized controlled trial published by Hillier et al. in *Ophthalmology* in 2018. The study enrolled 176 patients, who were randomly assigned to either a pneumatic retinopexy group or a PPV group and were then followed regularly for 12 months.

The inclusion criteria for the study were as follows: (1) The patient must have a single retinal break or a group of breaks within the detached area spanning no more than 1 clock hour (30°). (2) All breaks in the detached area must be located above the 8 and 4 o'clock meridians (i.e., the superior 8 clock hours of the retina, leaving the inferior 4 clock hours uninvolved). (3) The presence of any breaks (e.g., from lattice degeneration) in the attached retina was permitted, regardless of their location or size

The exclusion criteria were as follows: (1) Any break within the detached area located in the inferior retina, (2) significant media opacities, (3) proliferative vitreoretinopathy (PVR) of grade B or higher, (4) history of retinal detachment in the study eye, (5) history of PPV in the study eye, (6) age < 18 years, (7) presence of psychiatric disorders, (8) inability to read or understand English, (9) concurrent ocular diseases that could affect visual outcomes, and (10) inability to comply with postoperative positioning.

The study results demonstrated that among patients meeting the above criteria, the primary surgical success rates at the 12-month follow-up were 80.8% in the pneumatic retinopexy group and 93.2% in the PPV group—a difference that was statistically significant. The final success rates after secondary surgeries were 98.7% and 98.6%, respectively. The pneumatic retinopexy group exhibited slightly better visual recovery, as well as lower incidences of postoperative monocular diplopia and cataract formation, compared to the PPV group.

(3) Surgical Steps

1. Comprehensive fundus examination: all patients were examined under scleral indentation before and after surgery.
2. Treatment of abnormalities in the nondetachment area: before gas injection, laser photocoagulation of all breaks and lattice degeneration in the nondetachment area.
3. Treatment of breaks in the detachment area: before gas injection, cryotherapy was performed around breaks in the detachment area, and laser photocoagulation was applied within 24–48 h after gas injection.
4. Intravitreal gas injection: anterior chamber paracentesis to release as much aqueous humor as possible (generally $\geq$0.3 mL), and then inject 100% SF_6 (preferably $\geq$ 0.6 mL) into the vitreous cavity.
5. Postoperative position maintenance: according to the specific location of the break, require the patient to maintain a specific head position so that the gas can fully contact the break and prevent the subretinal fluid from invading the undetached area.
6. Repeat gas injection: if necessary, a secondary operation can be performed to supplement SF_6 to help retinal reattachment.

(4) Advantages and Disadvantages

From the results, pneumatic retinopexy has certain advantages in visual prognosis and secondary cataracts. However, it must also be recognized that intravitreal gas injection has the following limitations. When choosing, we must comprehensively weigh its pros and cons.

1. Fundus examination is relatively complex. A thorough evaluation with comprehensive scleral indentation is essential both preoperatively and during follow-up to identify all retinal breaks and areas of degeneration. This examination is performed using indirect ophthalmoscopy. Insufficient proficiency with the indirect

ophthalmoscope may compromise the ability to thoroughly assess the peripheral retina and may lead to missing subtle pathological changes in the far peripheral retina.

2. Multiple examinations can cause considerable patient discomfort, especially when a scleral indentation device is used. Some patients may experience significant pain, which can lead to apprehension about or even refusal of subsequent diagnostic and treatment procedures.
3. The success rate of the initial surgery is relatively modest. Although it exceeds 80%, it remains below that of the PPV group, which has achieved over 90%. For both surgeons and patients, the first-operation success rate plays an important role in strengthening the doctor-patient relationship. If retinal reattachment fails or more postoperative complications (e.g., PVR) occur, more time and effort may be required for communication and explanation before the subsequent secondary surgery, and the procedure may also become more technically challenging.

Therefore, when PPV is feasible, we should approach the choice of pneumatic retinopexy with both optimism and caution. We must strictly adhere to its indications and have a management plan ready for the higher likelihood of first-operation failure compared to PPV.

3.3.3 Other Indications for Gas Tamponade

Although considerable attention has been devoted to pneumatic retinopexy, the primary clinical utility of intraocular gas lies in the management of the following conditions: macular hole, RRD, proliferative diabetic retinopathy, and myopic macular schisis associated with high myopia. As these applications will be discussed in detail in subsequent chapters, they will not be further elaborated upon here.

3.3.4 Gas Injection Techniques

In China, in addition to filtered air, the most frequently used gas in vitreoretinal surgery is C_3F_8. Other types of inert gases are rarely mentioned in our literature reports. Here we take C_3F_8 as an example to introduce two commonly used injection techniques.

(1) Direct Injection Method

Based on long-standing surgical practice, we routinely inject approximately 0.6 mL of C_3F_8 using a 0.38-mm syringe needle. This injection is performed after completing fluid–air exchange, suturing the sclerotomies, and confirming wound integrity. The injection site is conventionally located 3.5–4 mm posterior to the limbus (Fig. 3.5). Assuming a vitreous cavity volume of approximately 4.5 mL, injecting 0.6 mL of pure C_3F_8 yields an immediate intraocular concentration of approximately 13%. Because the sclerotomy wounds are securely closed, the inert gas is retained,

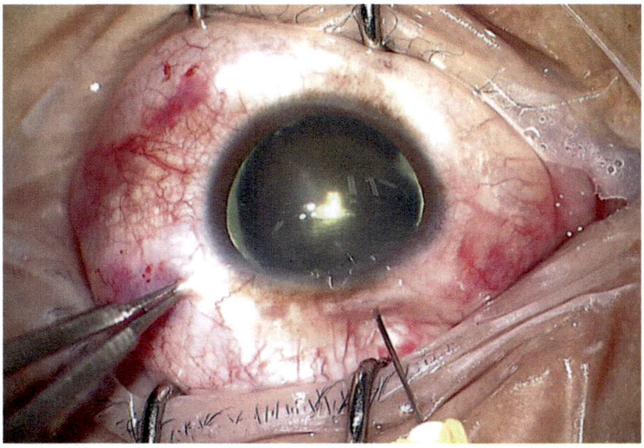

Fig. 3.5 Inert gas is injected using a fine needle at a site 3.5–4 mm posterior to the limbus. The needle should be directed away from the lens to prevent inadvertent injury to the posterior lens capsule

thereby maintaining adequate intraocular pressure and an optimal gas concentration. In eyes with longer axial lengths, such as those with high myopia, the injected volume of C_3F_8 may be increased to 0.8–1.0 mL.

(2) Dilution-Replacement Injection Method
First, draw 6.0–8.0 mL of pure C_3F_8 into a 50-mL syringe. Plug the syringe tip with a gauze block, then draw filtered air into the syringe until the total volume reaches 50 mL. This yields a C_3F_8 concentration of approximately 12%–16%. Next, close one of the superior scleral incisions. The assistant then connects the syringe to the infusion line and slowly injects about 20–25 mL of the gas mixture into the vitreous cavity to replace the existing gas. Simultaneously, the surgeon closes the other superior scleral incision. Throughout this process, the assistant must gently advance the plunger to maintain normal intraocular pressure. Finally, the surgeon closes the infusion incision to complete the procedure.

3.3.5 Precautions when Preparing for and Performing Intravitreal Gas Injection

(1) Control of the Total Amount and Concentration of Long-Acting Gas
Unlike other intraocular tamponade agents, inert gases undergo exponential expansion over a defined period due to Fick's law of diffusion. Therefore, when deciding on the volume of inert gas to inject, the surgeon must estimate both the patient's vitreous cavity volume and the gas's peak expansion ratio. The guiding principle should be: "Get it right the first time, aim for precision, maintain strict control over the total amount, and err on the side of less rather than more."

(2) Causes and Treatment of Intraoperative Abnormalities
The following situations may result in a low concentration of injected inert gas: (1) excessive axial length and large vitreous cavity volume, particularly when direct injection is used; (2) premature extraction of inert gas without timely sealing of the

syringe, allowing gas leakage and consequent concentration reduction; (3) calculation error; (4) leakage from the scleral incisions.

The following situations may cause excessive inert gas concentration: (1) short axial length and small vitreous cavity volume, such as microphthalmos; (2) when a large amount of BSS or vitreous remains, the effective volume of the vitreous cavity is not fully released; (3) inappropriate multiple replenishment of inert gas; and (4) calculation error.

If errors are found in the total amount and concentration of inert gas during the operation, for safety reasons, liquid perfusion can be restarted, and after all the gas in the vitreous cavity is expelled, gas/liquid exchange can be performed, and finally inert gas can be reinjected.

When the surgeon, assistant, and nurse repeatedly verify the injection parameters, errors resulting in severe overfilling with inert gas are exceedingly rare. Nevertheless, the literature contains case reports of extreme instances where excessive inert gas injection caused a sharp postoperative rise in intraocular pressure ($\geq$60 mmHg) and complete flattening of the anterior chamber.

3.3.6 Precautions After Intravitreal Gas Injection

Overall, intraocular gas is ultimately absorbable and is considered the safest of all intraocular tamponade agents. It is associated with a relatively low incidence of complications, and management of any that arise is comparatively straightforward. These characteristics explain why gas tamponade is favored by both surgeons and patients. Nevertheless, close postoperative monitoring of the following aspects remains essential to ensure its safety and efficacy.

(1) Correct Postoperative Position

Based on the location of the retinal pathology, patients should be instructed on the correct postoperative positioning to ensure that the gas bubble remains in contact with the target area for the longest possible duration and with the maximum surface area, thereby improving the anatomical success rate. Proper face-down positioning is especially critical in cases involving multiple or large retinal breaks, or when breaks are located in the inferior retina.

(2) Visual Recovery

Unlike infusion fluid or silicone oil, gas has a refractive index that is markedly different from that of the lens. When gas occupies the visual axis, both phakic and pseudophakic eyes develop a high degree of myopia (Fig. 3.6), typically reducing visual acuity to hand motion or counting fingers. Surgeons should thoroughly inform patients of this effect preoperatively, including the expected duration of blurred vision. Once the gas bubble descends below the visual axis, and provided the baseline visual potential is good, the patient's vision will improve substantially. Some patients may report a large, shifting shadow in the lower visual field or even

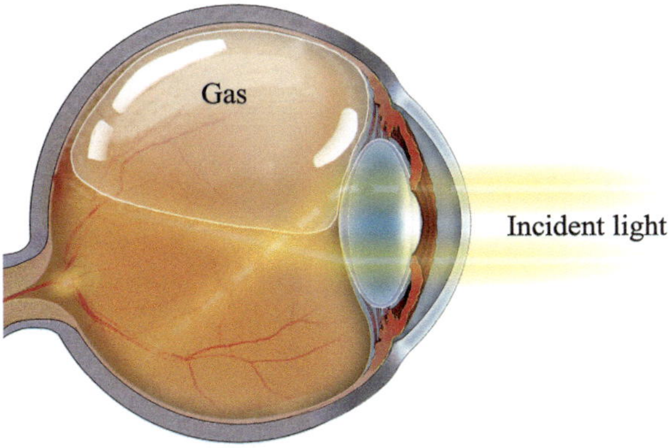

Fig. 3.6 In phakic eyes, the presence of gas within the vitreous cavity induces a highly myopic refractive state

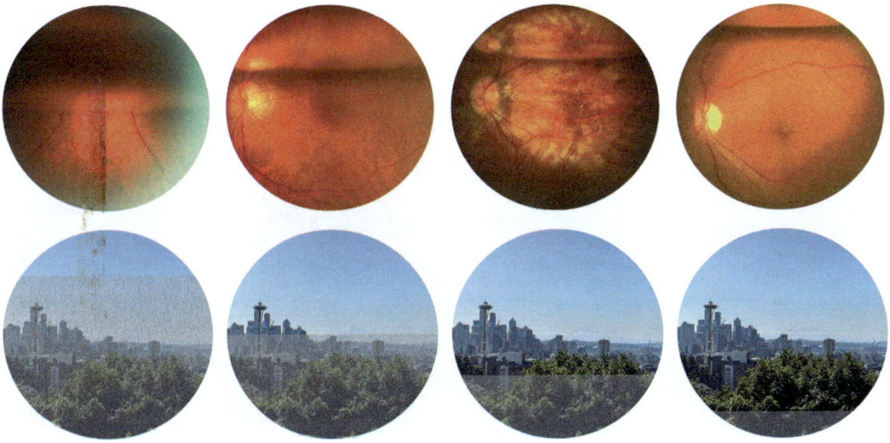

Fig. 3.7 The correspondence between the height of the gas bubble within the eye and the patient's visual field is as follows: when the gas occupies approximately 75%, 45%, 35%, and 20% of the vitreous cavity (from left to right), the corresponding visual field defects or refractive changes vary accordingly

dizziness. In such cases, the surgeon should explain—according to the specific gas used—that the shadow will gradually descend day by day and completely disappear within several weeks, thereby alleviating patient concerns (Fig. 3.7).

(3) Lens Transparency

In the postoperative period following gas tamponade, a small subset of patients may develop feathery opacities on the posterior lens capsule as early as postoperative day one (Fig. 3.8). As long as no iatrogenic lens damage occurred during the procedure, these opacities typically resolve spontaneously.

If iatrogenic lens damage occurs, the lens opacity will progressively worsen, leading to significant opacification that hinders clear fundus visualization. In the absence of other complications such as lens expansion (Fig. 3.9a), the condition may be

Fig. 3.8 Feather-like opacity in the posterior lens capsule on the first day after PPV with intraocular gas tamponade

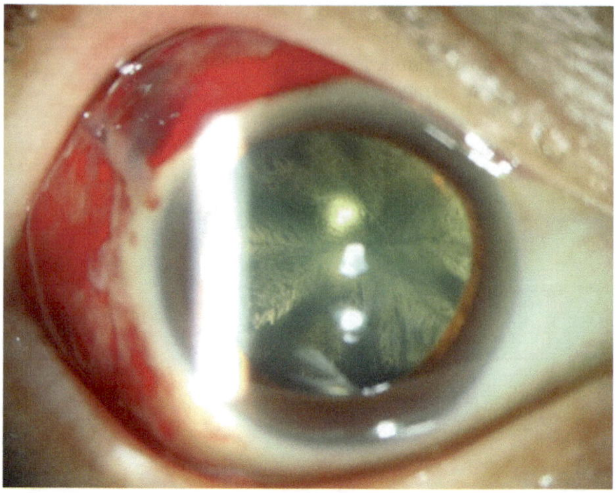

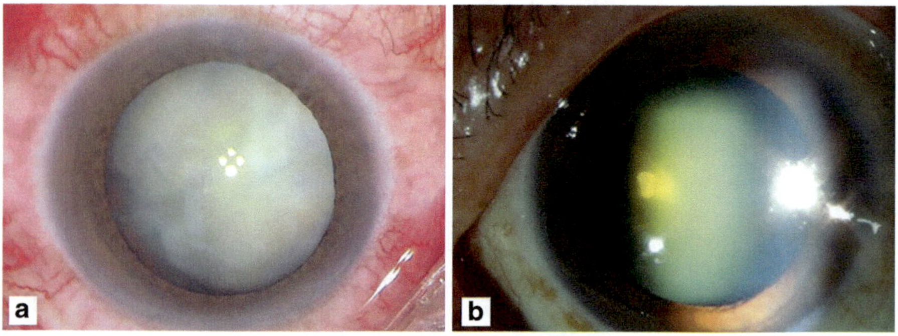

Fig. 3.9 Lens opacification secondary to vitrectomy. (**a**) The vitrectomy probe damaged the posterior lens capsule during surgery. After gas tamponading, the lens was obviously cloudy 2 weeks after. (**b**) The posterior lens capsule was not damaged during surgery, but nuclear cataracts appeared 3 months after the operation

temporarily observed without intervention; however, fundus changes must be monitored using B-scan ultrasonography. For instance, if significant lens opacification develops after retinal detachment surgery, cataract extraction with intraocular lens implantation may be performed once the intraocular gas has been largely absorbed and retinal reattachment has been confirmed by B-scan ultrasound. The earliest appropriate timing for such surgery is approximately 10 days after the initial procedure. During the operation, care should be taken to prevent a sudden intraocular pressure drop due to gas escape. Additionally, concurrent fundus examination may be performed, with further intervention carried out as clinically indicated.

Middle-aged and elderly patients may develop or show progression of nuclear cataracts approximately three months after surgery (Fig. 3.9b). At this stage, cataract surgery may be considered. In eyes with small pupils, such cataracts are easily overlooked, and the patient's postoperative vision loss may be erroneously attributed to ongoing deterioration of underlying fundus disease.

(4) Changes in the Patient's Altitude (e.g., Travel to High Altitude)
According to Boyle's law, the volume of intraocular gas varies with changes in atmospheric pressure (see Chap. 2 for details). After surgery, when a patient with a gas-filled eye travels to a lower altitude, the gas volume decreases. If aqueous humor production cannot compensate for this reduction, intraocular pressure may drop (hypotony).

Conversely, when a patient with a gas-tamponaded eye ascends to a high altitude, the intraocular gas volume expands. If aqueous humor outflow cannot compensate for this expansion, the anterior chamber becomes compressed. The resulting elevation in IOP affects the entire ocular wall, compromising ocular perfusion. This can ultimately lead to optic nerve atrophy, severe lens opacification, and other complications, resulting in serious and irreversible visual impairment (Fig. 3.10).

Below we summarize the management protocol for elevated IOP caused by rapid altitude change in patients with intraocular gas.

1. Preoperative Clear Instruction
   For patients scheduled to undergo intraocular gas tamponade, it must be clearly explained that air travel is absolutely contraindicated until the gas has been

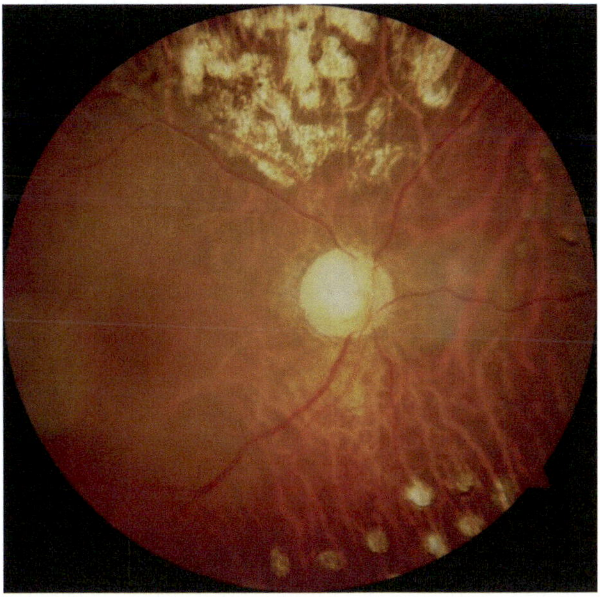

Fig. 3.10 Case of optic nerve atrophy secondary to intraocular gas expansion. The patient with a history of chronic hypertension and diabetes underwent vitrectomy with filtered air tamponade for vitreous hemorrhage. On postoperative day 1, prior to discharge, intraocular pressure (IOP) was measured at 12 mmHg. The patient then traveled by high-speed train from Guangzhou to Guiyang. During the journey, the patient experienced significant headache and nausea. IOP measured at a local hospital was 48 mmHg. After two days of topical medication, IOP returned to normal, but visual acuity had decreased to hand motion

fully absorbed, and high-speed rail travel to regions of significantly higher altitude (e.g., Guangzhou to Kunming) should also be avoided. If a patient must return to a high-altitude area (elevation difference >800 m) shortly after surgery, travel by conventional train or automobile is recommended. During the journey, the patient should closely monitor for symptoms such as ocular distension, headache, nausea, vomiting, or visual decline. Should such symptoms develop, the patient should immediately return to the original lower altitude and await gradual symptom resolution, or seek emergency care at a local hospital. (Note: Inexperienced practitioners may misdiagnose this condition as routine acute IOP elevation, potentially delaying appropriate management.) In special circumstances, silicone oil tamponade may be considered as an alternative.

2. Postoperative Emergency Management

   Aside from an immediate return to lower altitude, if the patient presents to a local hospital, treatment should not follow the protocol for acute angle-closure glaucoma (attack phase). The rapid IOP elevation is caused by acute expansion of intraocular gas, not by obstruction of aqueous outflow from the lens-iris diaphragm. Therefore, simple anterior chamber paracentesis should be avoided, as it may further collapse the anterior chamber and exacerbate lens opacification (Fig. 3.11). Relying solely on topical or systemic IOP-lowering medications is also not advisable, because their onset of action may be too slow to prevent irreversible vision loss during this critical window.

   The recommended approach is to insert a fine needle connected to a syringe through the pars plana—4 mm posterior to the limbus—into the vitreous cavity, and then slowly and controllably aspirate a portion of the intraocular gas. During aspiration, IOP should be monitored by digital palpation. The needle is withdrawn once IOP returns to the normal range.

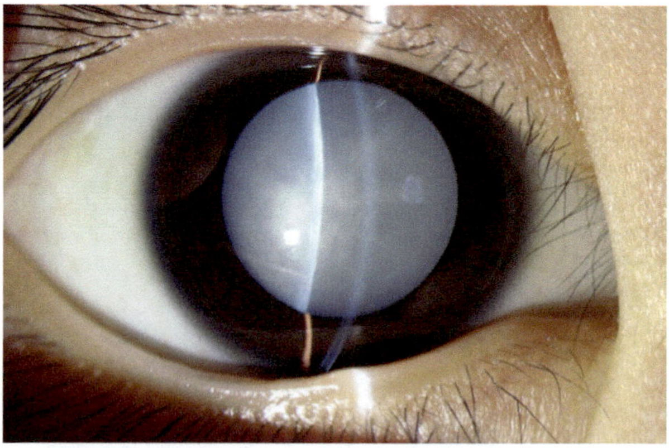

Fig. 3.11 A patient with a gas-filled eye developed intraocular gas expansion and a sharp intraocular pressure rise after traveling from a low-altitude area to a high-altitude region. Emergency anterior chamber paracentesis was performed at a local hospital, leading to rapid further collapse of the anterior chamber and ultimately resulting in complete lens opacification

3.4 Silicone Oil

3.4.1 Physical and Chemical Properties

Silicone oil, chemically designated as polydimethylsiloxane (PDMS), is a linear synthetic polymer composed of repeating siloxane (Si–O) units. It is chemically similar to silicone gel but differs in that its polymer chains are shorter and not cross-linked. As the liquid form of silicone gel, silicone oil is widely used in vitreoretinal surgery. It is chemically stable, non-absorbable by the body, colorless, and transparent, allowing it to remain in the eye for an extended period. This provides reliable time and space for both anatomical reattachment and functional recovery of the retina.

Clinically used silicone oil is available primarily in two viscosity grades: 1000 cSt and 5000 cSt. According to an international survey conducted in 2020, 59.0% of US retina specialists preferred 1000 cSt silicone oil, compared with 38.7% of specialists outside the United States. In China, surgeons tend to prefer 5000 cSt silicone oil, as higher-viscosity oil is less prone to emulsification and carries a lower risk of migration. Given the complexity and challenges associated with managing silicone oil-related complications, we advocate the use of higher-viscosity silicone oil to reduce the occurrence of such complications.

3.4.2 Silicone Oil Usage Rate

Recent years in China, the increased patient awareness of seeking timely care, along with a rise in the number and expertise of vitreoretinal surgeons, has enabled prompt treatment for most non-complex retinal diseases. This has reduced the technical difficulty of vitreoretinal surgery and led to a declining trend in the use of silicone oil.

We reviewed fresh RRD cases (duration 1–14 days) treated by our team over 2 months. Of the 61 patients who underwent PPV with C_3F_8 tamponade, the primary anatomical success rate at 6 months was 98.4%. Only one patient required a second surgery with silicone oil tamponade due to recurrent detachment.

We should always keep in mind that the retina is re-apposed rather than pressed back into place. Complications associated with silicone oil tamponade are not uncommon, making it a true double-edged sword. Overreliance on silicone oil to achieve short-term retinal reattachment should be avoided. A sound clinical decision should be based on the following two key factors: (1) intraoperative retinal mobility, and (2) the number, location, and size of retinal breaks (including both primary and iatrogenic breaks).

3.4.3 Effects and Indications of Silicone Oil Tamponade

Intraocular silicone oil tamponade serves both preventive and therapeutic roles in the management of complex vitreoretinal conditions. It offers distinct advantages in the following scenarios:

(I) Complex but Short-Duration Retinal Detachment

Since silicone oil is not absorbed by the body and generally does not induce retinal toxicity, it can maintain prolonged and stable contact with pathologic retinal tissues. Silicone oil may be preferentially considered under the following circumstances:

1. Multiple retinal breaks: Silicone oil can provide comprehensive tamponade of nearly all breaks for a sufficient duration.
2. Large retinal breaks, such as giant retinal tear (GRT): The presence of silicone oil maximally limits the dispersion of exposed retinal pigment epithelial (RPE) cells into the vitreous cavity, thereby helping to prevent PVR.
3. Retinal detachment secondary to chronic uveitis: Silicone oil helps maintain intraocular pressure and restricts the accumulation of inflammatory mediators in the vitreous cavity.
4. Poor vision in the fellow eye due to various reasons (e.g., prior failed retinal detachment surgery): Silicone oil tamponade in the operated eye can enable relatively rapid partial visual recovery, assisting patients in resuming work and daily activities in the short term.

(II) Retinal Detachment with Significant PVR

In retinal detachment associated with marked epiretinal and subretinal proliferation, the retina often becomes extensively edematous or even shortened. Traction from proliferative membranes or strands reduces overall retinal mobility and particularly impairs the compliance of break edges. Silicone oil tamponade offers the following clear advantages in such cases:

1. It maintains retinal apposition to the RPE layer over an extended postoperative period, allowing sufficient time for restoration of retinal elasticity and maturation of laser photocoagulation scars.
2. It hinders the dispersion of RPE cells within the vitreous cavity, thereby limiting the initiation of secondary PVR.
3. By occupying the vitreous cavity, silicone oil reduces the total volume of intraocular fluid, making the environment less favorable for the accumulation of inflammatory factors that can provoke PVR.

(III) Proliferative Diabetic Retinopathy

Silicone oil provides the following benefits:

1. As a stable tamponade agent, it maintains a vitreous cavity environment that resists accumulation of inflammatory factors, thereby helping to prevent recurrent retinal contraction and PVR development.

2. Because blood is immiscible with silicone oil, the pressure exerted by the oil tamponade produces a hemostatic effect on retinal vessels.
3. To some extent, it blocks the diffusion of VEGF from retinal tissues toward the anterior segment, thereby reducing or preventing iris neovascularization.

(IV) Complex Vitreoretinal Abnormalities Caused by Ocular Trauma
In addition to causing common retinal detachment, ocular trauma may simultaneously result in retinal incarceration, choroidal detachment, scleral rupture, vitreous hemorrhage, and ciliary body disorders. In such complex cases, silicone oil tamponade creates favorable conditions for ocular functional reconstruction, effectively prevents the onset and progression of PVR, and reduces the incidence of postoperative hypotony.

3.4.4 Techniques of Silicone Oil Injection

Both oil/air exchange and oil/fluid exchange can be performed. The former is more commonly used, less difficult, and applicable in a broader range of situations. The latter is typically employed to replace heavy liquid, aiming to prevent slippage and curling of the tear edge during fluid/air exchange—especially in giant retinal tears (GRTs) and cases requiring extensive retinectomy. The specific steps for each procedure are outlined below.

(1) Oil/Air Exchange Method
1. Fluid/air exchange: Increase the gas perfusion pressure to 30–50 mHg, and use a flute needle or vitrectomy probe to completely remove the liquid (BSS or heavy liquid) from the vitreous cavity.
2. Inject silicone oil: Reduce the gas perfusion pressure to 20–30 mmHg, and inject silicone oil into the vitreous cavity at a pressure of 70–80 psi. It is recommended to inject the silicone oil under direct visualization of the vitreous cavity in order to prevent inadvertent perfusion into the subretinal space.
3. Close the perfusion: When the silicone oil reaches the horizontal level of the inner opening of the trocar, clamp the perfusion tube or reduce the perfusion pressure to 0 to prevent gas from entering the silicone oil.
4. Continue to fill with silicone oil: When the silicone oil surface contacts the posterior capsule of the lens, the surgical field suddenly becomes clear under the wide-angle lens. At this point, silicone oil injection can be suspended.
5. Add a small amount of silicone oil as needed: When the silicone oil surface contacts the posterior capsule of the lens, the surgical field suddenly becomes clear under the wide-angle lens. At this point, silicone oil injection can be suspended.
6. Adjust intraocular pressure and close the incisions.

(2) Oil/Fluid Exchange Method
1. Inject part of the silicone oil: While maintaining the original water perfusion, inject a small amount of silicone oil through the upper trocar. The silicone oil

floats on the surface of the heavy liquid, preventing overflow of heavy liquid and preventing a sudden drop in intraocular pressure.

2. Remove the lower perfusion tube: Withdraw the perfusion tube from the lower trocar. This trocar is then used for silicone oil filling. The assistant inserts the silicone oil syringe.
3. Place the light fiber and flute needle in the upper trocar: Using a wide-angle lens, note that the tip of the flute needle should be positioned below the silicone oil/heavy liquid interface to avoid silicone oil blocking the flute needle (Fig. 3.12).
4. Continue to fill with silicone oil: During silicone oil filling, closely monitor the changes at the silicone oil/heavy liquid interface and observe whether the optic disc blood vessels pulsate due to excessive intraocular pressure. Adjust the speed of silicone oil injection accordingly. If the flute needle is not draining smoothly, replace it promptly. While inserting the flute needle, the thumb should occlude the outer opening of the flute needle to minimize clogging by silicone oil.
5. Aspirate heavy liquid droplets remaining in the posterior pole: This is a critical step in oil/fluid exchange. The flute needle tip should be positioned within the heavy liquid droplets without dispersing them. Finally, employ the siphon effect to drain the residual heavy liquid from the posterior pole in a single maneuver. If any heavy liquid droplets remain adherent to the retina, they can be actively aspirated using a flute needle connected to a syringe.
6. Adjust intraocular pressure and close the incisions.
7. Postoperative observation: Since the patient remains in a face-down position after surgery, it is possible to observe whether there is residual of heavy liquid in the anterior chamber.

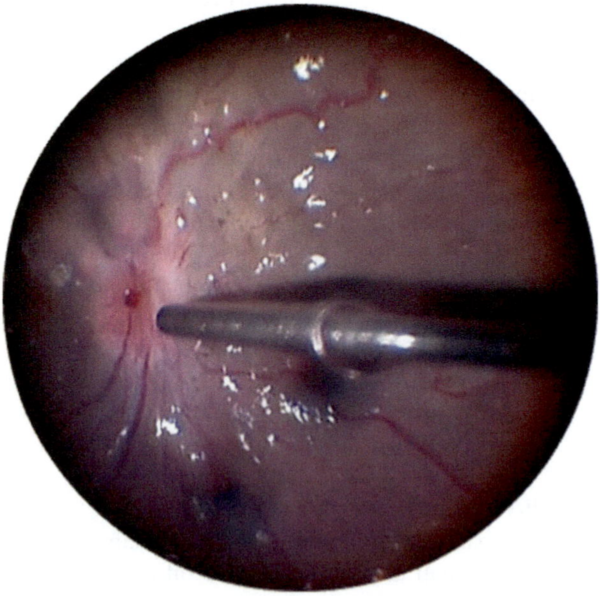

Fig. 3.12 When performing oil/fluid exchange, pay attention to the interface changes between silicone oil and heavy liquid, and keep the tip of the flute needle always below the interface to avoid blocking

3.4.5 Complications and Management of Silicone Oil

(1) Lens Opacity

In silicone oil-filled eyes, normal lens metabolism is disrupted because the posterior capsule remains in continuous contact with the silicone oil interface. When silicone oil tamponade is prolonged (e.g., beyond three months), it may result in nuclear cataract and posterior lens capsule opacification (Fig. 3.13a, b). If lens opacity was present preoperatively or the lens was injured during surgery, it may rapidly progress to significant opacification in the early postoperative period, compromising fundus visualization.

Cataract phacoemulsification with intraocular lens implantation can be performed simultaneously with silicone oil removal. This combined procedure is generally less technically demanding. If the posterior capsule is densely opacified, a vitrectomy probe may be used to create a window in the posterior capsule during the same surgery, thus avoiding the need for postoperative laser capsulotomy (Fig. 3.14a–d).

During combined silicone oil removal, phacoemulsification, and IOL implantation, three points require strict attention.

1. Protect the corneal endothelium. Silicone oil (especially if emulsified or in the anterior chamber) damages the endothelium. Nuclear cataracts require more ultrasonic energy and longer operation time. Strictly adhere to phacoemulsification principles: timely viscoelastic supplementation and nuclear chopping to minimize postoperative endothelial decompensation.
2. Maintain anterior chamber depth. Depth fluctuates more significantly in silicone oil-tamponaded eyes. Causes and management:
   (a) Buoyant force on the posterior capsule: Without stable irrigation or viscoelastic support, the capsule bulges upward, reducing working space and risking rupture. Adjust irrigation and inject viscoelastic to reposition the capsule.

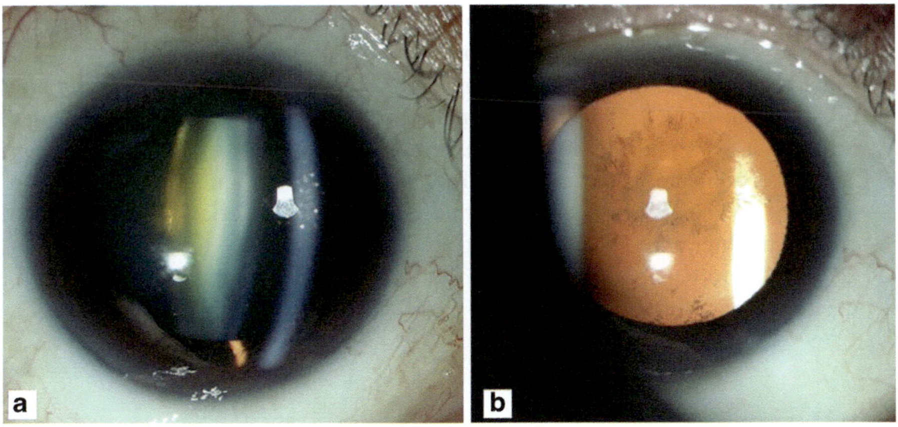

Fig. 3.13 Nuclear cataract (**a**) and posterior lens capsule opacity (**b**) caused by silicone oil filling

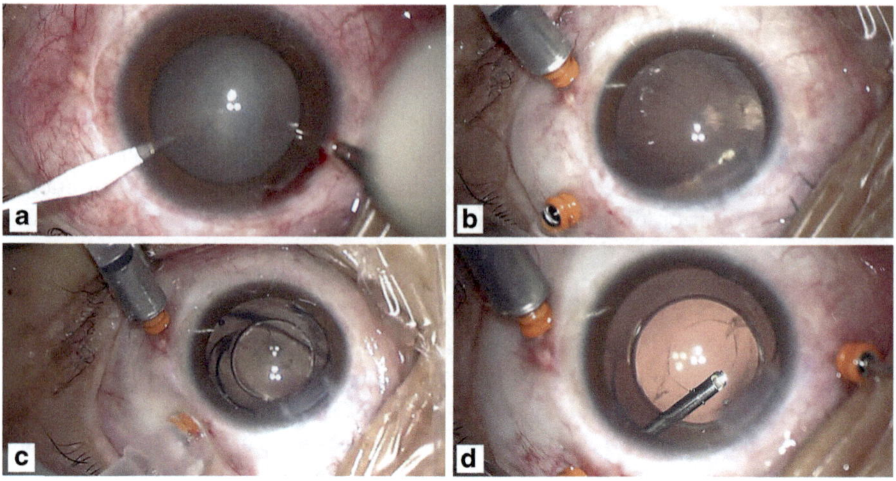

Fig. 3.14 Silicone oil removal combined with phacoemulsification. (**a**) Perform phacoemulsification first; (**b**) place trocar, remove part of the silicone oil first, and ensure the depth of the anterior chamber; (**c**) place an intraocular lens and completely remove the silicone oil; and (**d**) use a vitrectomy cutter to open a round window in the posterior capsule (approximately 4 mm in diameter)

(b) Poor posterior capsule elasticity or defects: Due to long-term silicone oil contact or prior iatrogenic damage. Inject viscoelastic at the capsule-oil interface to prevent oil migration. If the defect is large, avoid forced phacoemulsification; instead, enlarge the corneal incision for intact nucleus delivery, or remove oil first then extract nuclear fragments with a vitrectomy cutter.

(c) Lax zonular fibers: Anterior chamber fluctuations allow oil droplets to enter the anterior chamber, and fluid reflux from hydrodissection/phacoemulsification increases intraocular volume, narrowing working space. Insert a trocar to remove a small amount of oil, then maintain depth with viscoelastic. Keep the phaco tip within the capsular bag to protect the endothelium.

3. Rational Selection of Intraocular Lens
   Since residual silicone oil droplets inevitably remain in the vitreous cavity after oil removal, an IOL with low affinity for silicone oil should be implanted. Silicone IOLs should be avoided, as they adhere to oil droplets, causing lens surface opacification that compromises visual recovery and complicates management. When using a new IOL model, review its material composition and consult the literature for any reported adverse events related to silicone oil interaction. Where feasible, conduct in vitro testing for silicone oil adhesion before deciding on its suitability.

(2) Corneal Lesions

In aphakic, pseudophakic, and highly myopic eyes, the likelihood of silicone oil migrating into the anterior chamber after surgery is increased. Prolonged contact between silicone oil and the corneal endothelium impairs normal corneal metabolism and predisposes the eye to endothelial decompensation. Some patients may also develop band keratopathy (calcium carbonate deposition in the anterior elastic layer of the cornea; Fig. 3.15a, b).

The following preventive measures can be adopted: (1) Induce miosis during oil injection: In the final stage of silicone oil injection, dilute pilocarpine may be injected into the anterior chamber to induce miosis. Since pupil constriction takes 5–10 minutes, excessive injection to accelerate miosis should be avoided to prevent corneal endothelial damage. (2) Maintain face-down positioning postoperatively: Strict face-down positioning should be maintained. Short-term use of miotics may be considered, but anterior chamber depth and intraocular pressure must be closely monitored to promptly detect and manage any pupillary block induced by miosis. (3) Remove oil droplets early: During follow-up, silicone oil droplets in the anterior chamber should be identified early and irrigated promptly. If retinal reattachment is satisfactory, silicone oil removal from the vitreous cavity should be performed as early as possible. (4) Adjust head positioning for minimal residual droplets: If the amount of silicone oil in the anterior chamber is minimal, or if droplets continue to enter after repeated irrigation, patients may be advised to modify head positioning during daily activities and sleep. For example, alternating head positions during sleep (e.g., left lateral–supine–right lateral) can reduce the total duration of contact between silicone oil droplets and the superior corneal endothelium. (5) Remove band keratopathy deposits: Calcium carbonate deposits on Bowman's layer can be partially removed with a blade. Complete removal is often difficult and risks damaging the stromal layer. (6) Refer for corneal surgery if severe: If severe corneal endothelial decompensation has occurred, timely referral to a cornea specialist is necessary for penetrating keratoplasty or endothelial keratoplasty.

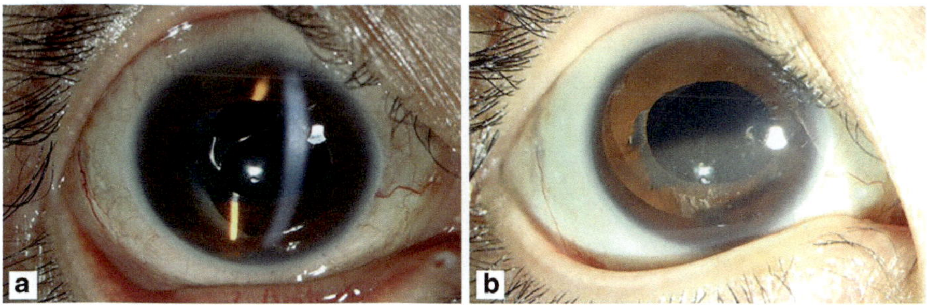

Fig. 3.15 Band-like keratopathy caused by silicone oil migration into the anterior chamber in aphakic eyes. (**a**) Two weeks after surgery, the inferior iris incision was intact, silicone oil had not migrated into the anterior chamber, and the cornea was transparent. (**b**) Two months after surgery, the inferior iris incision was blocked, silicone oil had migrated into the anterior chamber, and the cornea had band-like degeneration

(3) Elevated Intraocular Pressure

This is a relatively common (approximately 30%) yet often overlooked complication. Due to longer follow-up intervals and the typically gradual IOP rise, patients may easily overlook pressure abnormalities. High-risk patients should be closely monitored: ① High myopia; ② history of glaucoma; ③ postoperative hyphema; ④ pupillary block; ⑤ iris neovascularization; ⑥ posterior synechiae; ⑦ silicone oil migration into the anterior chamber; ⑧ significant silicone oil emulsification; and ⑨ long-term corticosteroid use. Management depends on retinal status and may involve silicone oil removal or exchange, combined with medical or surgical interventions in collaboration with a glaucoma specialist based on anterior segment findings.

(a) ***Early Postoperative Period*** During the period from the first postoperative day to approximately two weeks after surgery, careful assessment of the anterior chamber is essential to determine the cause of elevated IOP. This includes evaluating whether the anterior chamber has significantly shallowed, whether the angle is closed, and whether silicone oil has migrated into the anterior chamber (Fig. 3.16a–c). The main contributors to early postoperative IOP elevation include: (1) preexisting glaucoma or angle dysgenesis; (2) severe inflammatory reaction induced by surgery and silicone oil tamponading; (3) pupillary block (large oil droplet obstructing aqueous flow); (4) trabecular meshwork damage (postoperative free radicals); (5) Ciliary body edema (inflammatory), and (6) excessive silicone oil tamponading.

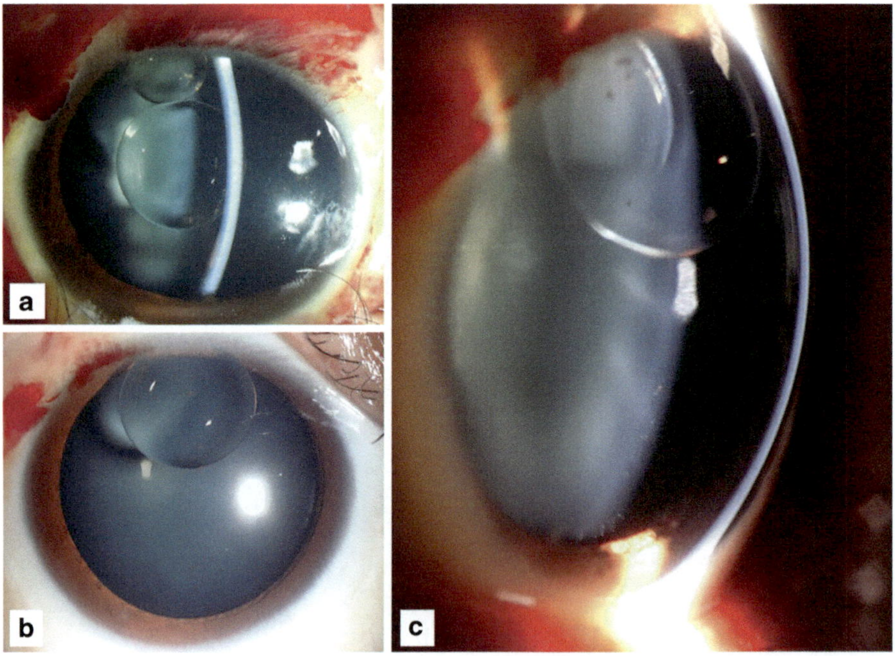

Fig. 3.16 Silicone oil overflows into the anterior chamber. **(a)** On the first postoperative day, silicone oil droplets are visible in the anterior chamber with an IOP of 35 mmHg. The patient was instructed to maintain face-down positioning with mydriasis for 14 days, then alternate left and right lateral positioning. **(b)** At two months, the cornea was clear, oil droplets were slightly reduced, and IOP was 15 mmHg. **(c)** Side view shows minimal contact between oil droplets and the corneal endothelium

(b) ***Mid- to Long-Term Elevated Intraocular Pressure (1–12 Months Postoperatively*** This is a relatively common (approximately 30%) yet often overlooked complication. Due to longer follow-up intervals and the typically gradual IOP rise, patients may easily overlook pressure abnormalities. High-risk patients should be closely monitored: (1) high myopia; (2) history of glaucoma; (3) postoperative hyphema; (4) pupillary block; (5) iris neovascularization; (6) posterior synechiae; (7) silicone oil migration into the anterior chamber; (8) significant silicone oil emulsification; and (9) long-term corticosteroid use. Management depends on retinal status and may involve silicone oil removal or exchange, combined with medical or surgical interventions in collaboration with a glaucoma specialist based on anterior segment findings.

The main causes of early postoperative IOP elevation are silicone oil entry into the anterior chamber and surgery-induced inflammation. The following management principles apply: (1) Anti-inflammatory therapy: Use corticosteroid and nonsteroidal anti-inflammatory eye drops at frequent intervals (e.g., every 2 hours), combined with mydriatics to maintain pupil mobility. If severe, add systemic corticosteroids (e.g., prednisone 30 mg once daily for 7 days). (2) Monitor and irrigate the anterior chamber: If a large silicone oil droplet is seen, promptly irrigate the anterior chamber. At the end of the procedure, inject filtered air into the anterior chamber to help prevent oil reentry (Fig. 3.17). (3) IOP-lowering medications: Use topical agents concurrently. Avoid prostaglandin analogues, as they may exacerbate inflammation. (4) Use systemic agents with caution: Systemic IOP-lowering agents offer limited effectiveness and potential side effects. Mannitol reduces aqueous humor volume by increasing plasma colloid osmotic pressure, but the intraocular silicone oil volume remains unchanged. Inappropriate use of mannitol can rapidly lower anterior chamber pressure, increasing the likelihood of silicone oil migration from the vitreous cavity into the anterior chamber.

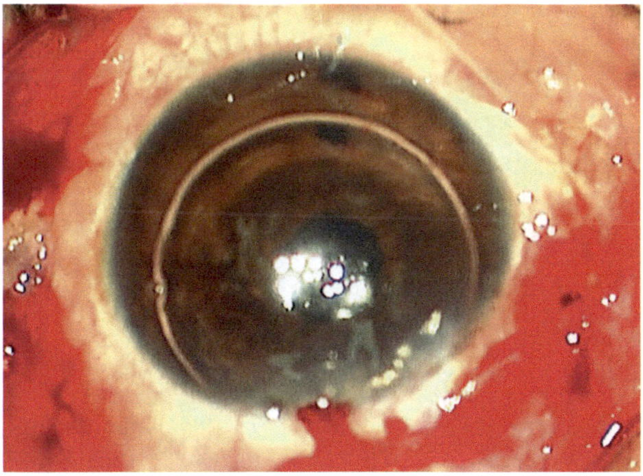

Fig. 3.17 Filtered air injection into the anterior chamber to prevent silicone oil migration. This patient presented with several special circumstances: (1) only seeing eye; (2) pseudophakic eye with an incomplete posterior capsule; and (3) intraoperative observation of silicone oil droplets entering the anterior chamber. To minimize further oil migration, after irrigating the oil droplets, two adjacent peripheral iridotomies were created in the inferior iris, and filtered air was injected into the anterior chamber

(4) Silicone Oil Dislocation

Because silicone oil is a fluid, it can migrate outside the vitreous cavity during or after surgery. Due to its high viscosity and surface tension, it rarely flows back on its own. Dislocation may occur in the following locations:

1. Anterior chamber High-risk patients: (1) high myopia; (2) aphakia; (3) zonular laxity; (4) pseudophakia; (5) poor postoperative face-down positioning.
   (a) Prevention during surgery: For aphakic or pseudophakic eyes, an inferior peripheral iridotomy (Ando's iridotomy) can be created (Fig. 3.18a, b).

   For heavy silicone oil, peripheral iridotomies should be placed superiorly. Illustrative case: A patient with an unremarkable right eye underwent vitrectomy with silicone oil tamponade and was instructed to maintain face-down positioning. That night, the left eye developed severe distending pain, which subsided spontaneously during the hospital visit. Medical history revealed that the left eye had undergone vitrectomy with lens extraction, heavy silicone oil tamponade, and a superior peripheral iridotomy 10 years earlier; the oil had never been removed and showed no significant emulsification. UBM revealed complete angle closure and anterior chamber flattening (Fig. 3.19a–c). The diagnosis was pupillary block caused by heavy silicone oil entering the anterior chamber due to sustained face-down positioning. After discontinuing face-down positioning, the pain resolved and did not recur.

   Ando's iridotomy was first proposed by Fumitaka Ando (Nagoya Medical University, Japan) in 1985. (He also invented the scleral nail for fixing retinal flaps, a valuable technique before the advent of heavy liquids.) In a correspondence published in *Am J Ophthalmol*, Ando first suggested that a circumferential incision at the iris base reduces silicone oil migration into

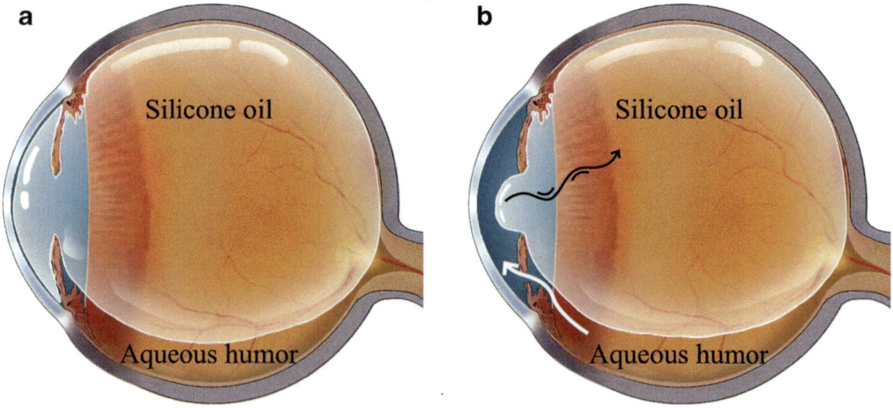

Fig. 3.18 Mechanism of action of Ando iridotomy. (**a**) Pupillary block caused by silicone oil. (**b**) Ando iridotomy (inferior peripheral iridotomy) creates an alternate pathway for aqueous humor, bypassing the pupillary block and preventing silicone oil migration into the anterior chamber

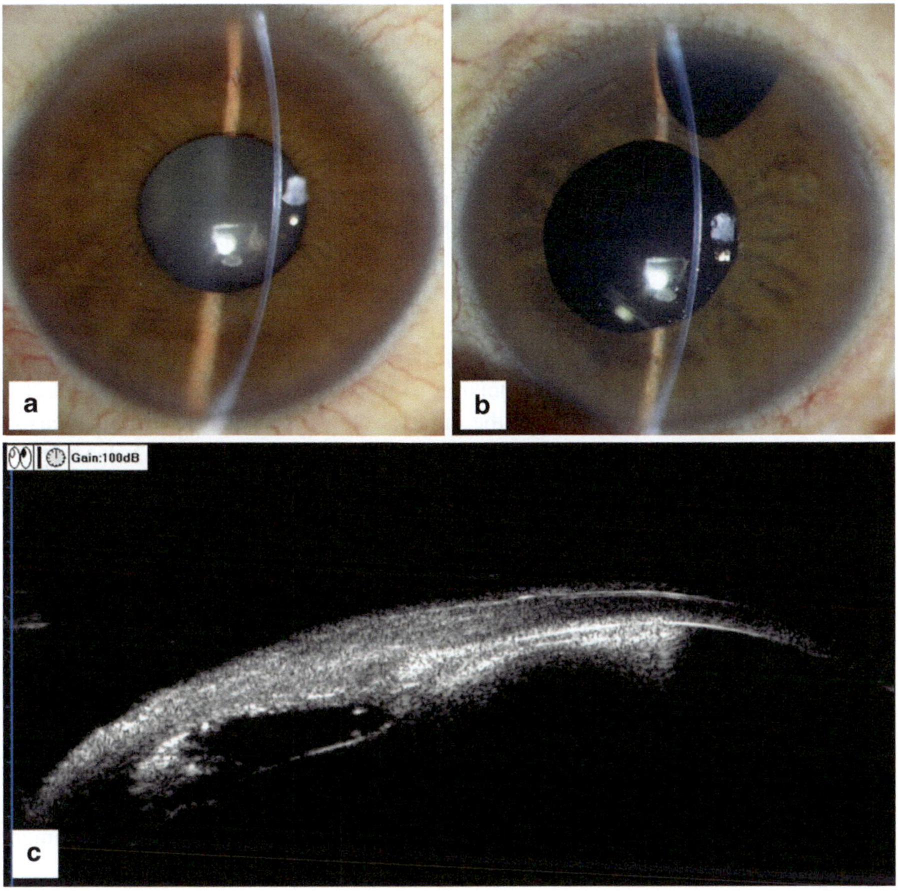

Fig. 3.19 An interesting case with concomitant tamponade of heavy and light silicone oils in each eye. (**a**) No abnormality in the anterior segment of the right eye. (**b**) The left eye shows an open superior iridotomy and a flat anterior chamber. (**c**) UBM examination reveals complete angle closure and pupillary block

the anterior chamber. The formal results were published in *Br J Ophthalmol* in 1987. Among 62 aphakic eyes with Ando's iridotomy, only four (6.5%) developed anterior chamber silicone oil dislocation after 7 months of follow-up.

When performing Ando's iridotomy with a vitrectomy cutter, maintain intraocular pressure to prevent iris bleeding. Spontaneous closure occurs in approximately 20% of cases, most commonly in younger patients and those with multiple prior surgeries. The main cause is postoperative inflammation leading to fibrin exudation at the iridotomy. Combined postoperative miosis and anti-inflammatory therapy may act to maintain the patency. If closure occurs, laser iridotomy under slit lamp or surgical revision may be performed; however, this may aggravate iris inflammation and often leads to re-closure. Close follow-up is required.

(b) Postoperative treatment: For phakic and pseudophakic eyes, if silicone oil overflows into the anterior chamber and causes acute intraocular pressure elevation, the anterior chamber can be flushed in the operating room. The surgical pearls are as follows: (1) If the anterior chamber becomes significantly shallower, it indicates the presence of malignant glaucoma. Before flushing the silicone oil in the anterior chamber, a trocar should be inserted to release the excessive pressure in the vitreous cavity; otherwise, silicone oil will continue to flow into the anterior chamber. (2) Use miosis to increase the blockage of the lens-iris septum against silicone oil in the vitreous cavity. (3) Corneal incisions can be made at the 6:00 and 12:00 positions. Inject viscoelastic into the lower incision, squeeze the silicone oil droplet toward the edge of the upper incision, and then gently press the posterior lip of the upper incision to release the silicone oil droplets. (4) Rinse the viscoelastic from the anterior chamber. Because fluid can easily flow back into the vitreous cavity, attention should be paid to releasing the pressure in the vitreous cavity at this time. If necessary, some silicone oil should be removed. (5) Finally, filtered air can be injected into the anterior chamber. The surface tension of the gas prevents silicone oil from overflowing again; on the other hand, it helps check whether the viscoelastic in the anterior chamber has been sufficiently removed.

2. Subretinal space: Subretinal silicone oil dislocation is rare but carries serious consequences and greater treatment difficulty. During oil injection, sudden globe collapse can fold the trocar opening. If a large peripheral tear is present, especially with anterior PVR, oil may enter the subretinal space. Sometimes, the management requires a large peripheral retinotomy to drive out the high-viscosity oil droplets.

   Postoperative subretinal oil dislocation occurs in recurrent retinal detachment with significant PVR, due to traction from fibroproliferative membranes that enlarge new or existing tears. Prognosis is poor. Prevention focuses on the first surgery: ensuring complete posterior vitreous detachment and adequate vitreous resection.
3. Suprachoroidal space: Suprachoroidal dislocation is extremely rare.It occurs when trocar dislocation or choroidal bulge causes the trocar opening to lie in the suprachoroidal space during oil injection. If it occurs, first remove the trocar and enlarge the scleral incision. Then, use silicone oil buoyancy and a cotton swab to express the suprachoroidal oil through the scleral incision. This process is very time-consuming, and IOP should be maintained stable throughout. To prevent this rare accident, inject silicone oil under direct visualization with a wide-angle lens.

(5) Toxicity to the Retina and Optic Nerve

Although the overall safety of silicone oil has been widely recognized, a small number of silicone oil toxicity cases still occur. Clinically, it presents as severe postoperative visual acuity loss and central scotoma. Morphologically, it often manifests as retinal ganglion cell apoptosis and optic nerve atrophy. Unfortunately, no effective prevention or treatment currently exists. Studies have shown that the retina is more susceptible to phototoxic damage when the eye is filled with silicone oil; therefore, excessively strong light should be avoided during silicone oil injection and removal. In addition, other contributing factors should be excluded, such as accidental retrobulbar anesthesia and excessive intraoperative intraocular pressure.

(6) Silicone Oil Removal

Silicone oil removal can be performed via an anterior or posterior approach, both of which are relatively straightforward. The anterior approach involves creating a capsulotomy in the posterior capsule after lens removal and expressing the silicone oil through a corneal incision; intraocular lens implantation may be considered depending on the clinical situation. The posterior approach uses negative pressure from a vitrectomy machine or a standard syringe to actively aspirate silicone oil through a scleral incision.

In China, we often use the machine-independent method to remove the silicone oil. The following is a brief description of its steps and precautions (Fig. 3.20a–d).

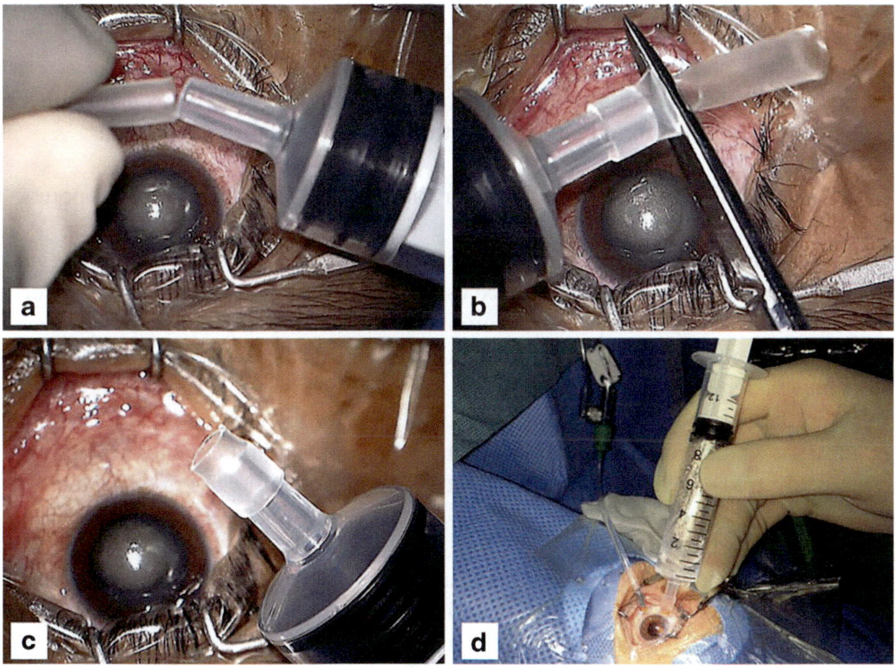

Fig. 3.20 Machine-independent method to have silicone oil removal. (**a**) Insert the polyethylene tube into the tip of a 10-mL syringe. (**b**) Use scissors to cut until 2~3 mm is exposed. (**c**) Pay attention to keep the cross-section smooth and flat. (**d**) Put the polyethylene tube on the trocar, retract the syringe plunger, and drain off the silicone oil

The approach is demonstrated below:

1. Prepare the silicone oil removal equipment. Insert a prepared polyethylene tube into a 10-mL syringe, leaving approximately 2–3 mm exposed. Cut the tube so that the cross-section is smooth and flat to ensure airtightness and avoid conjunctival trauma.
2. Insert the trocars. Insert the upper and lower trocars as usual. Use the temporal trocar for fluid infusion and the upper trocar for silicone oil removal.
3. Start fluid perfusion. To prevent low intraocular pressure and silicone oil droplets from blocking the inner opening of the trocar, temporarily increase perfusion pressure to 35–40 mmHg, then adjust to 20–25 mmHg after IOP stabilizes.
4. Aspirate silicone oil. Place the syringe (with the pre-covered polyethylene tube) perpendicular to the scleral surface and buckle it onto the outer opening of the trocar. Pull the syringe plunger by hand to generate negative pressure. A vascular clamp may be used to kept the plunger in postion.
5. Continue to aspirate. When the oil-fluid interface is observed through the pupil, fine-tune the position of the upper scleral incision toward the apex of the eyeball to ensure smooth silicone oil extraction and reduce sudden IOP changes.
6. Remove residual silicone oil droplets. The following methods can be used to further ensure the complete removal of silicone oil: (1) Insert a flute needle to guide the oil droplets. (2) Segmentally withdraw the upper trocar to allow fluid flow to flush out oil droplets hiding at its inner opening. (3) Use a squint hook to depress the peripheral sclera. (4) Perform air/fluid exchange.
7. Fully examine the fundus. Confirm complete silicone oil removal and check whether additional treatment (e.g., further photocoagulation) is needed.

When using this method, we should pay attention to the following three points:

1. Avoid damaging the conjunctiva: The polyethylene tube is relatively hard and may compress the conjunctiva. Excessive force can cause conjunctival injury. Ensure the tube cross-section is smooth and flat (trim with scissors if needed). Do not apply excessive pressure to the conjunctival surface; only enough to achieve adequate sealing.
2. Keep the syringe airtight: After the polyethylene tube is buckled onto the conjunctiva with appropriate pressure, pulling the syringe plunger generates negative pressure. This negative pressure aspirates silicone oil while also drawing the conjunctiva tightly against the tube cross-section, creating a closed space that ensures sufficient suction.
3. Pay attention to intraocular pressure fluctuations. The syringe can generate negative pressure up to 650 mmHg, which is higher than machine-generated negative pressure (Fig. 3.21). When the trocar inner opening is blocked by silicone oil but infusion is unobstructed, IOP fluctuation is generally minimal. However, during the final stage of oil extraction, aspiration should be performed slowly. If IOP becomes too low, release the contact between the syringe and the conjunctiva promptly.

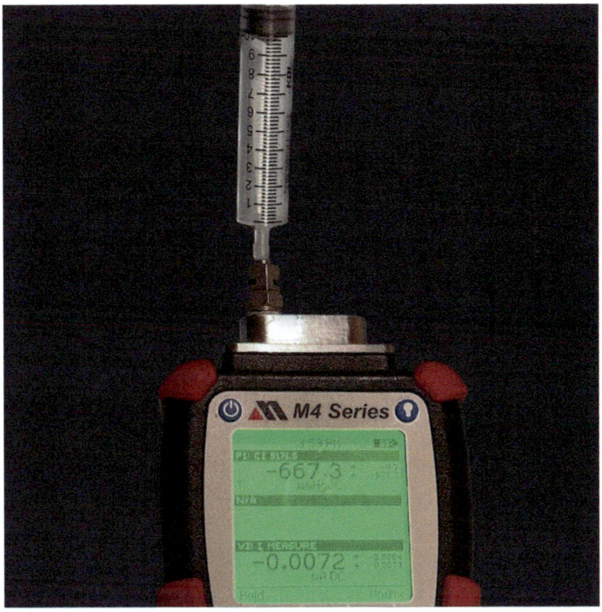

Fig. 3.21 The plunger of the 10-mL syringe is pulled up to the 10 mL mark, and the measured negative pressure is 667.3 mmHg

Finally, it must be noted that because silicone oil is hydrophobic and highly viscous, it can be "flushed" out of the vitreous cavity by perfusion fluid but cannot be "washed" clean. After most of the silicone oil is removed, a small amount remains adherent to the inner wall of the eyeball. Currently, no surfactant exists to help remove this residual oil more thoroughly. Therefore, regardless of the removal method used, some patients still complain of floaters postoperatively—these are caused by emulsified silicone oil droplets remaining in the vitreous cavity. This phenomenon is more common in highly myopic eyes and young patients. In a small number of patients, emulsified oil droplets may block the chamber angle and cause elevated IOP.

3.5 Heavy Liquid

3.5.1 Physical and Chemical Properties

The chemical name of heavy liquid is perfluorocarbon liquid (PFCL), a synthetic fluoride. The types commonly used in vitreoretinal surgery include perfluoro-octane (PFO), perfluoroperhydrophenanthrene (Vitreon), perfluorodecalin (PFD), perfluorotributylamide (PFTB), and perfluorooctylbromide (PFOB). PFD is the most commonly used type in China.

Heavy liquid is widely used in the chemical industry and has been gradually applied in clinical practice since the 1960s. Due to its strong oxygen-carrying capacity, it has been used as a blood substitute to save critically ill patients. Since the 1980s, heavy liquid has played an increasingly important role in vitreoretinal surgery, greatly reducing surgical difficulty and significantly improving success rates. It is known as the "third hand" of retina surgeons.

The characteristics of heavy liquid related to vitreoretinal surgery include the following:

1. High density: Approximately twice that of water. Since retinal density is roughly equal to water, gravity can flatten the retina, displace subretinal fluid, and facilitate removal of dropped lens fragments.
2. Colorless and transparent: Ensures a clear surgical field.
3. Low viscosity: Allows smooth injection onto the posterior pole and rapid removal from the eye.
4. Chemical inertness: Does not react with other intraocular substances in the short term, ensuring safety.
5. Refractive index: Close to water (1.33) but not identical, creating a refractive interface that allows the surgeon to distinguish the heavy liquid level in the vitreous cavity.
6. Vapor pressure: The vapor pressure indicates the ability of the molecules in the liquid to leave the liquid and vaporize or evaporate. The higher the vapor pressure, the easier it is for the liquid to vaporize (the vaporization of the intraocular fluid will cause turbidity of the posterior capsule of the lens); at 37 °C, the vapor pressure of the heavy liquid perfluorodecalin (PFD) we commonly use is 12.5 mmHg, while the vapor pressure of water is 47.1 mmHg, which means that heavy liquid is not easy to vaporize in the eye, which can further ensure the clarity of the surgical field.
7. Surface tension: Slightly lower than silicone oil, making it prone to form fish-egg-like droplets in the eye. This is a major disadvantage, as droplets can easily migrate through retinal breaks into the subretinal space. Therefore, droplet formation should be minimized during injection.
8. Interfacial tension: High interfacial tension between heavy liquid and water promotes a large, stable interface, which helps prevent intraocular fluid from re-entering the subretinal space.
9. Incompatibility: Under normal use, heavy liquid does not mix with water, silicone oil, blood, or other intraocular substances.

3.5.2 Indications and Usage of Heavy Liquid

With the popularization of wide-angle surgical lenses, the use of heavy liquid has declined significantly in recent years, especially in patients with fresh rhegmatogenous retinal detachment. As mentioned above, among the 61 patients with fresh rhegmatogenous retinal detachment who underwent PPV, only one patient required heavy liquid to reposition the retina (because the primary break spanned 5 clock hours). In the remaining patients, the wide-angle lens assisted with head positioning, and most subretinal fluid was drained through gas/liquid exchange. The small amount of residual subretinal fluid was completely absorbed by the first postoperative day.

Although the use of heavy liquid has declined significantly, it remains a powerful tool in certain vitreoretinal surgeries. Beginners should clearly understand its indications and strive to avoid complications during use.

3.5.3 Indications and Effects of Heavy Liquid

(1) Giant Retinal Tear

Because giant retinal tear (GRT) occurs mostly at the periphery, surgical treatment was very difficult before the advent of heavy liquid. The main problem was that the posterior edge of the tear was prone to slippage and curling during fluid/air exchange. Gas entering the vitreous cavity diffuses from the periphery to the posterior pole, generating a pressure difference that may cause the posterior edge of the tear to slip and curl.

Various improved surgical methods were used, such as an inversion bed, prone positioning, gas injection with retinal flattening from posterior pole to periphery followed by supine repositioning, and transscleral retinal nails to prevent edge slippage. Although these methods had certain advantages at the time, they were relatively difficult to perform. Understanding these challenges makes it easy to appreciate the important role of heavy liquid in GRT surgery.

Heavy liquid has revolutionized GRT treatment, and its advantages are clearly demonstrated during surgery: First, it fixes the retina at the posterior pole, improving the convenience and safety of delicate peripheral manipulations. Second, it can be gradually advanced from the posterior pole to the periphery, fixing the posterior edge and corners of the retinal tear against the RPE layer, thereby creating stable conditions for laser photocoagulation. This effect is known as the "steamroller effect" (Fig. 3.22a–c).

(2) Proliferative Vitreoretinopathy (PVR)

There are two major problems in the surgical treatment of PVR: first, a fibrous proliferative membrane at the posterior pole, which may present as a wide or narrow funnel; second, intraretinal PVR, characterized by a hardened retinal texture, poor mobility, and obvious shrinkage.

The role of heavy liquid in PVR surgery is reflected in the following aspects:

1. Expanding the posterior pole retina. After complete peeling of the fibrous proliferative membrane at the posterior pole, the retina often remains in a "pseudo-shrinkage" state due to poor mobility—i.e., although traction is relieved, the retina still cannot be adequately stretched. At this point, heavy liquid injection and its "steamroller effect" help flatten the posterior pole retina.

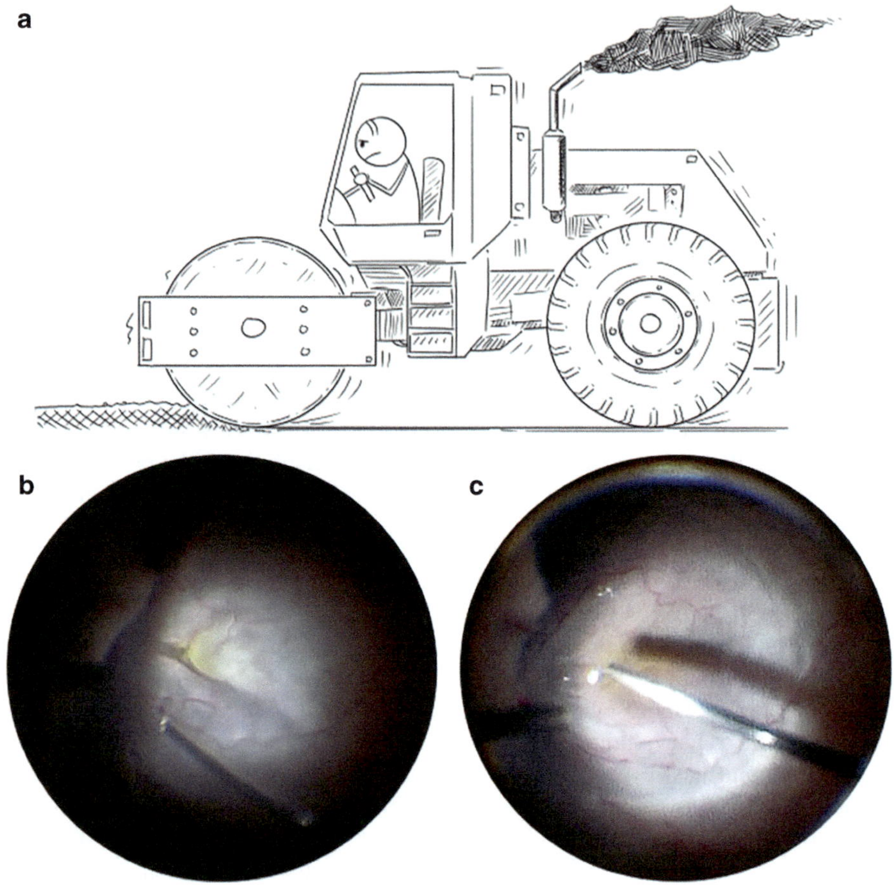

Fig. 3.22 The "steamroller" effect of heavy liquid. **(a)** Working principle of the steamroller. **(b)** After removal of the proliferative membrane at the posterior pole, retinal wrinkles remain. **(c)** After heavy liquid injection, the retinal wrinkles at the posterior pole are flattened

2. Reduce mobility of the peripheral retina. When the posterior pole is fixed with heavy liquid, the mobility of the peripheral retina will be significantly reduced, which will help the surgeon to use a vitrectomy cutter to remove the dense peripheral vitreous, and also provide a relatively stable force plane for the peeling of the proliferative membrane and bands.

(3) Retinal Detachment Without Macula Involvement or Secondary to Peripheral Tears

For retinal detachment without macular involvement, a small amount of heavy liquid may be injected onto the posterior pole before starting peripheral vitrectomy to prevent subretinal fluid from spreading under the macula. However, the injected volume should not be too large; it is best to keep the heavy liquid within the vascular arcades. Otherwise, heavy liquid may easily enter the subretinal space and leave residual droplets postoperatively.

If the retinal tear is located in the periphery, draining subretinal fluid using simple fluid/air exchange is difficult. Heavy liquid can be injected onto the posterior pole, up to just below the posterior edge of the tear. This displaces most of the subretinal fluid from the posterior pole through the tear into the vitreous cavity. The remaining subretinal fluid in the periphery is then aspirated using fluid/air exchange. This technique is known as the "sandwich technique" (Fig. 3.23a, b).

The obvious advantage of this method is that it prevents the surgeon from creating a retinal break to drain subretinal fluid and allows testing of the mobility and compliance of the mid-peripheral retina during surgery. If the peripheral retina remains incompletely flat after gas/liquid exchange, heavy liquid should not be injected in large quantities to try to "flatten" the retina. The following three problems must first be ruled out: (1) Whether the peripheral vitreous has been sufficiently removed. (2) Whether there are proliferative membranes or bands beneath or anterior to the retina. (3) Whether there is obvious retinal rigidity or shortening.

Heavy liquid may also be employed in the following scenarios: (1) Complex retinal abnormalities resulting from trauma, such as retinal incarceration or subretinal hemorrhage. (2) Dislocation of the lens or intraocular lens (though its use has been declining). (3) Subretinal or suprachoroidal hemorrhage secondary to various etiologies.

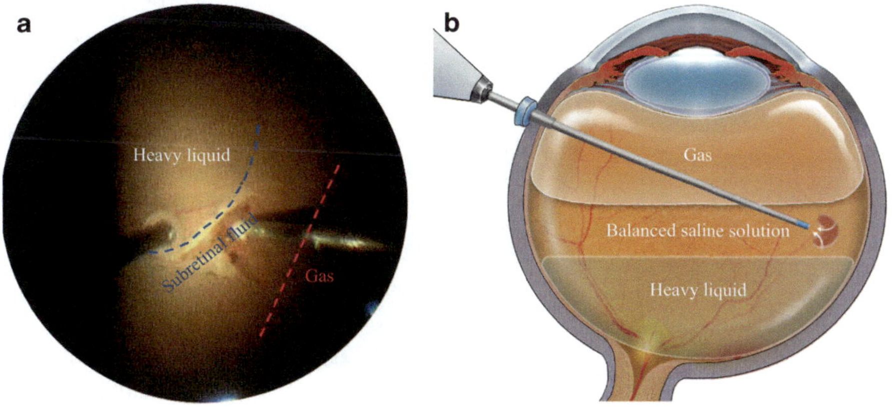

Fig. 3.23 "Sandwich technique" for retinal repositioning. (**a**) Surgical video screenshot. The red dotted line indicates the gas-water interface (subretinal fluid and perfusion fluid), and the blue dotted line indicates the water-heavy liquid interface. (**b**) Schematic diagram of the technique

3.5.4 Injection and Drainage of Heavy Liquid

(1) Injection

In some countries, a dual-bore cannula is often used to inject heavy liquid. The tip is placed within the heavy liquid droplet, while the side opening is kept above the heavy liquid level. The obvious advantage of this method is that, during heavy liquid injection, the side opening drains fluid from the vitreous cavity, thereby preventing an excessive rise in intraocular pressure.

In China, a blunt cannula (0.4 mm diameter) is commonly used. During injection, the cannula is first placed close to the posterior pole and should be positioned within the heavy liquid droplet to prevent the formation of fish-egg-like heavy liquid droplets (Fig. 3.24). The principle of "slow injection, multiple layers" should be followed to avoid compromising retinal blood perfusion due to excessive IOP. After injecting a certain amount of heavy liquid, the cannula should be withdrawn from the vitreous cavity to release pressure, then re-inserted for further injection. At the same time, observe the mobility of the mid-peripheral retina. If it appears relatively stiff, heavy liquid should not be injected forcibly, as this may cause heavy liquid to enter the subretinal space or induce retinal rupture.

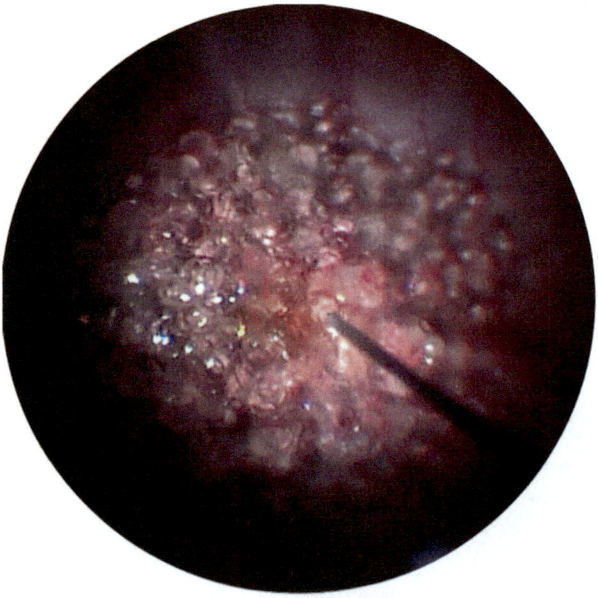

Fig. 3.24 During heavy liquid injection, fish-egg-like droplets may form. These droplets can easily enter the subretinal space and should be avoided or aspirated promptly

(2) Removal

Depending on the situation, heavy liquid can be removed by the following methods:

1. Drainage with a syringe. After heavy liquid injection, if retinal wrinkles have not been completely flattened, the heavy liquid in the vitreous cavity can be aspirated with a syringe for potential reuse.
2. Fluid/air exchange. This is the most commonly used method. Perfusion pressure in the gas-filled vitreous cavity can be increased to 50 mmHg, and heavy liquid is extracted using a vitrectomy cutter or flute needle.
3. Oil/fluid exchange. While under heavy liquid tamponade, first inject some silicone oil to stabilize intraocular pressure, then use a flute needle to aspirate the heavy liquid. During this process, closely monitor intraocular pressure changes.
4. Fluid/fluid exchange. If a large amount of heavy liquid remains or heavy liquid is being removed during a second-stage surgery, fluid/air exchange may not be necessary. Under BSS perfusion, a flute needle can be used to rapidly drain off the heavy liquid.

(3) Complications of Heavy Liquid

Complications of heavy liquid are the key reason hindering its wider application. These mainly include the following aspects:

1. Dislocation into the anterior chamber. When the patient is in the face-down position postoperatively, heavy liquid may cross the lens-iris septum (in phakic or pseudophakic eyes) or directly (in aphakic eyes) enter the anterior chamber under gravity (Fig. 3.25a). If the amount of heavy liquid is large, it can damage the corneal endothelium. Most residual heavy liquid can be removed at the slit lamp through an inferior corneal incision. If the anterior chamber becomes significantly shallow during removal, the procedure may be performed in multiple sessions.
2. Preretinal residue. When lying flat, patients often experience subjective discomfort of small droplets shaking in the center of the visual field, especially when vision is good (Fig. 3.25b, c). The main cause is that during gas/liquid exchange, a small amount of heavy liquid remains layered on the posterior pole and mid-peripheral retina. This is more likely if the retinal surface is irregular. Prevention can be achieved by the following two methods: (1) "Eye-shake" technique: The surgeon uses both hands—an endoillumination probe and a flute needle—to gently shake the eyeball. The centripetal force overcomes friction between the heavy liquid droplet and the retina, allowing the droplet to fall to the posterior pole under gravity, where it is then aspirated with the flute needle. (2) BSS flush: Inject a small amount of BSS to flush heavy liquid from the retinal surface toward the posterior pole, then aspirate all liquid with a flute needle.
3. Subretinal residue. If a heavy liquid droplet lies outside the vascular arcades, it generally does not affect vision. However, if it is located beneath the macula, it causes significant visual disturbance (Fig. 3.25d, e). Various methods have been used to remove subretinal heavy liquid, primarily by creating a retinotomy with

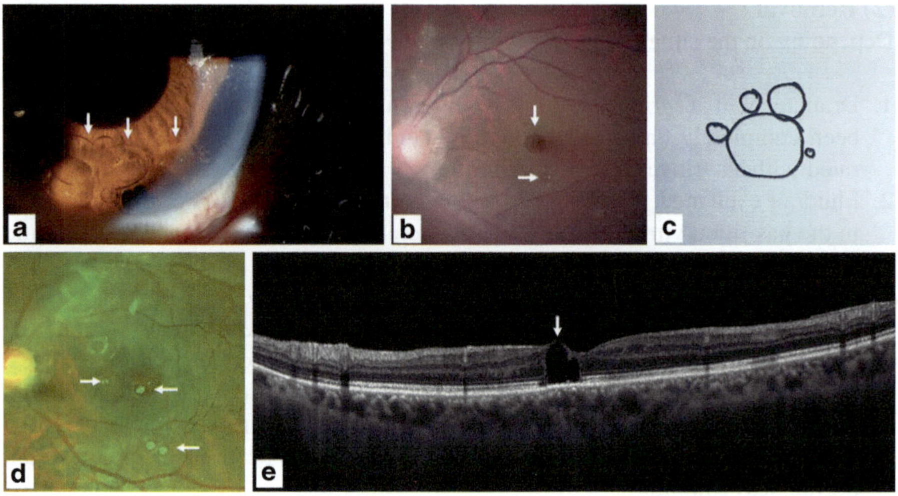

Fig. 3.25 Common postoperative complications of heavy liquid. **(a)** Heavy liquid enters the anterior chamber (white arrow). **(b)** During silicone oil removal, small heavy liquid droplets remain anterior to the retina (white arrow). **(c)** Patient complaint: when lying flat, small droplets rotate in front of the eyes; the patient drew the perceived image with a pen. **(d)** Heavy liquid retained in the neuroepithelial layer, involving the fovea (white arrow). **(e)** OCT image confirming heavy liquid retention in the fovea (white arrow)

a thin needle and then draining the droplet. However, secondary damage is almost inevitable, and symptoms may not improve substantially. (A simple technique is to use a 27-gauge diathermy to create a retinotomy, followed by passive drainage with a 27-gauge flute needle.)

(4) Foreign Body Inflammatory Reaction

Heavy liquid is a fluorine-containing synthetic substance with a certain amount of polar impurities. If too much heavy liquid remains in the eye for too long, it can stimulate a foreign body inflammatory reaction involving macrophages and multinucleated giant cells. In severe cases, it may cause dense macular epiretinal membranes (Fig. 3.26). Pathological examination can reveal transparent heavy liquid vesicles within macrophages in the vitreous cavity, beneath the posterior capsule, and within the retina. In silicone oil-filled eyes, heavy liquid droplets may interact with silicone oil, accelerating its emulsification. The resulting inflammatory reaction can further promote epiretinal membrane formation.

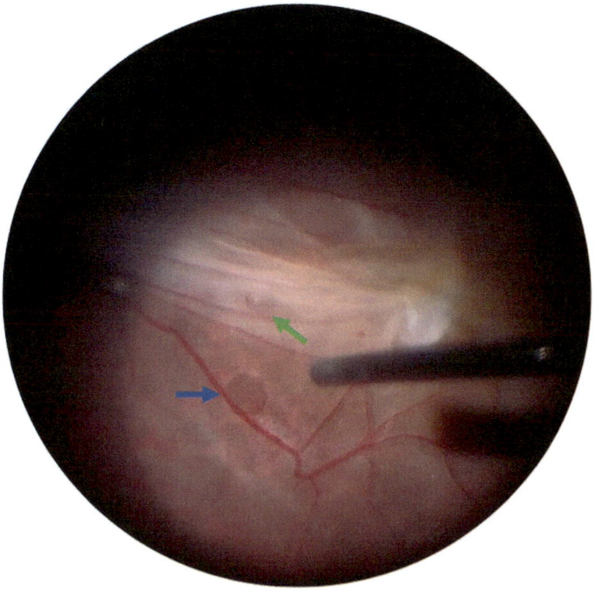

Fig. 3.26 Epiretinal membrane caused by heavy liquid residue. Heavy liquid droplets are visible anterior to the retina (blue arrow), and heavy liquid droplets wrapped by the epiretinal membrane (green arrow)

3.6 Summary

"A tool is only as good as the hand that wields it." In summary, intraocular tamponade agents—whether gas, silicone oil, or heavy liquids—remain indispensable pillars of vitreoretinal surgery, yet their success depends entirely on the surgeon's mastery of their behavior. For the beginner, these agents should not be viewed as simple "fillers," but as dynamic pharmacological and physical tools. Mastery begins with a rigorous understanding of their unique physical and chemical properties, such as surface tension, buoyancy, and viscosity. Only with this foundational knowledge can a surgeon identify the optimal scenarios and precise timing for their use, leveraging their specific advantages to solve complex clinical challenges like giant retinal tears or proliferative vitreoretinopathy.

Equally critical is the ability to look beyond the successful injection and understand the pathological and anatomical basis of potential complications. A skilled surgeon is defined not just by their ability to use a tool, but by their foresight to anticipate intraoperative shifts and postoperative risks, such as secondary glaucoma or emulsification. By learning to recognize the early warning signs of these complications, you can intervene before serious, irreversible consequences develop.

This chapter has laid the groundwork for that transition. By integrating the physical principles of these agents with a deep respect for ocular anatomy, the novice surgeon can move beyond mechanical repetition. Only through this disciplined approach can you gradually grow from a trainee into a master, wielding intraocular tamponade agents with the precision and skill necessary to achieve superior, life-changing surgical outcomes for your patients.

Part II

Vitrectomy in China

4 Preoperative Preparation and Anesthesia

Preoperative evaluation is an essential step in all surgeries, and vitreoretinal surgery is no exception. An accurate and objective preoperative evaluation helps surgeons better understand the patient's condition and expectations, develop an individualized treatment plan, and establish realistic expectations for surgical outcomes, thereby laying a solid foundation for a long-term, positive doctor-patient relationship.

Anesthesia for vitreoretinal surgery also has certain unique aspects, particularly local anesthesia, which is often administered by the surgeon. How to ensure the anesthetic effect while avoiding related complications is a topic that beginners in vitreoretinal surgery need to study in depth. This chapter will briefly describe preoperative evaluation and anesthesia precautions, aiming to create more favorable conditions for the smooth performance of vitreoretinal surgery.

4.1 Doctor-Patient Interaction

Before starting vitreoretinal surgery, the following points must be carefully confirmed.

1. The patient's general ocular condition. Do not rely solely on fundus examination findings or on reports from assistants. The surgeon must personally check the patient's vitreoretinal condition and confirm whether there are other ocular abnormalities, such as blepharitis, conjunctivitis, or dacryocystitis, which are high-risk factors that can easily cause postoperative intraocular infection.
2. The patient's demands and expectations. The complexity of vitreoretinal surgery makes the postoperative outcome highly uncertain. We should listen carefully to the patient's subjective complaints before surgery and accurately grasp their expectations when they are referred to us, and then make a decision on whether to perform surgery. For example, some patients come to the clinic only because of dry eyes and a foreign body sensation, but are found to have an epiretinal

Z. Zhang, U. Spandau, *Vitreoretinal Surgery*,
https://doi.org/10.1007/978-3-032-25271-5_4

membrane or a macular hole as an incidental finding. In this situation, we should inform the patient and decide whether to perform vitreoretinal surgery based on the severity of the disease.

3. Risk communication. Patients must be fully informed of the surgical objectives and potential risks through an objective, comprehensive preoperative consultation. This dialogue should encompass four critical pillars: (1) expected anatomical success rates; (2) the inherent uncertainty regarding functional visual recovery; (3) potential intraoperative and postoperative complications; and (4) the specific postoperative compliance required from the patient to optimize outcomes.

   For example, for non-complex rhegmatogenous retinal detachment, we not only need to explain why surgical intervention is the only option (because it is a sight-threatening disease) but also need to inform the patient which surgical approach will be taken and why (e.g., why pars plana vitrectomy is chosen instead of scleral buckling). We should then inform them about the anatomical success rate of the first surgery (approximately 90%), the uncertainty of postoperative visual recovery (individual outcomes vary considerably), possible complications during and after surgery (this should not be done with a "reading from a book" mentality; the surgeon should emphasize and fully inform according to the specific condition), and finally the tasks that patients need to cooperate with after surgery (such as maintaining a face-down position and attending scheduled follow-ups). Full and frank communication before surgery can lay a solid foundation for a good doctor-patient relationship.
4. Guarantee of objective conditions. Confirm whether the patient's pupil can be fully dilated and whether the refractive media are clear enough. Design the surgical procedures and their sequence in advance, and confirm with the operating room staff whether all required instruments and medications are available.
5. Ensuring the safety of patients. For patients with poor systemic conditions, ECG monitoring and rescue measures must be prepared in advance. It is best to schedule the operation during the time when medical staff at all levels in the hospital are most fully present.

4.2 Preparation of the Surgeon

The surgeon is definitely the key factor for surgical success. The surgeon is not only the planner of the surgery and the dispatcher of human and material resources but also the operator of the key steps of the procedure. In addition to non-replicable factors such as surgical experience, the surgeon's physical and mental states are also crucial in determining the final success or failure of the surgery.

1. Anticipate difficulties and propose solutions. The surgeon should carefully consider the patient's ocular condition, make a comprehensive estimate of the key points and possible complications during the surgery, and mentally rehearse the surgical steps.

For example, patients with retinal detachment concomitant with severe PVR or choroidal detachment are likely to experience inadvertent infusion at the early stage of surgery; they may also require retinectomy due to severe retinal shortening, resulting in significant bleeding from the retina; heavy liquid may accidentally enter the subretinal space, and slippage of the retinal flap may occur during silicone oil injection.

We should have an adequate knowledge base to manage this series of emergencies. The long-term accumulation of experience and extensive observation of surgeries can provide a solid foundation for the growth of novices.

Although we often emphasize that prevention is key, timely and appropriate interventions are also essential qualities and skills for surgeons.

2. Objectively evaluate your own surgical ability. Never start a procedure that you are not capable of completing without the guidance of a senior surgeon. Note that this refers to your "ability" rather than "confidence."

   Under normal circumstances, the first vitreoretinal surgery for an individual patient often has the best outcome. If the first surgery fails due to lack of experience or shortage of instruments, the subsequent intervention will become more complicated, and the outcome will often be poor.

   For example, when a young patient with fresh rhegmatogenous retinal detachment presents and the surgeon decides to perform PPV. Novice surgeons sometimes overlook the key step of creating posterior vitreous detachment. Because the patient's vitreous body is relatively transparent, the surgeon may mistakenly believe that the vitrectomy can be completed in a very short time, when in fact a large amount of transparent vitreous remains. If the retina is directly reattached at this point, proliferative changes and recurrent detachment may occur postoperatively. As a result, the difficulty of the second operation will increase significantly, and the prognosis will be greatly worsened.

   Another example is severe proliferative diabetic retinopathy with condense fibrovascular membranes. Without rich experience and delicate skills, the surgeon is very likely to be unable to finish the surgery well, ultimately causing excessive iatrogenic breaks and severe hemorrhage.

3. Reasonable arrangement of surgeries. Surgeries should be scheduled in an order that reflects their difficulty. When beginning to perform vitreoretinal surgery independently, the surgeon must estimate the difficulty and duration of each case and strive to balance challenging and routine cases within each surgical session.

   For example, we can place noncomplex rhegmatogenous retinal detachment at the beginning of the surgical day, which can improve our confidence and flexibility in subsequent operations in a very short time. Macular holes and epiretinal membranes can be arranged subsequently, which require very precise operations. And finally, to deal with proliferative diabetic retinopathy and other time-consuming surgeries. This arrangement not only allows us to concentrate on completing simple cases but also allows us to focus on solving complex problems without distraction.

4. Always maintain optimal psychological and physiological readiness. Ophthalmic surgery has a near-zero tolerance for error; even a minor lapse in judgment or

focus can result in severe, irreversible ocular damage. This demanding environment requires the surgeon to possess unwavering concentration and exceptional manual stability.

Prior to surgery, adequate rest and restorative sleep are mandatory. Surgeons should limit the intake of stimulants, such as caffeine and strong tea, and avoid strenuous physical activities like heavy lifting to minimize physiological tremors. These precautions are essential to ensuring the fluid and precise execution of delicate intraocular procedures.

When managing high-stakes cases or complex pathologies, maintaining a composed and objective mindset is vital. A disciplined mental state ensures that the surgeon's cognitive agility and manual dexterity remain uncompromised by psychological pressure, even in the most challenging surgical scenarios (Fig. 4.1).

5. Always maintain a good mental and physiological state. Ophthalmic surgery has a very low tolerance for error. Any carelessness may lead to serious, irreversible damage, which requires the surgeon to have good concentration and hand stability.

   We must ensure adequate rest and sleep before surgery, avoid excessive coffee and strong tea intake, avoid lifting heavy objects, and minimize hand tremor during surgery to ensure high-quality completion of delicate procedures. For patients with special conditions, the surgeon must maintain a normal mindset to ensure optimal performance. When encountering difficult situations, one should not allow mental factors to reduce the agility of thinking or the dexterity of the hands (Fig. 4.1). The distance between the operating table, operating chair, and microscope jointly determines whether the surgeon can achieve good sitting posture. The surgeon must ask the nurse to adjust the height of the operating table and then adjust the height of the operating chair accordingly, keeping the head and back naturally straight and the shoulders naturally relaxed (Fig. 4.2a).

   The most common mistake that surgeons make is to bend over unconsciously to accommodate the height of the microscope and the operating table. This causes the muscles of the waist and back to become overstretched. Long-term strain can lead to chronic pain, which may ultimately affect the successful completion of surgeries. When using microscopes, the surgeon's head and neck must inevitably maintain a fixed posture. To relieve fatigue, joints can be moved and

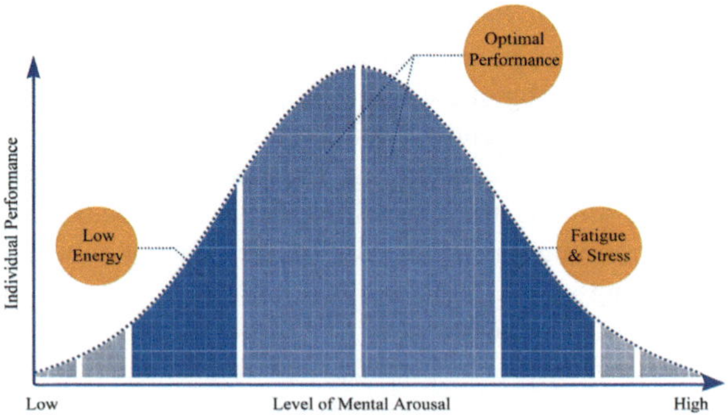

Fig. 4.1 Relationship between mental stress and surgical performance

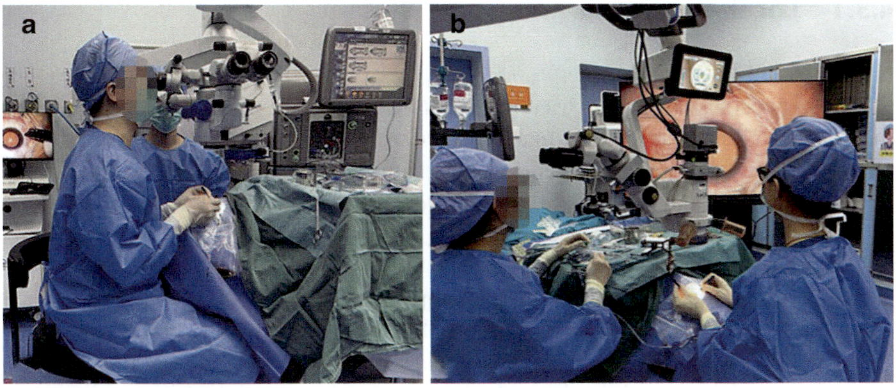

Fig. 4.2 Correct sitting posture under different microsurgery systems. (**a**) Correct sitting posture when using a microscope for vitreoretinal surgery. (**b**) When using a head-up three-dimensional imaging system, the surgeon's sitting posture is relatively comfortable, but the assistant sometimes has to turn his head to face the screen, which increases his fatigue

relaxed during intervals between surgeries. Studies in recent years have shown that the application of head-up three-dimensional imaging systems can significantly improve surgeon comfort and effectively reduce muscle and joint fatigue (Fig. 4.2b).

In scleral buckling, using an indirect ophthalmoscope to locate retinal breaks is a step that is particularly likely to cause surgeon fatigue. Almost all beginners will unconsciously move their heads closer to the indirect ophthalmoscope and the patient in an attempt to observe the vitreous and retina more clearly. Excessive bowing and bending will aggravate fatigue. The surgeon should gradually find the most comfortable working distance through daily practice.

4.3 Choice of Anesthesia

Anesthesia is a key component of all surgeries, and vitreoretinal surgery is no exception. Good anesthesia not only relieves the patient's pain but also ensures the normal performance of the surgeon. If the patient cannot cooperate well due to pain, it will greatly affect the surgeon's attention and skill level, resulting in an inability to optimally manage various possible complex conditions.

Anesthesia methods are divided into local anesthesia and general anesthesia, each with different advantages and disadvantages. The choice is primarily determined by multiple factors, including the patient's systemic condition, the complexity of the surgery, and the surgeon's preference.

4.3.1 Local Anesthesia

(I) Commonly Used Methods

Common anesthesia methods used in vitreoretinal surgery include retrobulbar anesthesia, peribulbar anesthesia, and sub-Tenon block. As retrobulbar anesthesia remains the most commonly used local anesthesia method in China, we will focus on its injection technique and precautions here.

(II) Retrobulbar Anesthesia

Retrobulbar anesthesia involves injecting anesthetic drugs into the intraconal space (the posterior muscle cone) to block the ophthalmic branches of cranial nerves III, IV, V, and VI; to immobilize the eyeball; and to eliminate sensation in the conjunctiva, cornea, and uvea, while also reducing extraocular muscle tension.

1. Injection method. Generally in China, a retrobulbar injection needle with a total length of 38 mm and a diameter of about 0.4 mm is used. The needle is initially inserted vertically at the junction of the lateral and middle thirds of the inferior orbital rim. The needle tip's bevel and the barrel's markings should be aligned and face the globe. Once the needle reaches a depth of 20 mm—passing the equator of the eyeball (noting that highly myopic eyes have a longer axial length)—or when the tip gently contacts the orbital floor, the needle is redirected approximately 30° superiorly and nasally. As the needle reaches a total depth of 30–35 mm (measured from the skin surface), the tip should be positioned within the muscle cone, between the optic nerve and the lateral rectus muscle. Before injection, aspiration is mandatory to confirm the absence of blood reflux. Upon confirmation, 3–4 mL of anesthetic is injected. The total insertion depth must not exceed 35 mm, and excessive nasal angulation must be avoided to prevent injury to the optic nerve or major orbital vasculature (Fig. 4.3).
2. Retrobulbar anesthesia in high myopia. Given the high prevalence of high myopia in East Asia, surgeons must account for the characteristic elongated axial length and the potential presence of posterior staphyloma in these patients. During retrobulbar injection, in addition to following standard protocols, it is crucial to avoid premature redirection of the needle. Upon entering the muscle cone, the angulation should be more acute (flatter) than usual; excessive nasal or superior tilting increases the risk of globe perforation at the site of the staphyloma. Such an injury often involves the macula, leading to devastating and irreversible visual loss (Fig. 4.4).
3. Choice of anesthetic drugs. Two percent lidocaine is commonly used for retrobulbar anesthesia. It can also be mixed with 0.75% bupivacaine in a 1:1 ratio to prolong intraoperative analgesia or relieve postoperative pain. The mixture must be thoroughly blended before injection. The onset time of lidocaine is 4–6 minutes, and its duration of action is 40–60 minutes. The onset time of bupivacaine is 5–11 minutes, and its duration of action is 4–12 hours. For non-complex vitreoretinal surgeries, most of which can be completed within one hour, lidocaine

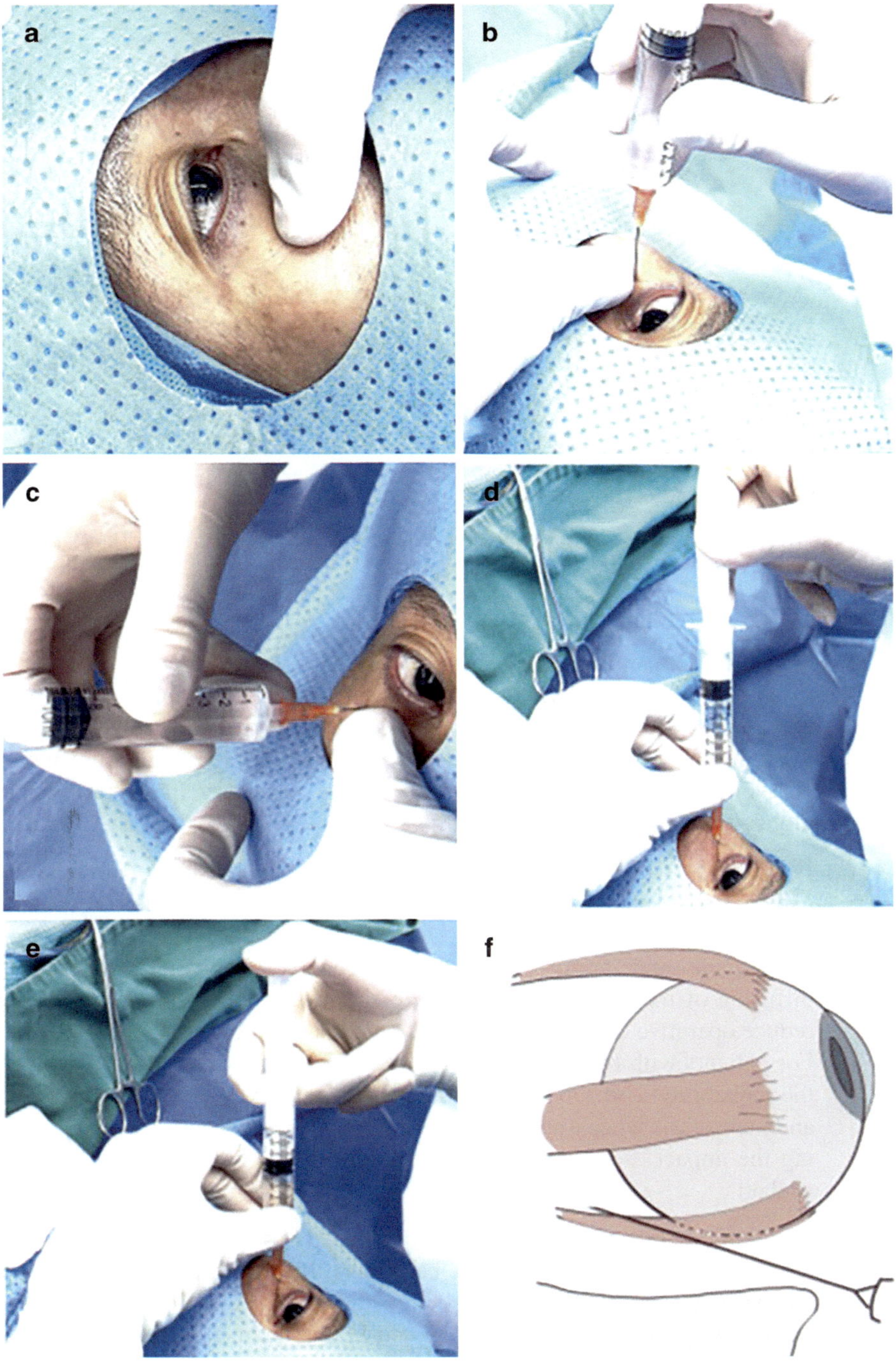

Fig. 4.3 Retrobulbar anesthesia. **(a)** Insert the needle at the junction of the outer and middle thirds of the lower orbital margin. **(b)** Insert the needle vertically. **(c)** After inserting the needle vertically for approximately 20 mm, change the direction of the needle to tilt 30° upward and nasally. **(d)** After the total length of the needle entering the orbit reaches 30–35 mm, aspirate the syringe to confirm no blood reflux. **(e)** Hold the syringe firmly with the left hand and inject the anesthetic with the right hand. **(f)** Side view of retrobulbar injection

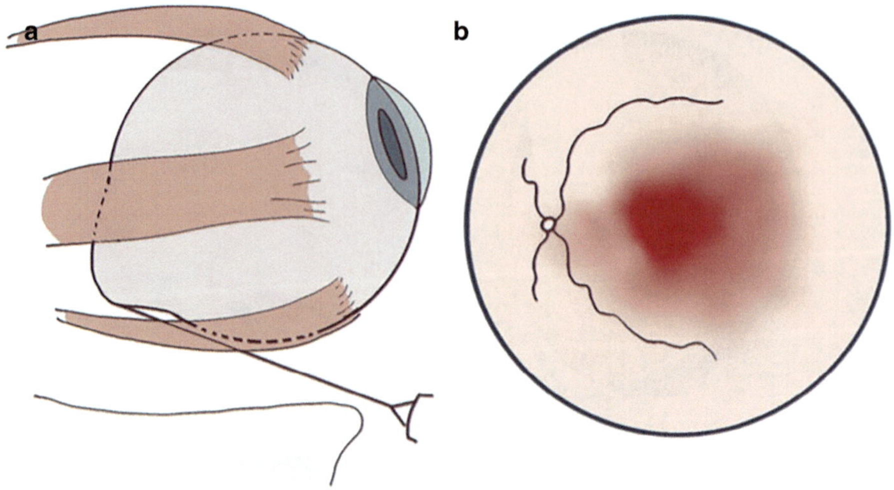

Fig. 4.4 High myopia with posterior staphyloma: retrobulbar injection carries a risk of macular injury. (**a**) Side view (**b**) Posterior-pole view

can be used alone. If intraoperative analgesia is insufficient, a small additional dose of anesthetic can be administered.

4. Eye compression. After injecting the anesthetic, use gauze to apply pressure to the eyeball for 5–10 minutes, releasing pressure every 10–15 seconds, to promote diffusion of the anesthetic, reduce intraocular pressure, and minimize retrobulbar bleeding. Oculopression is particularly necessary in the following situations:

   (a) For patients with a low pain threshold and emotional tension, oculopression can reduce the anxiety caused by sudden pain when cutting the conjunctiva or depressing the sclera.
   (b) For patients undergoing macular surgery, oculopression can promote full diffusion of the anesthetics, more effectively immobilize the eyeball, and reduce operative errors caused by the patient's eye movements.
   (c) For patients with hypertension or diabetes, oculopression not only reduces the probability of retrobulbar bleeding but also provides timely compression and hemostasis when a small amount of bleeding just occurs, thereby avoiding the impact of excessive orbital pressure on the blood perfusion of the eyeball.

5. Treatment of complications. If the eyeball gradually protrudes, orbital pressure is excessively elevated, eyelid closure becomes difficult, or upper eyelid ptosis occurs, the operation should be stopped immediately. The eyeball should then be bandaged with pressure, and surgery should be rescheduled (usually after 2–3 days). If bleeding is minimal with no obvious proptosis or persistent elevation of orbital pressure, the operation may be continued. For patients with diabetes or hypertension that may compromise intraocular blood perfusion, scleral incision

or anterior chamber paracentesis should be performed promptly, and vitrectomy may be used to remove part of the vitreous or release aqueous humor to lower intraocular pressure and restore normal intraocular blood perfusion as soon as possible.

6. Cooperation during surgery. During local anesthesia, the patient may experience the most noticeable pain during the following steps: (1) lifting the rectus muscle (during scleral buckling, if this step causes the patient significant pain, the patient must be calmed before subsequent scleral external fluid injection; gentle language and movements are essential to help avoid choroidal hemorrhage); (2) scleral indentation (especially when depressing the nasal sclera); (3) subconjunctival injection; and (4) removal of the surgical patch.

Patients with good vision can observe the movement of surgical instruments above the retina. When performing delicate macular operations, patients should be informed and comforted in advance to alleviate their nervousness and avoid sudden eye rotation while grasping the epiretinal membrane or internal limiting membrane, which could damage the neuroepithelial layer and cause holes or bleeding.

Based on our experience, after the surgeon uses intraocular forceps to remove part of the epiretinal membrane or internal limiting membrane, he or she can gently shake the tissue within the vitreous cavity a few times and tell the patient that these white membranes are the lesions that have been successfully removed. This positive interaction can greatly improve patient compliance, allowing subsequent delicate maneuvers to be performed more effectively (Fig. 4.5).

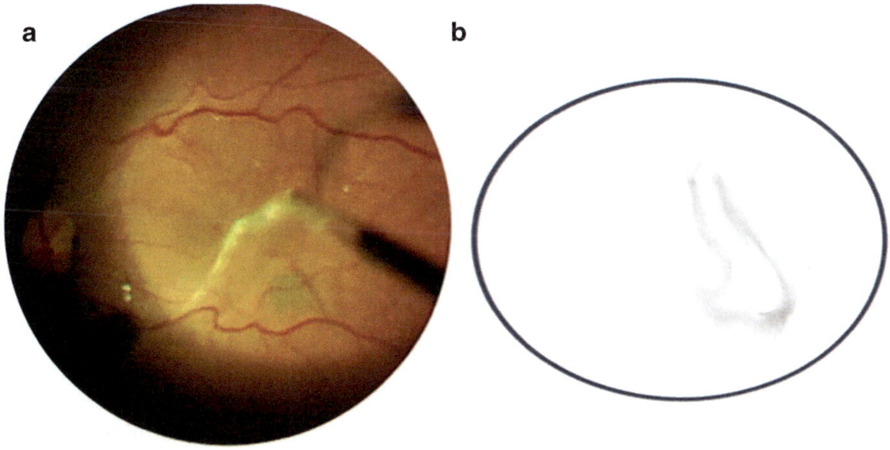

Fig. 4.5 Interaction during epiretinal membrane surgery. (**a**) Gently shaking the removed epiretinal membrane within the eye. (**b**) The patient describing the scene he or she sees at that moment

4.3.2 General Anesthesia

Compared with local anesthesia, general anesthesia is more expensive and requires the cooperation of anesthesiologists and nurses, but its advantages are very significant.

The following patients can consider general anesthesia.

1. Young or mentally immature.
2. Easily nervous and agitated, with poor cooperation.
3. Sensitive to pain and require prolonged muscle traction or external scleral pressure during surgery.
4. Have undergone multiple recent eye surgeries and are more sensitive to pain due to tissue edema and inflammation.
5. The surgery is expected to take a long time and be more complicated.
6. Suffering from claustrophobia.
7. With communication difficulties.

It should be noted that for patients who may undergo fluid/air exchange during vitreoretinal surgery or who still have residual gas in the eye, nitrous oxide (N_2O) should be avoided as a general anesthetic; otherwise, intraocular pressure in the operated eye may rise sharply, potentially leading to irreversible visual impairment.

4.4 Summary

"By failing to prepare, you are preparing to fail." In the realm of vitreoretinal surgery, where the threshold for error is near zero, meticulous preoperative planning is not merely a preference but a prerequisite for success. Given the intricate nature of intraocular maneuvers and the irreversible consequences of technical lapses, surgical preparation must extend far beyond the operating table.

A truly comprehensive plan begins with transparent and empathetic communication with patients and their families, ensuring that expectations are managed and informed consent is deeply understood. Furthermore, seamless collaboration within the surgical team is vital; this involves synchronizing with attending physicians, anesthesia staff, and nursing teams to anticipate every possible intraoperative requirement.

Beyond interpersonal coordination, strict adherence to medical regulations and standardized safety protocols serves as the final safeguard. By fortifying every link in this preparatory chain—from clinical assessment to logistical readiness—the surgeon can navigate the complexities of the posterior segment with confidence, ensuring the smooth execution of the procedure and the highest standard of patient safety.

Basic Steps and Techniques of Vitrectomy

5

Vitreoretinal surgery refers to a series of procedures that alter the pathological state of the vitreous and retina to achieve anatomical reattachment and functional repair, including various surgical methods and their combinations. The patient's condition and the surgeon's experience jointly determine the most suitable combination of approaches. Pars plana vitrectomy (PPV) is the most complex and important component of vitreoretinal surgery, with significant individual variability. In this chapter, we will focus on PPV to introduce the basic steps and precautions of vitreoretinal surgery.

5.1 Common Terms and Instruments

5.1.1 Instrument Diameter

In vitreoretinal surgery, gauge (G) is commonly used to indicate the diameter of instruments. Although it is not a standard international unit of measurement, it remains widely used in medicine—for example, to indicate the caliber of syringe needles. This unit originated from the British wire industry. At a time when no universal thickness standard existed, gauge was conventionally used for thickness measurement and commercial transactions. There is no fixed linear conversion between gauge size and metric units. The corresponding relationship between the diameters of commonly used vitrectomy instruments and millimeters (mm) is shown in Fig. 5.1.

5.1.2 Trocar-Cannula System

The trocar-cannula system is a fundamental instrument in vitreoretinal surgery. Its function is to use a puncture knife to penetrate the scleral wall and retain the cannula in place, serving as a channel for fluid, gas, and instruments to enter and exit the

Z. Zhang, U. Spandau, *Vitreoretinal Surgery*,
https://doi.org/10.1007/978-3-032-25271-5_5

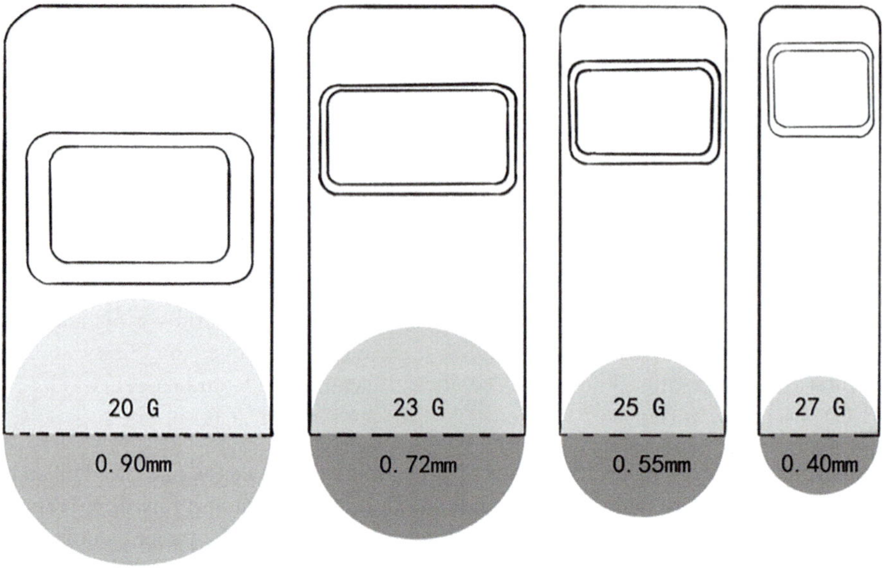

Fig. 5.1 Correspondence between vitreoretinal instrument gauges and millimeters (mm)

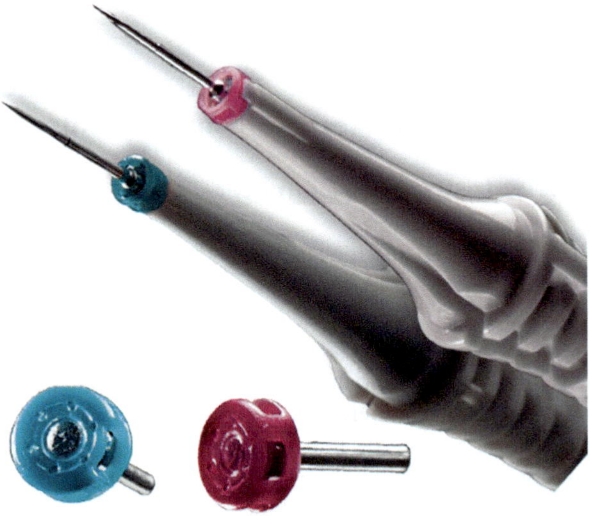

Fig. 5.2 The trocar-cannula system: "trocar" refers to the cannula at its tip (indigo and purple parts). (Photo courtesy of Alcon)

vitreous cavity (Fig. 5.2). The word "trocar" (also spelled "trochar" in British English) comes from the French "trocart," which has been in use since 1694. It is composed of two elements: "trois," meaning three, and "carré," meaning sides or faces, referring to the instruments three-sided shape.

In vitreoretinal surgery, for convenience of expression, "trocar" is often used to refer to the cannula retained in the scleral wall. This convention is also adopted in this book.

5.1.3 Vitrectomy Machine

The vitrectomy machine mainly provides cutting power and an illumination source for ophthalmic surgery. There are various brands and series available, which have undergone multiple upgrades. Existing vitrectomy machines have greater stability and more complete functions, and can support multiple intraocular operations simultaneously, such as retinal laser photocoagulation, intraocular electrocoagulation, and cataract phacoemulsification. Most vitrectomy machines employ venturi pumps, which must be connected to high-pressure gas to provide power. The most prominent advantage of using a venturi pump is that the on-off state of the negative pressure at the cutter opening can be flexibly and immediately controlled by the surgeon, avoiding accidental injury to intraocular tissues due to machine delay.

5.2 Basic Steps

First, it is necessary to ensure that the patient has a good and stable head position, and that the periorbital skin is routinely disinfected. To better prevent infection, topical anesthetics and 5% povidone-iodine can be instilled into the conjunctival sac in sequence and left in place for at least one minute. According to domestic and international research reports, as well as our years of experience, this method can effectively prevent the occurrence of infectious endophthalmitis.

5.2.1 Selection of PPV

Before deciding to perform PPV, the surgeon should objectively evaluate the risks and benefits and carefully consider the following three questions:

1. What vitreoretinal disorder does the patient expect to address?
2. What other treatment methods are available besides PPV to solve this problem?
3. Can you handle or, with prompt help from others, resolve the difficulties and possible complications during the surgery?

5.2.2 Basic Objectives of PPV

1. Ensure unobstructed entry of fluid and gas into the vitreous cavity.
2. Facilitate subsequent intraocular operations.
3. Avoid iatrogenic injuries, especially protecting the retina and lens.
4. Achieve good wound closure and rapid healing.

5.2.3 Basic Operation of PPV

(1) Surgical Draping and Eyelid Speculum Placement

The purpose is to enclose the upper and lower eyelashes within the drape, secure the surgical field, and avoid contamination caused by overflow of the perfusate. Special attention must be paid to sealing the nasal orbital margin and nasal root to prevent water vapor exhaled by the patient from condensing on the surgical contact lens and compromising the clarity of the surgical field (Fig. 5.3).

(2) Creating Transconjunctival Scleral Incision

For 23G and 25G vitrectomy, scleral incisions may be created either vertically or obliquely, depending on the surgeon's preference, provided the wound remains self-sealing and architecturally sound. Achieving a high-quality incision becomes significantly more challenging in the following scenarios: (1) profound hypotony (low intraocular pressure); (2) pediatric patients due to increased scleral elasticity; (3) coexisting choroidal detachment or suprachoroidal effusion; and (4) re-operation (previous vitrectomy) where the vitreous cavity is fluid-filled. In cases of severe hypotony, intraocular pressure should be restored prior to incision to prevent globe collapse; this can be achieved by injecting balanced salt solution (BSS) into the vitreous cavity via a 30-gauge needle, 3.5–4.0 mm posterior to the limbus.

For PPV beginners, it is especially important to maintain a relaxed, natural wrist position with the wrist slightly extended to ensure the puncture knife always advances centripetally (Fig. 5.4). Excessive tension during trocar insertion may

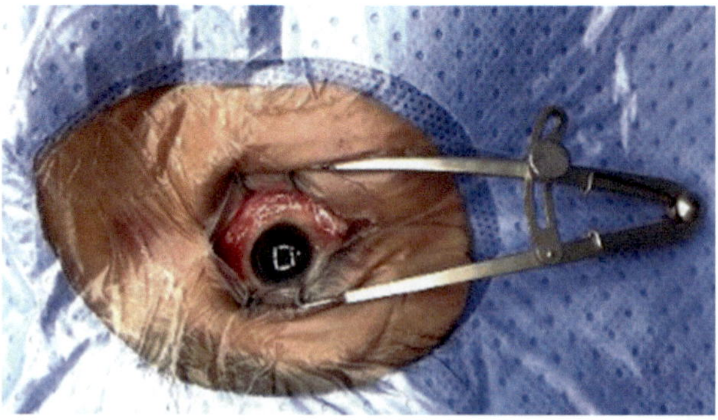

Fig. 5.3 Standard surgical draping

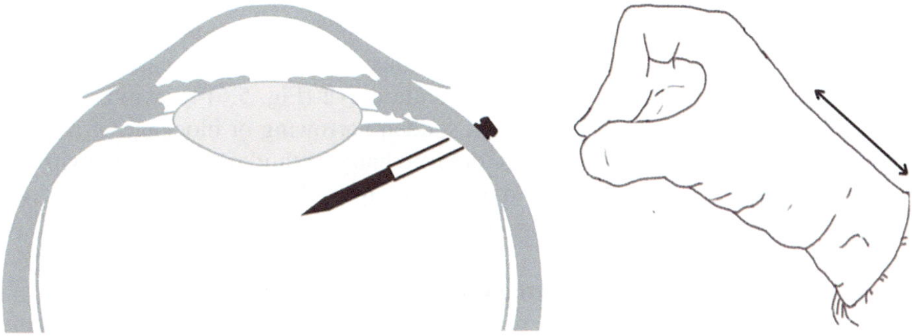

Fig. 5.4 Correct wrist angle for trocar insertion

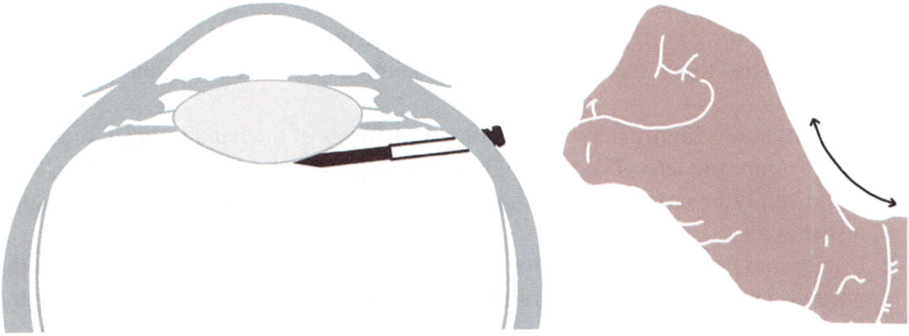

Fig. 5.5 Incorrect wrist angle for trocar insertion

cause involuntary wrist stiffness and overextension, potentially leading to lens injury from the puncture tip (Fig. 5.5).

(3) Connecting the Perfusion Line to the Lower Trocar

First, confirm that the inner opening of the trocar has fully entered the vitreous cavity. When intraocular pressure is low (≤9 mmHg) or the retina is highly detached, before turning on the perfusate, it is essential to verify complete entry of the trocar's inner opening. The simplest method is to gently push the outer opening of the trocar slightly upward toward the center of the vitreous cavity (taking care to avoid contact between the inner opening and the posterior lens capsule). If the inner opening is visible through the pupil, perfusion can be turned on. Alternatively, using a surgical wide-angle lens and a light pipe inserted through the trocar opposite the perfusion trocar, if the metal reflection of the inner opening is clearly visible, perfusion can be turned on. We will elaborate on how to eliminate risk factors and ensure safe entry of the perfusion cannula into the vitreous cavity in the presence of choroidal detachment with low intraocular pressure in the following chapters.

(4) Securing and Arranging the Perfusion Line

Use the surgical drape to secure the proximal end of the perfusion tube and arrange the tube from the vitrectomy machine to the inner opening of the trocar. First, ensure that the proximal perfusion tube has a gentle curve (Fig. 5.6) to avoid excessive kinking. This reduces friction, prevents sudden narrowing or blockage of the tube lumen, and helps avoid insufficient or delayed entry of fluid or gas into the vitreous cavity, which could otherwise lead to ocular collapse, choroidal detachment, or even expulsive choroidal hemorrhage.

(5) Inserting the Light Pipe Through the Upper Trocar

Beginners are particularly prone to errors during this step and must pay special attention. The surgeon's hand-eye-foot coordination may decrease due to mental tension, mainly manifested in the following aspects:

1. The surgical field suddenly shifts from the ocular surface to the intraocular space, requiring corresponding adjustments to microscope focus and magnification. At this time, the surgeon must maintain hand stability and foot pedal flexibility.
2. The surgeon is highly nervous, leading to stiffness of the hand joints, which may easily injure the lens. The surgeon should keep the hand joints naturally relaxed while applying appropriate force to maintain a firm grip on the intraocular instruments.
3. Due to inexperience or excessive tension, the depth of the light pipe entering the vitreous cavity cannot be accurately estimated, which may lead to puncturing the

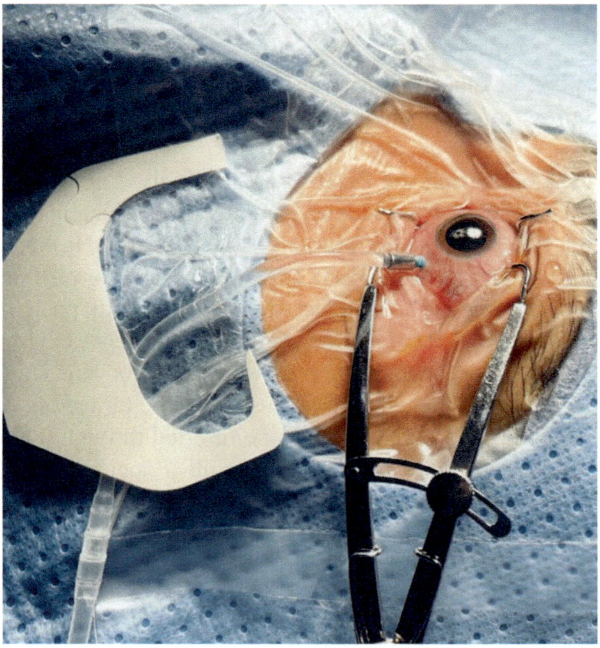

Fig. 5.6 Ideal curvature of the proximal end of perfusion line

posterior pole retina, causing bleeding and retinal tears. If the macula is involved, the patient's visual recovery will be seriously affected. The surgeon should accurately determine the allowable intraocular length of the instrument by observing the length of the outer end that has not yet entered the vitreous cavity.

After the light pipe safely enters the vitreous cavity and aligns with the surgical wide-angle lens, the surgeon observes the intraocular light through the eyepiece. The surgeon should first maintain hand stability (avoiding large movements of the light pipe) and then adjust the microscope foot pedal for focus. Once the optic disc and retinal vessels are clearly visualized, the next step can proceed.

(6) Inserting the Cutter to Start Vitrectomy

Beginners should proceed to this step only after properly adjusting the microscope and light pipe, as improper handling of the cutter tip may cause iatrogenic injuries. "Never operate if you cannot see clearly"—this is one of the fundamental principles of intraocular surgery. The cutter should first be activated in the central vitreous cavity. After removing part of the central vitreous, posterior vitreous detachment (PVD) is induced. Creating PVD and accurately determining whether any vitreous remains at the posterior pole are key skills that beginners need to master, and will be elaborated on later.

(7) Removing Adequate Vitreous

Adjust the depth and angle of the light pipe to fully visualize the vitreous in different regions using the Tyndall phenomenon, and remove as much vitreous as possible with the cutter (Fig. 5.7). When shaving off peripheral vitreous or vitreous around retinal breaks, where the vitreous cortex is denser and adheres more tightly to the retina, use high-speed cutting (e.g., 5,000 cpm) with low vacuum (100–250 mmHg). The foot pedal can be tapped to achieve slow, controlled shaving. In

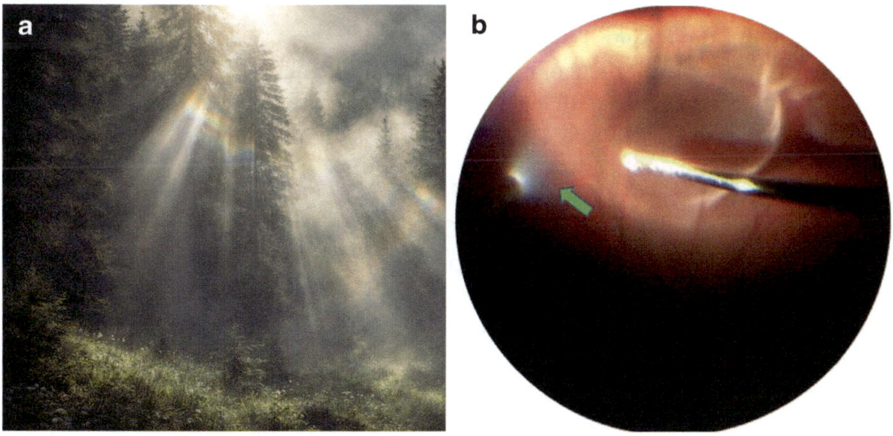

Fig. 5.7 Tyndall phenomenon. (**a**) Tyndall phenomenon in nature. (**b**) Inducing Tyndall phenomenon with a light pipe during vitreoretinal surgery

addition, iatrogenic lens injury must be strictly avoided. In phakic eyes, the surgeon should always keep both hands coordinated and stay clear of the "unsafe zone" near the posterior lens capsule.

(8) Other Intraocular Operations
After removing an adequate amount of vitreous, the surgeon may proceed with other intraocular procedures, such as fluid/air exchange, internal limiting membrane peeling, and retinal laser photocoagulation. These techniques will be detailed in the following chapters.

(9) 360° Scleral Indentation
The importance of scleral indentation is self-evident, but it also places high demands on both the surgeon and the assistant. Beginners should proceed step by step and may first familiarize themselves with the technique in pseudophakic eyes.

There are three main methods of scleral indentation:

1. The assistant holds a strabismus hook or scleral depressor, while the surgeon holds a light pipe to illuminate the indented area. This is the most commonly used method, offering a short learning curve and high safety.
2. One of the upper trocars is kept closed (if the trocar lacks a self-sealing valve, a scleral plug is inserted). The surgeon holds the depressor and examines the depressed vitreous and retina using external microscope illumination through the pupil.
3. Under chandelier illumination, one upper trocar is also kept closed, and the surgeon holds the depressor to expose the peripheral retina.

Each of these three methods has its own advantages and disadvantages. The surgeon may choose based on the specific situation and personal preference. If an assistant is unavailable or inexperienced, the latter two methods are good options to learn.

(10) Removing the Upper Trocar
Regardless of whether vertical or oblique incisions are made, the surgeon must carefully inspect each incision. If leakage is detected and adequate tightness is not achieved, suturing is required to reduce the risk of postoperative hypotony and infectious endophthalmitis.

(11) Removing the Lower Trocar and Checking for Incision Leakage
If intraocular pressure is low, an appropriate amount of balanced salt solution or filtered air can be injected 4 mm posterior to the superior limbus using a fine needle to rapidly elevate the pressure. If the eye is soft, the needle may easily injure the lens during injection. In such cases, micro-toothed forceps can be used to grasp the conjunctiva around the injection site before inserting the needle.

The above mainly describes the conventional steps and precautions of PPV. The surgeon may adjust according to personal preference, but must keep three key principles in mind throughout the procedure: (1) stable intraocular pressure; (2) a clear surgical field; and (3) appropriate instrument distance. Standard three-port PPV accounts for an increasing proportion of vitreoretinal surgeries. Although the technology and instruments have matured, and their safety and efficacy have been widely recognized in long-term clinical practice, beginners must adopt a step-by-step learning approach, strictly follow the vitreoretinal surgery learning curve, and ultimately master this skill with confidence.

5.3 Practical Skills and Detailed Illustration

5.3.1 Creation of Scleral Incision

(1) Position and Direction of Scleral Incision

In standard three-port PPV, the trocar should be placed 4 mm posterior to the limbus in phakic eyes and 3.0-3.5 mm behind the limbus in aphakic or pseudophakic eyes. This positioning ensures that the blade passes through the pars plana, which is avascular; therefore, bleeding does not occur from the incision. The pars plana adheres tightly to the underlying choroid and will not detach due to sharp trauma. The ora serrata, located approximately 1–2 mm away, is also tightly adherent, further preventing subretinal fluid from spreading to this area. The trocar placement must always avoid iatrogenic damage to the long ciliary arteries and nerves.

For oblique incisions, it's recommended that the direction of the incision be parallel to the tangential direction of the limbus (Fig. 5.8).

(2) Sequence and Precautions for Trocar Placement

The lower trocar should be placed first, typically in the inferotemporal quadrant. In special cases, such as significant choroidal detachment or a temporal silicone buckle, the inferonasal quadrant may be chosen first. The lower trocar should not be placed too close to the eyelid margin. Taking the right eye as an example, it is generally

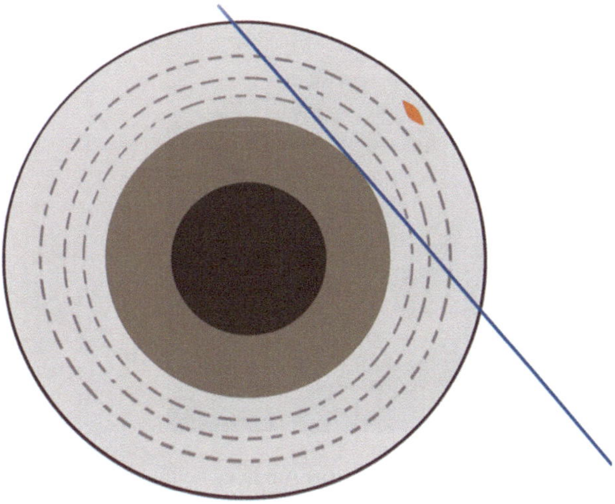

Fig. 5.8 Recommended incision direction (at the red dot); the blue line is the tangential direction of the limbus

positioned at the 7:30 to 8:00 o'clock position to avoid contact with the eyelid speculum, which could cause trocar slippage or interfere with scleral indentation.

In the following situations, special attention should be paid to ensuring prompt connection of perfusion to the lower trocar:

1. Preoperative low intraocular pressure: After confirming that the inner opening of the trocar has entered the vitreous cavity, perfusion should be turned on promptly to maintain intraocular pressure.
2. Previous vitrectomy with intraocular fluid or gas tamponade: After trocar placement, if perfusion is not turned on promptly, a large amount of intraocular fluid or gas will escape from the eye, causing a sudden drop in intraocular pressure.
3. Elderly patients: Vitreous liquefaction is often significant. If perfusion is not turned on promptly, the liquefied vitreous will overflow through the trocar, leading to a drop in intraocular pressure.

In the above situations, valved trocars may also be used to improve surgical safety.

The upper trocars are recommended to be placed at the 2:00 and 10:00 o'clock positions (with a 120° angle between them) for the following three reasons:

1. Ergonomically, when both hands cooperate at this angle—similar to holding a steering wheel—the wrist is in a naturally extended position, offering the greatest range of motion and optimal stability for intraocular movements (Fig. 5.9).
2. The two upper trocars serve as stable fulcrums, allowing the surgeon to slightly adjust eye position using intraocular instruments. If the angle is too small, the range of motion is reduced; if too large, the eyeball is prone to horizontal rotation.
3. This configuration not only maximizes the reach of intraocular instruments within the eye but also maximizes protection of the posterior lens capsule when both hands are coordinated. If the angle is too large, the posterior lens capsule is very likely to be touched during peripheral vitreous removal (Fig. 5.10).

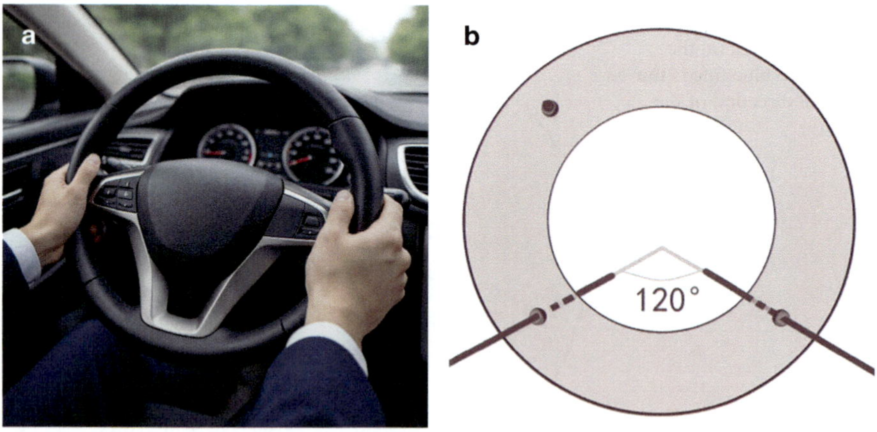

Fig. 5.9 Wrist ergonomics. (**a**) Angle of holding the steering wheel. (**b**) The two upper trocars maintain a 120° angle

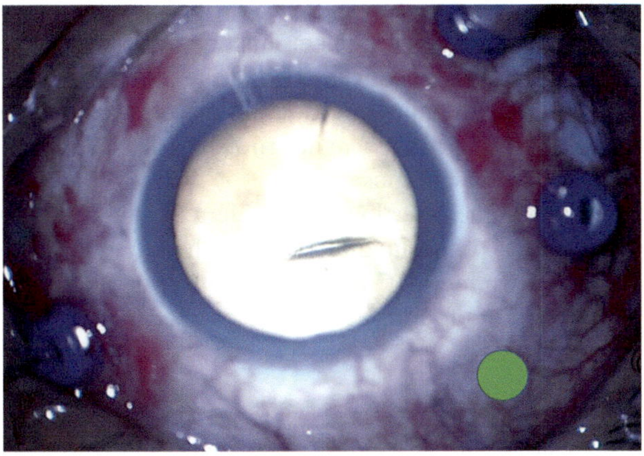

Fig. 5.10 A superotemporal trocar placed too inferiorly with an excessively large angle may cause the cutter to injure the posterior lens capsule when cutting the superior vitreous; the correct position is shown by the green dot in the figure

(3) Creation of Self-Sealing Sclerotomy

1. Advantages and Disadvantages of Non-Self-Sealing and Self-Sealing Incisions

   If self-sealing is not a consideration, the incision perpendicular to the scleral surface is the safest. This is because the trocar's trajectory through the scleral wall is the shortest, the inner end of the trocar extends farthest into the vitreous cavity, and the elastic force from the scleral collagen fibers is evenly distributed around the trocar, making it less likely to slip during eye movements.

   Although non-self-sealing incisions possess certain clinical merits, we recommend that beginners prioritize mastering the creation and management of self-sealing (sutureless) scleral incisions. These techniques offer several distinct advantages: (1) optimized operative efficiency with shorter surgical times; (2) enhanced patient comfort through a reduction in postoperative foreign body sensation; and (3) a minimized risk of suture-induced inflammation and surgically induced astigmatism.
2. Anatomical Principles of Self-Sealing Incisions

   The creation of self-sealing scleral incisions is governed by two fundamental principles: (1) The three-dimensional nature of tissue entry: An incision is not a simple linear cut on a two-dimensional plane, but a dynamic tunnel through the scleral architecture. Its length, depth, and angle must be synchronized to create a valvular effect. (2) The utilization of spherical geometry: The eyeball is a curved surface rather than a flat plane. By accounting for this natural curvature during trocar insertion, the surgeon can create a longer, tangential tunnel that leverages intraocular pressure to facilitate a secure, self-sealing closure.

   For example, in cataract phacoemulsification, we understand why the incision is not made perpendicular to the corneal surface but rather as a trapezoidal incision. The reason is that this configuration provides good self-sealing and effectively prevents postoperative wound leakage. By extension, the self-sealing of a scleral incision is also closely and directly related to the trajectory of the puncture knife through the ocular surface tissues.

3. Methods of Creating Self-Sealing Incisions
   Conjunctival displacement must be performed first, after which the scleral incision can be created using one of the following three methods (Fig. 5.11):
   (a) Direct oblique insertion of the trocar-cannula into the vitreous cavity.
   (b) First, make vertical insertion into the sclera, and then make oblique insertion into the vitreous cavity.
   (c) Oblique insertion of the sclera to half depth, followed by oblique puncture in the opposite direction into the vitreous cavity.

   As shown in Fig. 5.12, the third insertion method is the most stable because the forces from four directions are balanced, and the wound will not shift.

Fig. 5.11 Schematic diagrams of different self-sealing scleral incisions. (**a**) Oblique incision; (**b**) vertical-oblique incision; and (**c**) forward-reverse oblique incision (V-shaped incision)

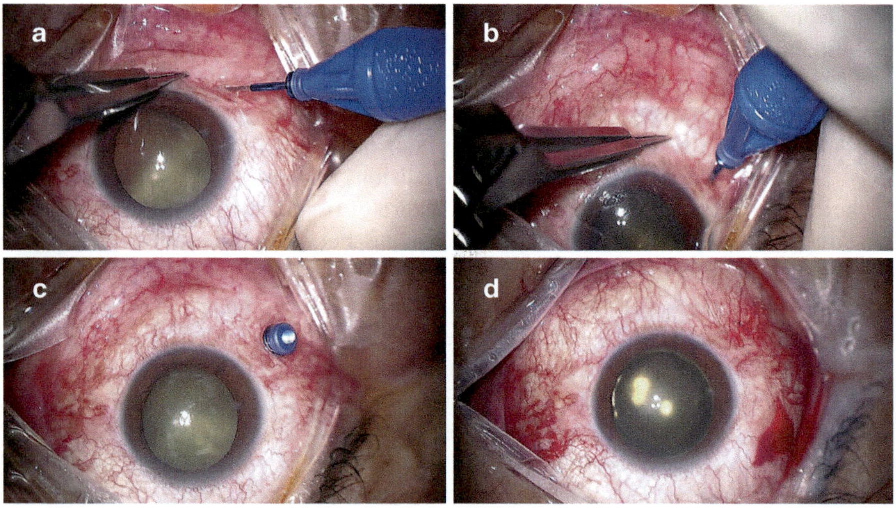

Fig. 5.12 Creation of V-shaped incision. (**a**) First, perform conjunctival displacement, and then insert the blade obliquely along the tangential direction of the limbus into the scleral lamella. (**b**) After the tip enters the lamella, insert the blade obliquely in the opposite direction along the tangential direction of the limbus to the vitreous cavity. (**c**) The trocar has been inserted into the scleral. (**d**) All trocars are removed after the surgery, and no obvious leakage is found

5.3.2 Safety of the Perfusion Line

Maintaining a stable perfusion pressure is essential for the safety of vitreoretinal surgery. Beginners must understand the specific causes of perfusion abnormalities and quickly master their solutions.

After connecting the tip of the perfusion line to the trocar, a small piece of drape can be used to secure the perfusion line to the zygomatic region, slightly outside and below the trocar. At the same time, the proximal end of the perfusion line should maintain a gentle curve, not too high or too low (see Fig. 5.6).

When the assistant indents the peripheral sclera, or when the surgeon moves the patient's eyeball, the inner opening of the perfusion cannula may sometimes tilt upward and enter the anterior chamber through the angle or iris (Fig. 5.13). This is particularly concerning under high-pressure gas perfusion (e.g., 50 mmHg), where the anterior chamber will deepen sharply, the surgical field under the wide-angle lens will become immediately blurred, and magnification will decrease accordingly. This phenomenon should be identified and corrected promptly.

When the lower perfusion cannula becomes displaced from the scleral, the surgeon should promptly detect the following signs:

1. Soft eyeball: Due to the lack of continuous supplementation of perfusate or gas, intraocular pressure will continue to drop to near atmospheric pressure, and the outward pressure exerted by intraocular contents on the scleral will decrease. Treatment is relatively simple, just promptly reconnect the infusion line or inject fluid into the vitreous cavity to maintain intraocular pressure and eliminate the risk.
2. Localized choroidal elevation: Due to the sudden drop in intraocular pressure, if not handled promptly, this may further lead to ocular collapse and even choroidal detachment (Fig. 5.14). As long as intraocular pressure is promptly maintained, the choroidal detachment can also subside within a short time.
3. Explosive choroidal hemorrhage: If intraocular pressure remains low without prompt treatment, choroidal detachment is likely to progress to extensive choroidal hemorrhage. At this stage, management becomes very difficult, and it may be necessary to close the incision and perform a second-stage operation. When

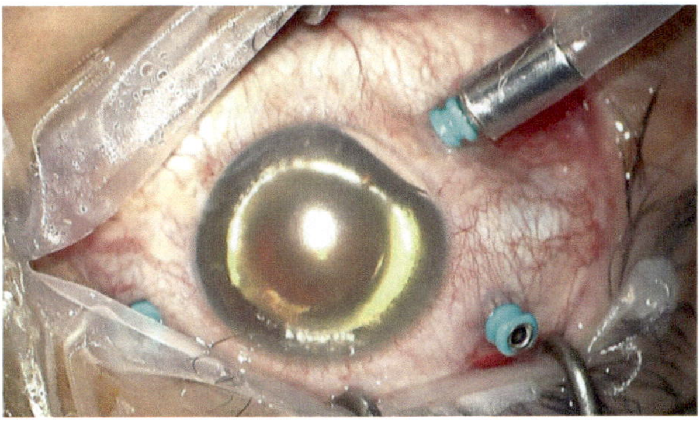

Fig. 5.13 The inner opening of the infusion trocar pierces the iris and enters the anterior chamber, with gas filling the entire anterior chamber

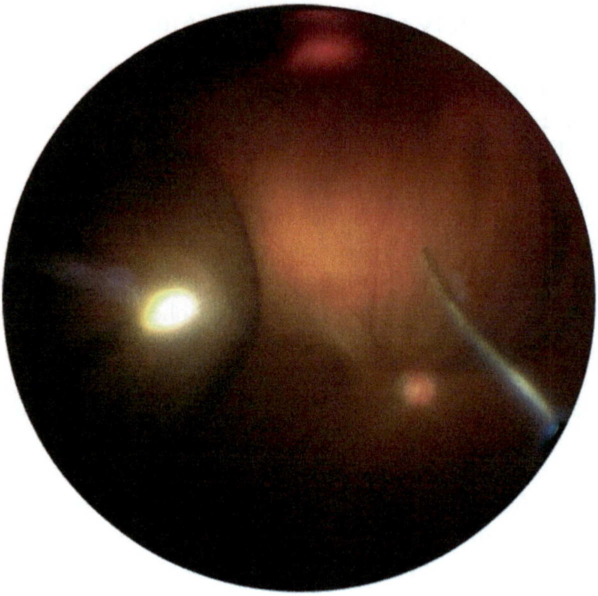

Fig. 5.14 Choroidal detachment caused by displacement of perfusion line

choroidal hemorrhage begins, the patient may sometimes complain of obvious ocular distension and pain, followed by uncontrollable breath-holding and eyelid closure, which will increase the difficulty of the surgeon's management.

If no obvious complications occur, the solution for perfusion cannula displacement is shown in Fig. 5.15. The key factor is maintaining normal intraocular pressure throughout the procedure to avoid a cascade of adverse events caused by hypotony.

Next, we list the causes and solutions of perfusion pressure abnormalities in the following table (Table 5.1).

5.3.3 Posterior Vitreous Detachment (PVD)

(1) Importance of Posterior Vitreous Detachment

Posterior vitreous detachment (PVD) refers to the loss of adhesion between the posterior vitreous cortex and the internal limiting membrane. In the general popu-MatchCaseReplacelation, the vitreous gradually liquefies with age, manifested by collapse and condensation of the collagen fiber scaffold, degradation of hyaluronic acid molecules, and gradual formation of internal cavities. The normal gel-like structure of the vitreous progressively disappears, ultimately leading to PVD. During preoperative fundus examination, the surgeon must carefully determine whether PVD is already present in the eye. The most intuitive sign is the presence of a Weiss ring (Fig. 5.16).

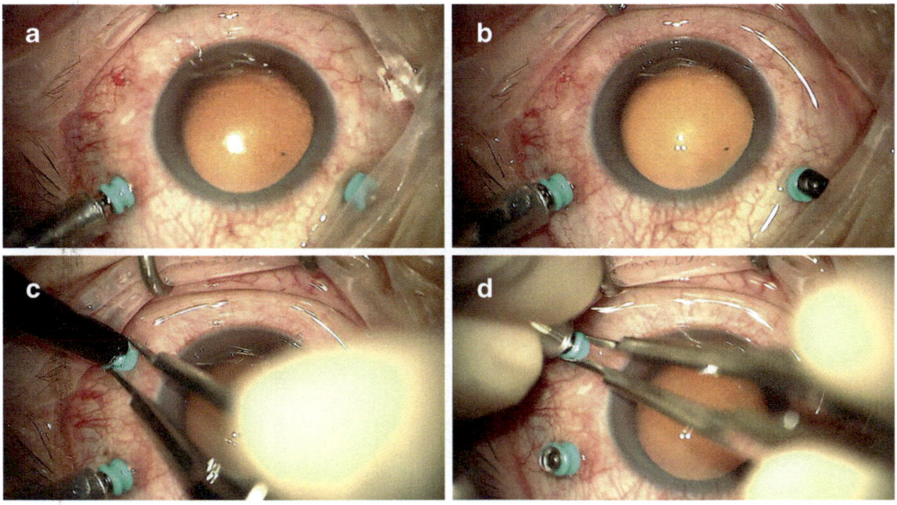

Fig. 5.15 Treatment of perfusion line displacement. (**a**) Connect the perfusion tube to the upper trocar to maintain intraocular pressure. (**b**) Insert a scleral plug into another trocar to ensure no eyeball collapse during insertion of the trocar-cannula. (**c**) Re-insert the lower trocar, and at this time, the intraocular pressure can be temporarily increased to maintain the hardness of the eye wall for the ease of insertion. (**d**) Reconnect the perfusion line to the lower trocar

For example, in fresh rhegmatogenous retinal detachment, the presence of PVD often indicates that the difficulty of PPV is relatively low, and the surgeon may be more inclined to choose PPV as the preferred treatment. The presence (or intraoperative creation) of PVD is a prerequisite for effective vitrectomy and an important guarantee of long-term surgical success. Unless the Weiss ring is clearly visualized during surgery, the surgeon must repeatedly confirm whether PVD has been successfully induced—this is particularly important in young patients (Fig. 5.17).

Beginners should always remember a fact: when you think you have removed most of the vitreous quickly and well, the truth is often that most of the vitreous is still adhering to the retina (Fig. 5.18).

(2) Principles of Creating PVD

Beginners can adopt a step-by-step approach to inducing PVD intraoperatively, following these four principles:

1. First remove the central vitreous to disrupt the internal vitreous structure. The inflow of perfusate will further liquefy the posterior vitreous, creating favorable conditions for subsequent PVD.
2. Begin inducing PVD above the optic disc. Use gentle negative pressure to aspirate the vitreous (typically holding for 2–3 seconds before pulling the cutter peripherally to allow the cutter port to better engage the posterior vitreous cortex). Then, follow the direction of the nerve fiber layer into the four quadrants to minimize transverse traction on the nerve fiber layer.

Table 5.1 Causes and treatment methods of perfusion pressure abnormalities

Intraocular pressure	Concomitant circumstances	Possible causes	Management
Too low	① Noncomplex macular hole/epiretinal membrane surgery ② No other complex abnormalities	(1) Forgot to turn on infusion on the vitrectomy machine's control panel (2) Accidentally entered the wrong perfusion pressure setting value (such as 30 mmHg was entered as 3 mmHg) (3) The perfusion line was excessively bent (4) The inner opening of the trocar was blocked by the peripheral dense vitreous *The above situations can occur in any cases	(1) Ask the assistant to confirm whether the panel of the vitrectomy machine is properly operated (2) Comb the perfusion line from the distal to proximal (3) Withdraw the infusion line from the trocar to observe whether there is liquid outflow from the tip (4) If there is liquid outflow from the tip, reconnect the infusion line, and the surgeon can use a vitrectomy probe to remove some of the peripheral vitreous around inner opening of the infusion trocar *The above situations can occur in any cases
	① With extensive choroidal detachment and/or obvious suprachoroidal fluid ② Existing hypotony before surgery	(1) Inner opening of the trocar has not been inserted into the vitreous cavity (2) The trocar is surrounded by dense peripheral vitreous and other intravitreal tissues (such as proliferative membranes)	Stop the perfusion immediately and inject some balanced saline solution into the vitreous cavity to increase the intraocular pressure. Indent the trocar to check whether the inner opening is well located in the vitreous cavity
	① During or shortly after scleral indentation ② The patient has small palpebral fissure ③ The patient has deep eye socket	(1) The scleral depressor has dragged out the infusion line (2) The infusion trocar is too close to the lower eyelid margin, causing it to be squeezed and displaced	(1) If there is no obvious choroidal detachment, reinsert the perfusion trocar (2) If obvious choroidal detachment has occurred but does not deteriorate, connect the perfusion line to one of the upper trocars as soon as possible; the infusion pressure can be adjusted to be higher than normal now (3) If the choroidal detachment is deteriorating but there is still enough space in the vitreous cavity, use a syringe to inject balanced saline solution into the vitreous cavity to increase intraocular pressure (4) If the choroidal detachment is extensive and operating space in the vitreous cavity is limited, it is safer to suture the sclerotomies and wait 1–2 weeks for a second stage of surgery

	(1) When gas/liquid exchange is just performed (2) After gas/liquid exchange, balanced salt solution is infused into the vitreous cavity (3) Gas/liquid exchange is performed after heavy liquid is injected	(1) Failure to accurately switch the three-way channel, the assistant may sometimes make mistakes and close the channel that was supposed to be opened, or even completely close the fluid/gas channel (2) Segmental gas/water exists in the infusion line, blocking the fluid/gas from entering the vitreous cavity (3) The proximal end of the perfusion line may be overfilled with heavy liquid, blocking the fluid/gas from entering the vitreous cavity *Small-caliber trocars, such as 27G, are more likely to have this problem	(1) Check the three-way channel (2) Increase the perfusion pressure to 40~50 mmHg in a short period of time, observe the changes in intraocular pressure and adjust it to normal value in time (3) Unscrew the proximal end of the perfusion line, and inject balanced saline solution to repel the residual heavy liquid from the tube
	(1) When silicone oil is being removed (2) After all silicone oil has been removed	Silicone oil droplets block the inner opening of the infusion trocar	(1) Increase the perfusion pressure to 40~50 mmHg in a short period of time, observe the changes in intraocular pressure, and adjust it to normal value in time (2) Unscrew the proximal end of the perfusion line, and inject balanced saline solution to repel the residual silicone oil
Too high	When injecting heavy liquid or silicone oil	When using valved trocar-cannulas, rapid injection of heavy liquid and silicone oil will induce rapid elevation of intraocular pressure	Drain off a small amount of heavy liquid and silicone oil, or remove the valve of the trocar

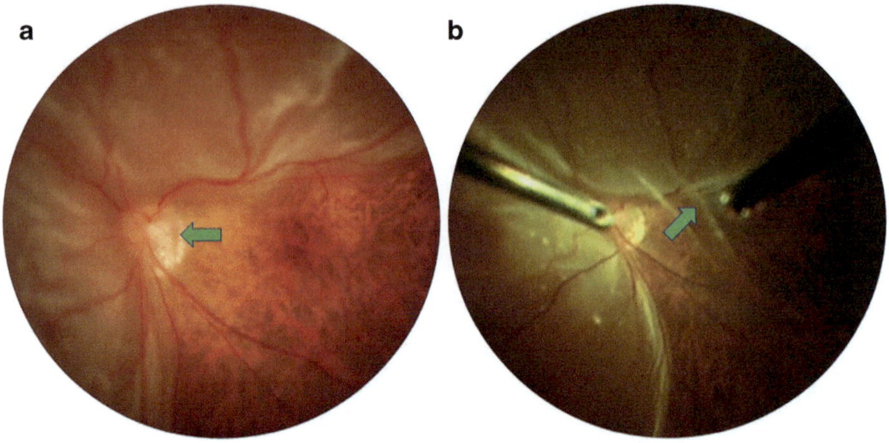

Fig. 5.16 Retinal detachment complicated with obvious posterior vitreous detachment. (**a**) Preoperative fundus photography shows the Weiss ring (green arrow). (**b**) Obvious posterior vitreous detachment is visible under endoillumination during the operation

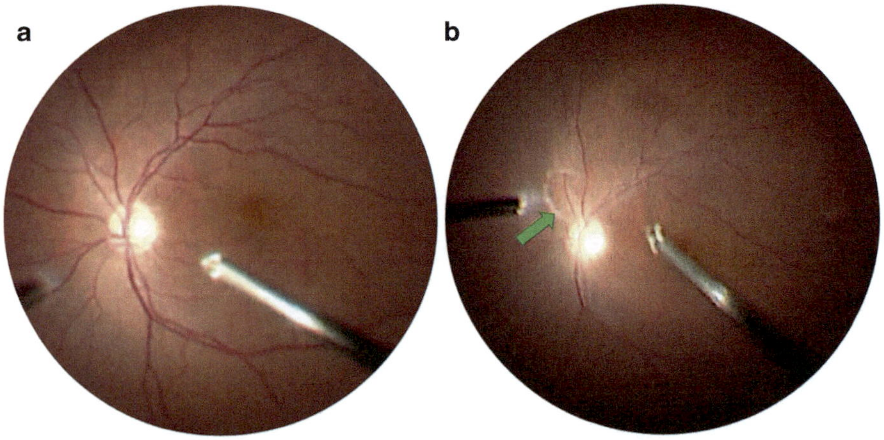

Fig. 5.17 Comparison before and after intraoperative posterior vitreous detachment. (**a**) Before PVD, the transparent vitreous adheres tightly to the posterior pole retina, and the surgical field is uniformly clear. (**b**) After creation of PVD, a large gap appears between the vitreous and the posterior pole retina, and the Weiss ring is visible (green arrow)

3. Avoid operating within the superior and inferior vascular arcades to prevent damage to the macula.
4. If a U-shaped tear already exists or if a mid-peripheral tear occurs during PVD induction, strictly control the vacuum. Use the cutter to first relieve vitreous traction at the periphery of the tear before continuing PVD, to avoid extending the tear.

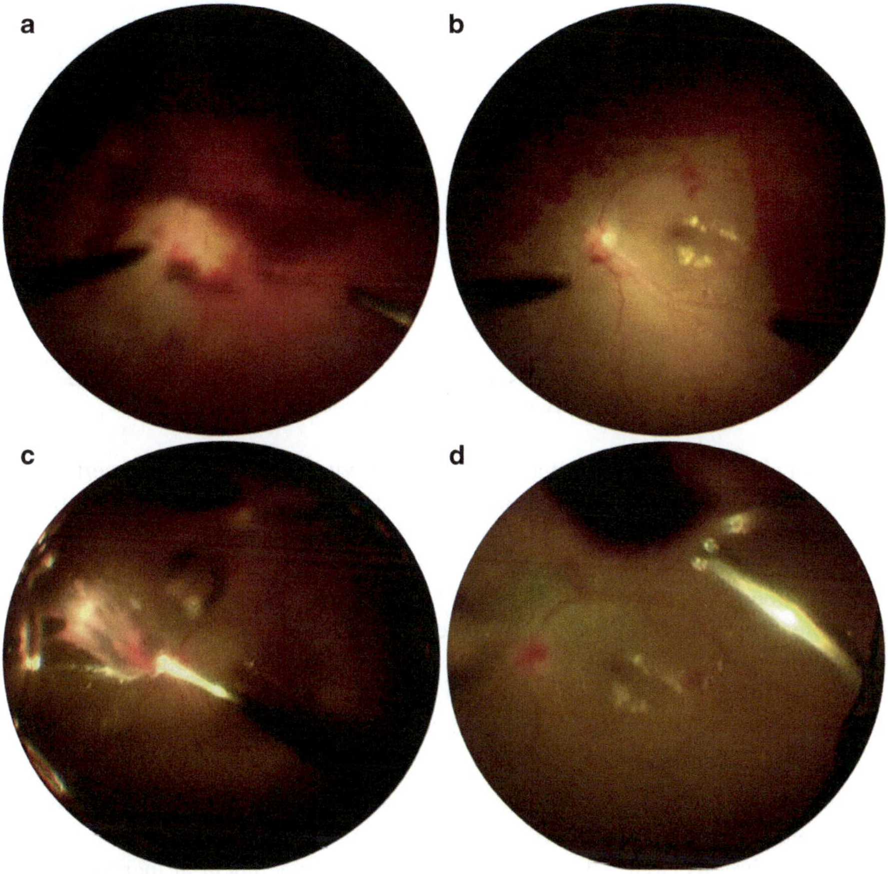

Fig. 5.18 Misunderstandings in judging posterior vitreous detachment. (**a**) Vitreous hemorrhage, using a cutter to clear the central vitreous hemorrhage. (**b**) After clearing the hemorrhage, the vitreous cavity becomes transparent, but there are still blood clots deposited around the lower vascular arcade, which are difficult to aspirate completely. This often indicates that PVD has not yet occurred. (**c**) After injecting triamcinolone acetonide, a large amount of residual vitreous is found. (**d**) After successful induction of PVD, posterior pole hemorrhage is completely cleared, and a flat, uniform retinal reflection is visible

(3) When Creating PVD Is Difficult

In the following patients, inducing PVD may be difficult: (1) patients under 40 years of age; (2) patients with high myopia—even if vitreous liquefaction is present, PVD may be incomplete, and a thin layer of tightly adherent vitreous cortex (vitreoschisis) may remain at the posterior pole; and (3) patients with proliferative diabetic retinopathy (PDR), where the posterior hyaloid is often pathologically adherent to the optic disc and along major retinal vessels, increasing the risk of iatrogenic complications.

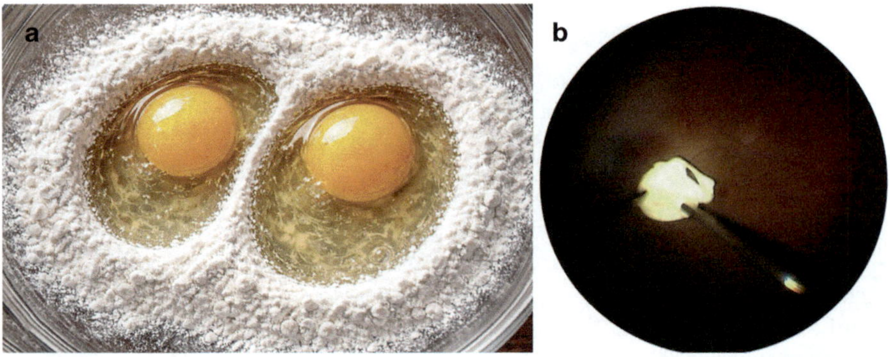

Fig. 5.19 Schematic diagram of vitreous coloring with TA. (**a**) Flour adheres to the surface of egg whites to show its boundaries. (**b**) TA adheres to the posterior pole vitreous

If PVD induction is difficult and the extent of vitreous removal is uncertain, triamcinolone acetonide (TA) can be injected to stain the vitreous. A concentration of 40 mg/mL is typically used, and only 0.1–0.2 mL is needed.

TA is a white powder that is insoluble in water. Because the vitreous contains collagen fibers, TA adheres to its surface, thereby outlining the vitreous cortex. This principle is similar to sprinkling flour on egg whites when making pastries—before being fully incorporated, the flour adheres to the egg whites, revealing their boundaries (Fig. 5.19).

The following details should be noted when injecting and aspirating TA suspension:

1. Position the needle as close to the posterior pole as possible. Observe whether TA reaches the macula immediately upon injection. If it spreads directly throughout the vitreous cavity, this indicates no vitreous attachment at that location. If TA initially attaches locally before spreading to the entire vitreous cavity, vitreous attachment may be present and should be carefully noted.
2. When TA spreads throughout the vitreous cavity, intraocular visibility decreases sharply. Pay attention to observing the metal reflection of the cutter to ensure that intraocular instruments remain in a safe position within the vitreous cavity, avoiding injury to the retina and lens during TA aspiration.
3. After completely aspirating TA and the vitreous cavity becomes transparent again, carefully observe whether any punctate TA deposits remain at the posterior pole. If the presence of PVD remains uncertain, TA can be reinjected and the above steps repeated.

In patients with high myopia and vitreoschisis, even after multiple TA stainings, the vitreous edge may sometimes be difficult to visualize clearly. In such cases, indocyanine green (ICG) can be injected for double staining to better mark the scattered residual vitreous at the posterior pole.

5.3.4 Safe Removal of Sufficient Vitreous

In the surgical treatment of various vitreoretinal disorders—such as rhegmatogenous retinal detachment, proliferative diabetic retinopathy, and proliferative vitreoretinopathy—the surgeon must remove sufficient vitreous to relieve traction of the pathological vitreous on the retina.

(1) Importance of Sufficient Vitreous Removal

Long-term and extensive clinical practice has demonstrated that thorough vitreous removal is critical for the following three reasons: (1) Relieving the traction of the dense peripheral vitreous on the retina to create more favorable conditions for anatomical reattachment; (2) Reducing the risk of postoperative proliferative vitreoretinopathy (PVR), as residual vitreous can serve as a nidus for the mesenchymal transformation of retinal pigment epithelium (RPE) cells that have migrated into the vitreous cavity; and (3) Preventing the formation of new retinal breaks, as the contraction of residual vitreous may exert renewed traction on the underlying retina, leading to secondary tears.

(2) How to Ensure Safe and Sufficient Vitreous Removal

1. Make full use of the light pipe. Adequate illumination is a necessary prerequisite for all intraocular procedures. When removing vitreous, fully utilize the Tyndall phenomenon generated as the light pipe irradiates the vitreous.
2. Introduce TA staining at an appropriate time. As noted above, TA helps the surgeon complete PVD. In many cases, TA staining also helps visualize residual peripheral vitreous.

   TA staining is particularly necessary in the following situations, even when obvious PVD is present: (1) High myopia; (2) Adolescents; (3) Postoperative PVR due to residual vitreous; and (4) Extensive peripheral retinal elevation with poor mobility.

   The purpose of TA injection is to help the surgeon more accurately assess the amount of residual vitreous and identify its clear margins, enabling precise, targeted resection—avoiding both significant residual vitreous and iatrogenic breaks.
3. Perform 360° scleral indentation. With the application and widespread use of wide-angle microscope systems, the difficulty of vitrectomy has been greatly reduced. Compared with contact lenses, although wide-angle lenses allow visualization of most peripheral areas, scleral indentation remains an essential step in most cases. In pseudophakic and aphakic eyes, if the pupil cannot be fully dilated or the lens capsule is opaque, scleral indentation must also be performed. Scleral indentation is also the most direct and accurate method of exploration, helping surgeons promptly identify and manage peripheral lesions while minimizing postoperative complications.

5.3.5 Common Mistakes in Light Pipe Operation

Common mistakes made by beginners in operating the light pipe include the following three aspects:

1. Improper depth control: If the light pipe enters too shallowly and remains only at the inner opening of the trocar, the entire vitreous cavity cannot be adequately illuminated due to the distance from the posterior pole and obstruction by the lens. If inserted too deeply, approaching the posterior pole, the light may not adequately transilluminate the mid-peripheral vitreous.
2. Inability to flexibly adjust the direction of the light pipe: Operating without a clear purpose—for example, directing the light pipe to shine directly onto the cutter—produces strong reflection, leading to glare and interfering with precise manipulation.
3. Entering dangerous areas: The surgeon may be overly eager to illuminate the peripheral vitreous, causing the light pipe to injure the peripheral retina or the posterior lens capsule, resulting in unnecessary iatrogenic trauma.

As shown in Fig. 5.20, both direct and indirect projection methods can be used to visualize the peripheral vitreous edges clearly by utilizing the Tyndall phenomenon generated when light irradiates the peripheral vitreous. We vividly describe the peripheral vitreous displayed by the Tyndall phenomenon as a "skirt."

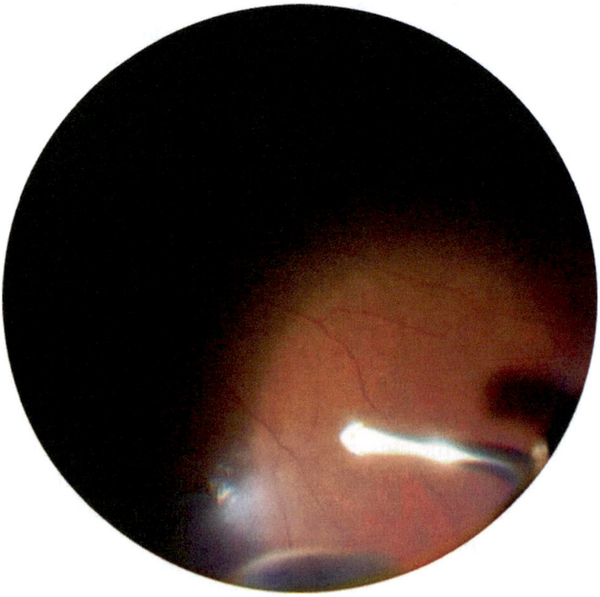

Fig. 5.20 Scleral indentation, adjusting the angle of the light pipe to see the peripheral vitreous

5.3.6 How to Perform Scleral Indentation Well

For beginners, removing peripheral vitreous under scleral indentation is challenging, time-consuming, and most likely to cause iatrogenic breaks—especially when the assistant is unfamiliar with the technique, the difficulty increases significantly.

As shown in Fig. 5.21, whether using a scleral depressor or a strabismus hook, scleral indentation should adhere to the following principles:

1. The depressor tip must be positioned close to the orbital margin and slid into the conjunctival sac from the limbus. This approach conforms to the curvature of the scleral wall, reducing resistance to deep movement of the depressor tip. It also minimizes the vertical downward force on the scleral, which could otherwise cause ocular depression or deformation, compromising the image quality under the microscope.
2. Keep the depressor as vertical as possible. When the operator maintains the depressor in a vertical orientation, the position and depth of its tip can be perceived more accurately, as the operator's fingertip and the depressor tip lie on the same vertical line (Fig. 5.21).
3. Avoid complications related to scleral indentation. When sliding the depressor in and out, the operator should act gently to avoid displacing the perfusion cannula. Also avoid contacting the surgeon's hands or the edge of the wide-angle lens, so as not to interfere with the normal progress of the procedure.
4. No indentation when intraocular pressure is low: When the operated eye is hypotonous, scleral indentation will sharply increase ocular deformation,

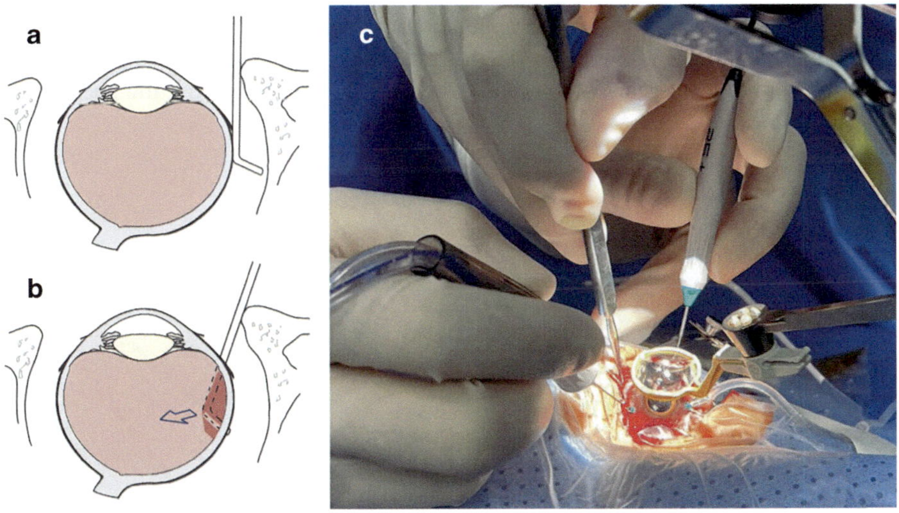

Fig. 5.21 Correct posture for scleral indentation. (**a**) The tip of the strabismus hook first reaches the target position along the orbital margin. (**b**) Use wrist movement to press the tip of the strabismus hook toward the center of the vitreous cavity. (**c**) Correct holding posture of the strabismus hook

potentially causing choroidal detachment or perfusion cannula displacement, and may even lead to explosive choroidal hemorrhage.

Indentation should be performed slowly, progressing from deep to shallow. A recommended technique is as follows: after the assistant slides the depressor along the orbital margin to the periphery of the equator, they then elevate the sclera toward the center of the vitreous cavity. This maneuver maximizes exposure of the peripheral vitreous. After the vitreous in this area has been removed, the assistant gently lifts the depressor toward the limbus to expose the more peripheral region, allowing the surgeon to resect the vitreous layer by layer.

5.3.7 Understanding the Safe Operation of Intraocular Instruments from a Geometric Perspective

Iatrogenic injury to the posterior lens capsule is like a footprint in our growth journey—an experience encountered by nearly every vitreoretinal surgeon during training. Nevertheless, we must always remember that any intraocular maneuver must avoid the posterior lens capsule. If an iatrogenic "mark" is observed on the lens during surgery, we should pause for a moment to reflect on which step went wrong. Prompt feedback and correction will help us grow rapidly.

To maximize protection of the posterior lens capsule from iatrogenic injury by intraocular instruments, we must understand it from a three-dimensional geometric perspective.

As shown in Fig. 5.22, the apex of the anterior lens surface lies approximately at the same horizontal plane as the limbus. The central thickness of the adult lens is approximately 4.5–5 mm, the scleral puncture for the trocar is located 4 mm behind the limbus, and the lens equator is fixed to the scleral wall by zonules approximately 1.5 mm from the limbus. We tentatively define the line connecting the apex of the

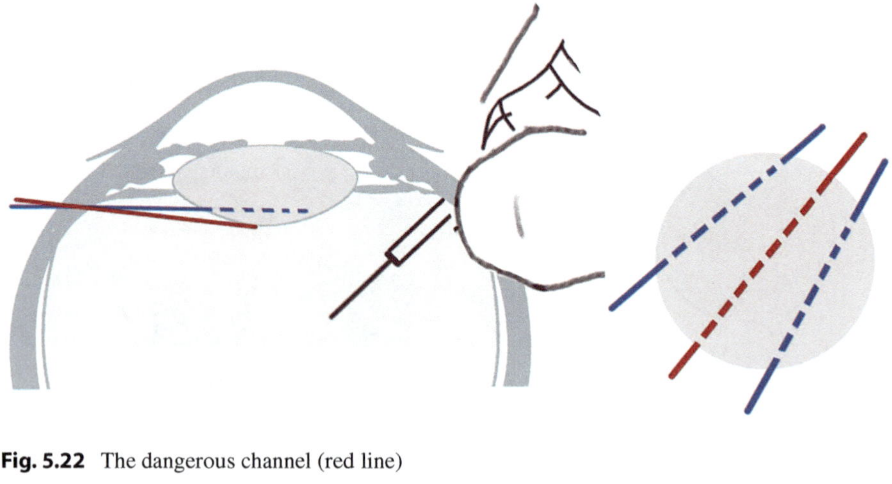

Fig. 5.22 The dangerous channel (red line)

posterior lens capsule to the upper scleral incision as the "dangerous channel". All intraocular instruments must strictly avoid this channel; otherwise, they are likely to contact the posterior lens capsule.

Once we understand this "dangerous channel," we can grasp how to operate the light pipe and cutter effectively. Beginners should recognize the importance of exchanging the light pipe and cutter between hands and should strengthen their practical training to ultimately achieve proficient bimanual coordination, thereby improving the safety and efficiency of vitrectomy.

Assuming the upper trocars are placed at the 2:00 and 10:00 o'clock positions, to resect an adequate amount of vitreous while ensuring lens safety, beginners must adhere to the following principles when performing PPV:

1. Strictly avoid the aforementioned "dangerous channel" and its adjacent areas.
2. All intraocular instruments must enter and exit the vitreous cavity in a centripetal direction.
3. The light pipe and cutter in the left and right hands should not cross the line between the 6:00 and 12:00 o'clock positions, especially when shaving off the peripheral vitreous in the arc area between 2:00 and 10:00.

In addition to lens protection, safe operation of intraocular instruments encompasses many other aspects, which we will elaborate on in subsequent chapters.

5.4 Summary

"Little by little, one travels far." This timeless proverb serves as a vital reminder for every surgeon embarking on the demanding path of vitreoretinal surgery. While continuous technological innovations—from advanced digital visualization to high-speed instrumentation—constantly expand our treatment indications, the core pillars of surgical excellence remain unchanged. Success in this field is never the result of a single factor; it requires the seamless integration of thorough preoperative examination, comprehensive planning, clear patient communication, and a resilient, stable mindset. None of these elements—including solid surgical skills and reliable instrumentation—can be omitted if one is to achieve consistent, superior outcomes.

For the beginner, the journey toward mastery is a marathon, not a sprint. It necessitates a disciplined, step-by-step approach, intentionally progressing from straightforward cases to the most daunting complexities. In your daily clinical practice, let precision, diligence, and a profound respect for scientific principles be your guiding lights. By focusing on these fundamentals and maintaining a consistent effort, you will move steadily toward your long-term goals, ensuring that every small step contributes to a lifetime of professional excellence and patient restoration.

6 Surgical Intervention of Rhegmatogenous Retinal Detachment: Part 1 (Scleral Buckling)

Rhegmatogenous retinal detachment (RRD) is the most important condition managed in vitreoretinal surgery. The term "rhegmatogenous" derives from the Greek word "rhegma," meaning discontinuity or break. From a pathophysiological perspective, "retinal detachment" is not entirely accurate, as the retina consists of the neurosensory layer and the retinal pigment epithelium (RPE); clinically, it refers to detachment between these two layers. Currently, the two most commonly used surgical methods for RRD worldwide are scleral buckling and vitrectomy—often referred to by ophthalmic surgeons as the "ab-externo" (external) approach and the "ab-interno" (internal) approach. "Ab," "externo," and "interno" are derived from Latin, corresponding to "from," "external," and "internal" in English, which parallel the Chinese concepts of "外路 (ab externo)" and "内路 (ab interno)."

As the name (ab-interno) suggests, scleral buckling for RRD refers to a series of surgical procedures performed via an external approach to achieve retinal reattachment and functional recovery. This chapter will focus on the basic steps and related surgical techniques of scleral buckling.

6.1 Current Status of Scleral Buckling

For several decades after the 1950s, scleral buckling was the mainstream treatment for RRD. Because of its high efficacy and safety, it was widely adopted worldwide and gave rise to a variety of modified surgical techniques.

Over the past 20 years, with the advancement and widespread adoption of vitrectomy, the popularity of scleral buckling has gradually declined. The reasons can be summarized as follows:

1. Patients often experience severe pain during surgery, which may lead to poor cooperation.
2. Overall, the postoperative retinal reattachment rate is slightly lower than that of vitrectomy.

Z. Zhang, U. Spandau, *Vitreoretinal Surgery*,
https://doi.org/10.1007/978-3-032-25271-5_6

3. Due to the relatively low number of training cases, beginners have low proficiency and tend to choose the more familiar approach (vitrectomy).
4. Difficulties in managing intraoperative complications, such as choroidal hemorrhage.
5. Unpredictable postoperative complications, including pain, refractive changes, diplopia, and explant extrusion.
6. Lack of publicity and education, as the proportion of scleral buckling in various academic activities has gradually decreased.

According to an international survey conducted in 2005 for phakic eyes without macular involvement and with a primary break (1.5 clock hours in size) at the 11:00 o'clock position, 35.36% of surgeons choose simple scleral buckling, while only 13.94% choose simple vitrectomy. By 2021, the proportion of surgeons choosing scleral buckling had decreased (23.9% in the United States, 30.5% outside the United States), while the proportion choosing simple vitrectomy had increased significantly (29.6% in the United States, 35.9% outside the United States). In the same 2021 survey, for elderly pseudophakic patients without macular involvement and with a primary break at the 8:00 o'clock position, the proportion choosing simple scleral buckling was low (4.8% in the United States, 11.4% outside the United States), and the majority chose simple vitrectomy alone (71.8% in the United States, 68.6% outside the United States).

The above data indicate that although the proportion of scleral buckling is decreasing, three major factors significantly influence the decision-making of retinal surgeons: ① the location of the primary break, ② lens status, and ③ patient age. This indirectly demonstrates that the unique advantages of scleral buckling—such as better lens protection and a higher success rate for retinal detachment caused by inferior breaks—are still recognized by many retinal surgeons. Therefore, it is unlikely to become "a lost art" in the near future.

Jules Gonin once said: "It is not with one and the same weapon that can win all the battles." Despite many controversies, scleral buckling remains an essential skill for beginners in clinical practice. How to identify the most suitable surgical strategy for oneself is a question that we must continually consider while learning scleral buckling.

6.2 Indications for Scleral Buckling

To fully understand the indications for scleral buckling, we must analyze them from two perspectives: first, the pathological mechanism of rhegmatogenous retinal detachment, and second, the unique characteristics of scleral buckling.

6.2.1 Pathological Mechanism of Rhegmatogenous Retinal Detachment

Retinal detachment occurs when the combined forces acting on the retina overcome normal retinal adhesion. Primary rhegmatogenous retinal detachment involves three important factors: ① abnormal vitreous movement or localized liquefaction; ② retinal breaks that are either pre-existing or caused by vitreous traction; and ③ entry of liquefied vitreous into the subretinal space through the breaks. (Fig. 6.1).

Since vitreous liquefaction is an irreversible process, RRD surgery targets the other two factors: (1) relieving vitreous traction on the retina to restore retinal mobility, and (2) sealing retinal breaks to isolate the passage between the vitreous cavity and the subretinal space. Both external and internal approaches aim to achieve these two goals.

Next, we examine how scleral buckling relieves vitreous traction and seals breaks, based on the formation mechanism of retinal breaks. Traditionally, retinal breaks are divided into three categories: ① holes, ② tears, and ③ dialyses. Holes are usually not closely related to vitreous traction; the key factor is

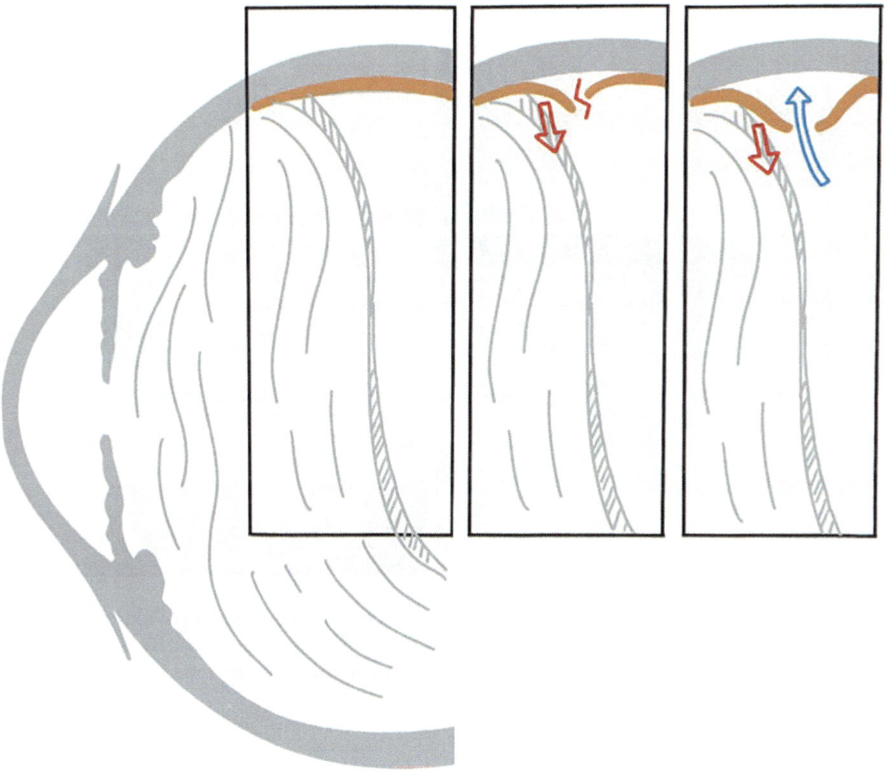

Fig. 6.1 Schematic diagram of the three major factors of rhegmatogenous retinal detachment

atrophic changes of the retina itself (Fig. 6.2a). Common underlying conditions include familial exudative vitreoretinopathy (FEVR). Tears are typically secondary to acute posterior vitreous detachment (PVD). The liquefied vitreous in the posterior pole loses its supporting effect on the retina, while the peripheral vitreous remains partially adherent. When the balance between support and traction is disrupted in a given area, a retinal tear occurs. Vitreous liquefaction and vitreous traction are the two key factors in tear formation, which often present as U-shaped tears (Fig. 6.2b). Another special type is the giant retinal tear (GRT) (Fig. 6.2c). Dialyses often occur at the peripheral ora serrata (Fig. 6.2d), usually secondary to trauma but may also be spontaneous. They mainly manifest as shallow peripheral detachment, making them difficult to detect on routine fundus examination. Circular centripetal traction caused by peripheral vitreous contraction is the key factor.

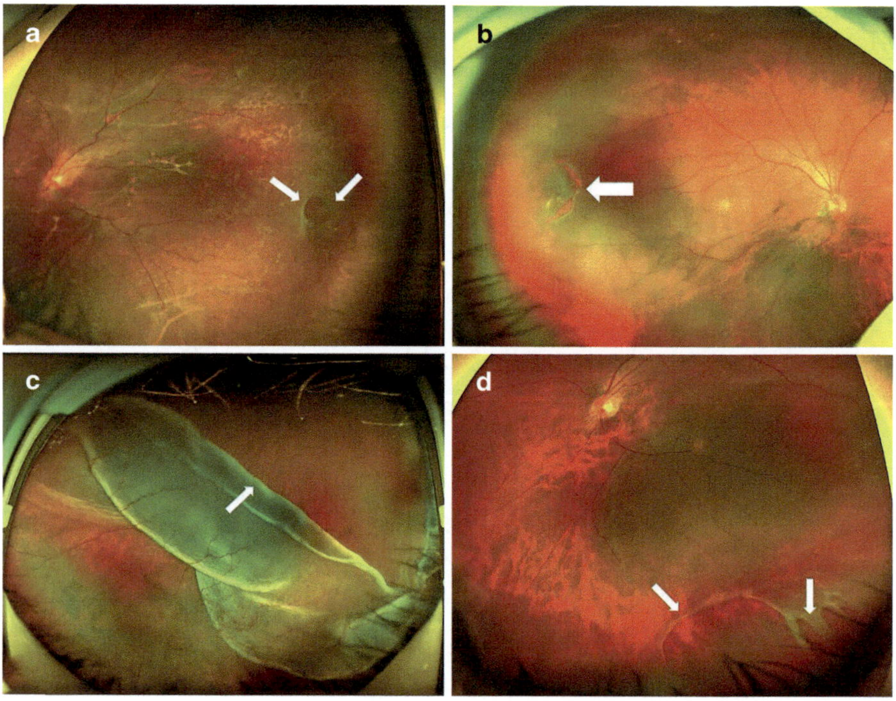

Fig. 6.2 Representative retinal breaks. (**a**) Temporal atrophic hole without obvious vitreous traction. (**b**) U-shaped tear caused by vitreous traction. (**c**) Giant retinal tear caused by peripheral vitreous shrinkage and traction. (**d**) Shallow retinal detachment caused by peripheral retinal dialysis

6.2.2 Functions of Scleral Buckling

Since it does not directly involve the vitreous, scleral buckling is often regarded as a "minimally invasive" procedure. This concept of minimal invasiveness stems from the fact that it preserves the entire vitreous and minimizes disruption to the original intraocular structures—aside from altering the inherent shape of the scleral.

From an anatomical and physiological perspective, scleral buckling exerts the following effects on the vitreous and retina:

1. Relieving vitreous traction: The explant on the scleral wall alters the shape of the sclera, pushing the retina closer to the center of the vitreous cavity. As a result, tension in the vitreous adherent to the break decreases, and vitreous traction on the retina is reduced or eliminated.
2. Dividing subretinal fluid: The scleral buckle partitions the originally continuous subretinal fluid into two compartments: anterior and posterior to the buckle. From a fluid mechanics perspective, this disrupts the balance between subretinal fluid production and absorption, creating the necessary conditions for RPE cells to completely absorb the subretinal fluid.
3. Promoting apposition between the break edge and the RPE layer: At the microscopic level, fluid in the vitreous cavity flows through the break at a certain rate. Without external intervention, this flow rate is relatively constant and linearly related to the amount of subretinal fluid absorbed by RPE cells per unit time. After scleral buckling, the cross-sectional area between the retina around the break and the underlying RPE layer is significantly reduced.

According to Bernoulli's equation, the flow velocity of fluid in the vitreous cavity will increase significantly when passing through the scleral buckle. Correspondingly, the pressure exerted by this fluid on its surroundings will decrease. At this point, the pressure balance between the preretinal and subretinal spaces is disrupted. As a result, the retina experiences a net outward force from the vitreous cavity, which pushes the break toward the RPE layer (Fig. 6.3). This force promotes closer apposition between the break and the underlying RPE layer, ultimately achieving complete break apposition. The passage of fluid from the vitreous cavity into the subretinal space is completely blocked, allowing RPE cells to absorb most of the subretinal fluid within a short period (typically 1 day).

6.2.3 Indications for Scleral Buckling

"Unfazed by floating clouds blocking the view, only because standing at the highest peak." When determining the indications for scleral buckling, the key is to integrate the pathological mechanism of RRD with the fundamental characteristics of scleral buckling and identify their intersection. As long as an intersection exists, indications are present. However, in clinical practice, other external factors also dynamically influence the surgeon's final decision. This is a choice that will continue to exist for the foreseeable future, and we must face it objectively.

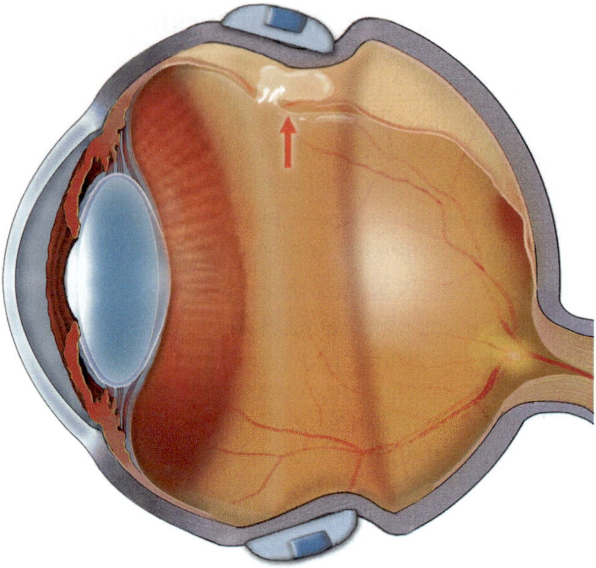

Fig. 6.3 Bernoulli's principle in scleral buckling surgery

In light of the development and refinement of the pars plana vitrectomy, the following indications for scleral buckling in clinical practice are proposed as a reference for RRD without retinal fixed folds (PVR < C1) (see Sect. 11.2 of Chap. 11 for classification).

1. No obvious PVD or predicted difficulty in inducing PVD intraoperatively: In some patients younger than 40 years of age, the adhesion between the posterior vitreous cortex and the posterior pole may still be relatively tight. Performing vitrectomy in such cases may pose significant challenges in inducing PVD and could even result in iatrogenic retinal damage (Fig. 6.4).
2. Primary break located in the peripheral retina: If the break is situated peripherally, there is no need for excessive extraocular muscle retraction when suturing the explant, allowing both the surgeon and patient to have a more comfortable surgical experience.
3. Young patients with phakic eyes: For patients who require near-vision work, preserving the crystalline lens is of great importance, as internal approach surgery can induce or accelerate cataract progression.
4. Primary break located in the inferior retina: Silicone oil and gas tamponades have relatively poor sealing effects for inferior breaks. If retinal reattachment is not achieved by pars plana vitrectomy, the success rate of subsequent procedures will also decrease accordingly. However, scleral buckling shows no significant difference in sealing effectiveness for breaks at different locations. Given the advantages mentioned above, scleral buckling is undoubtedly the better choice (Fig. 6.5).

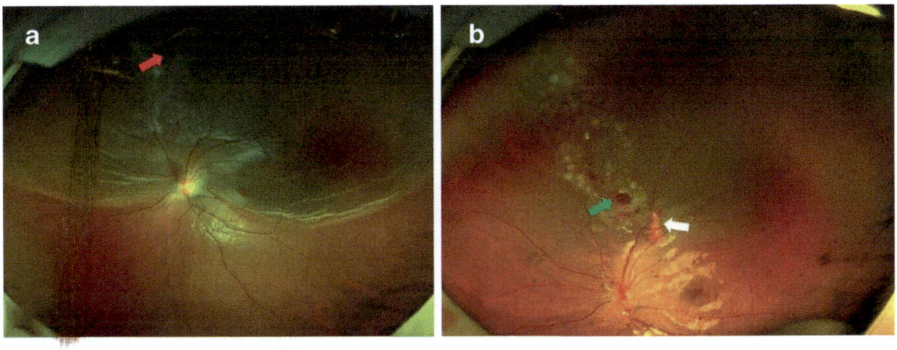

Fig. 6.4 Iatrogenic retinal break in the posterior pole caused by inducing posterior vitreous detachment in a young patient. The patient received silicone oil tamponade after surgery. Although the retina reattached well, persistent high intraocular pressure due to silicone oil led to a poor visual prognosis. (**a**) Traumatic retinal detachment with peripheral breaks (red arrow); the vitreous was not obviously liquefied. (**b**) During PVD induction, excessive suction by the vitrectomy probe caused a posterior pole retinal break (green arrow) and secondary subretinal hemorrhage (white arrow)

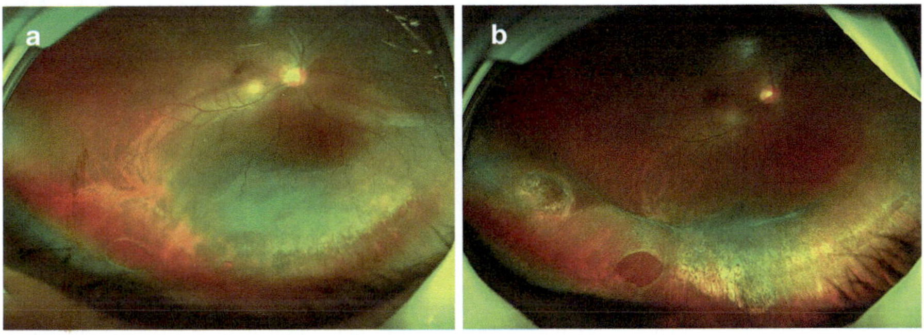

Fig. 6.5 Preoperative and postoperative fundus photographs of a patient with retinal detachment caused by an inferior break (patient age 22 years old, preoperative and postoperative corrected visual acuity were both 1.0). (**a**) Preoperative inferior retinal break without macular involvement. (**b**) Postoperative well-sealed break and attached retina

5. Presence of multiple subretinal bands: In some young patients with chronic retinal detachment, multiple subretinal bands may develop. Vitrectomy would require retinectomy to remove them, ultimately necessitating silicone oil tamponade. Moreover, the risk of postoperative proliferative vitreoretinopathy is high, and the patient may require multiple surgeries (Fig. 6.6). In such cases, scleral buckling may be the preferred option, as long as no retinal fixed folds are present.
6. Ora serrata dialysis: Due to the large extent of breaks and their peripheral location, scleral buckling can effectively seal them. Particularly for inferior ora serrata dialysis, scleral buckling offers dual advantages: low surgical difficulty and the ability to surround the break over a wide area (Fig. 6.7).

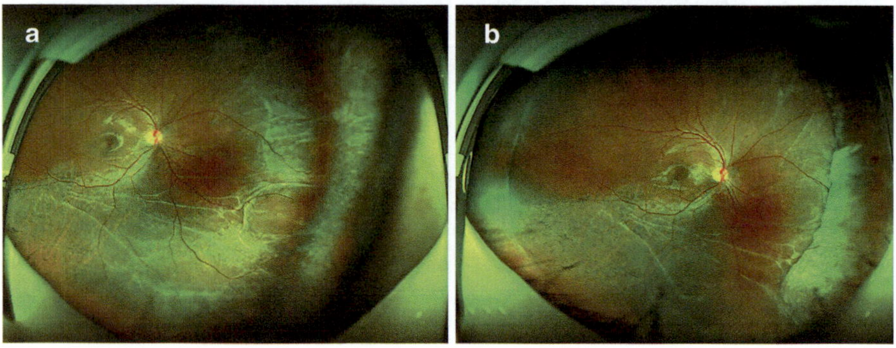

Fig. 6.6 Preoperative and postoperative fundus images of multiple subretinal bands caused by chronic retinal detachment. (**a**) Multiple subretinal strands in the nasal retina of the right eye; the macula is attached, with corrected visual acuity of 1.0. (**b**) Encircling with scleral buckling was performed. One day after surgery, the retina was attached, and corrected visual acuity remained 1.0

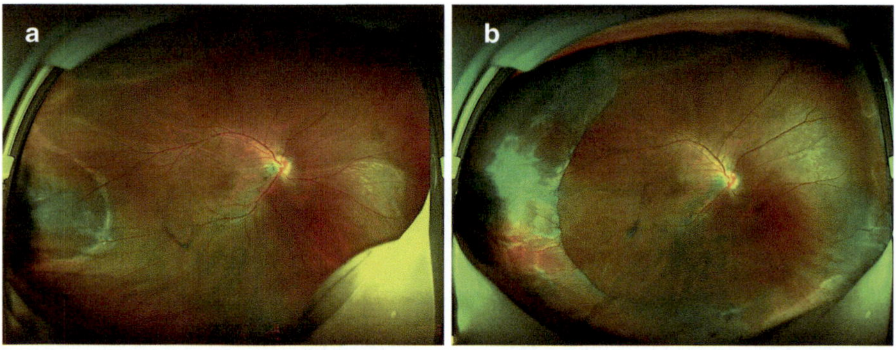

Fig. 6.7 Preoperative and postoperative fundus images of ora serrata dialysis. (**a**) No definite retinal break was identified on preoperative wide-field fundus photography. Retinal detachment was determined to be caused by superotemporal ora serrata dialysis on three-mirror lens examination. (**b**) One day after surgery, the retina reattached

7. With anterior segment abnormalities: In some patients with anterior segment abnormalities—such as lens abnormalities combined with pupillary displacement or deformation (Fig. 6.8)—vitrectomy may result in a compromised surgical field and a higher probability of postoperative complications. If objective conditions permit, scleral buckling may be preferred.
8. Auxiliary means for vitrectomy: For breaks located inferiorly, especially ora serrata dialysis (Fig. 6.9) and recurrent retinal detachment, scleral buckling can be used as an adjunct to vitrectomy to relieve possible traction on the peripheral retina and further improve the retinal reattachment rate.

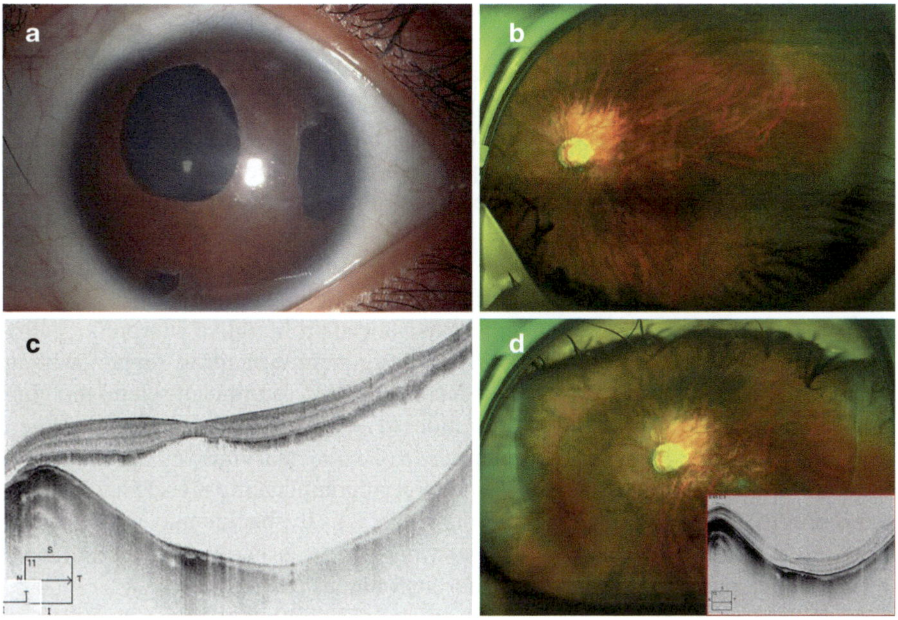

Fig. 6.8 Retinal detachment with significant anterior segment abnormalities. (**a**) The patient (11 years old) was diagnosed with Axenfeld-Rieger syndrome and had undergone antiglaucoma surgery 8 years prior. Findings included Haab's striae of the cornea, marked pupil and iris abnormalities, and mild lens opacity. (**b**) Wide-field fundus photography showed shallow temporal retinal detachment without an obvious primary break. (**c**) OCT confirmed that the retinal detachment had involved the macula. (**d**) One day after scleral buckling, retina reattached, and OCT demonstrated complete disappearance of the subretinal fluid (indicated by the red box in the figure)

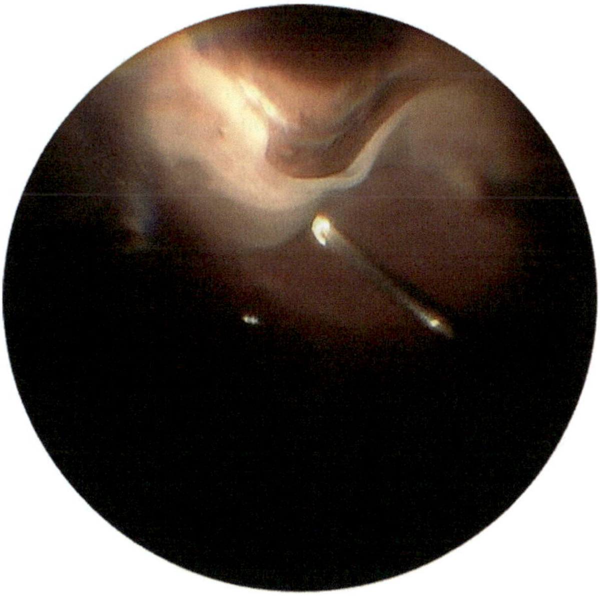

Fig. 6.9 Video snapshot showing inferior ora serrata dialysis, combining vitrectomy with scleral buckling can improve the long-term success rate for this kind of retinal detachment

6.2.4 Relative Contraindications for Scleral Buckling

Understanding the relative contraindications for scleral buckling requires a comprehensive evaluation of three aspects: (1) The intrinsic characteristics and limitations of the scleral buckling procedure; (2) Whether the patient's sclera can provide safe and stable structural support for the explant; and (3) Whether the specific shape and location of the retinal break are compatible with the geometric requirements of a scleral buckle.

"Forewarned is forearmed." Based on the preceding discussion, we summarize the relative contraindications for scleral buckling for clinical reference: (1) Presence of fixed retinal folds, which often indicate advanced proliferative vitreoretinopathy; (2) Breaks located relatively posteriorly, making them difficult to support with an external explant; (3) Long axial length accompanied by significant scleral thinning, which increases the risk of globe perforation; (4) Presence of a macular hole, where internal tamponade is generally preferred; (5) Extraocular muscles near the clock hour of the break having undergone prior surgery, complicating muscle hooking and exposure; (6) Previous glaucoma filtering surgery, as the buckle may interfere with the filtration bleb or drainage device; and (7) Poor transparency of the refractive media, which precludes the essential thorough fundus examination.

6.3 Preoperative Break Localization for Scleral Buckling

6.3.1 Emphasize the Application of Three-Mirror Lens Examination

Localization and sealing of breaks are key steps in treating RRD. This is a fundamental skill that beginners must diligently practice and an issue that retinal surgeons must take seriously throughout their careers.

The three-mirror lens is the most effective tool for locating peripheral retinal breaks. Beginners must become proficient in its use and strive to identify all breaks preoperatively without omission. Only by adhering to this rigorous approach can the efficacy of scleral buckling be maximized.

Wide-field fundus photography is capable of capturing a significant portion of the peripheral retina, yet it faces two major limitations in clinical practice: (1) It still cannot visualize the extreme periphery, as the area near the ora serrata remains difficult to image even with guided changes in eye position; and (2) Pseudocolor rendering can compromise image quality, which may lead to small degenerative lesions or subtle retinal breaks being overlooked.

"The starting point of scleral buckling is the three-mirror lens." Among all fundus examination methods, the three-mirror lens achieves the best balance between ease of use and retinal coverage. Other examinations may serve as supplementary tools. When using the three-mirror lens, the area corresponding to each mirror can be remembered using the following rules demonstrated in Fig. 6.10.

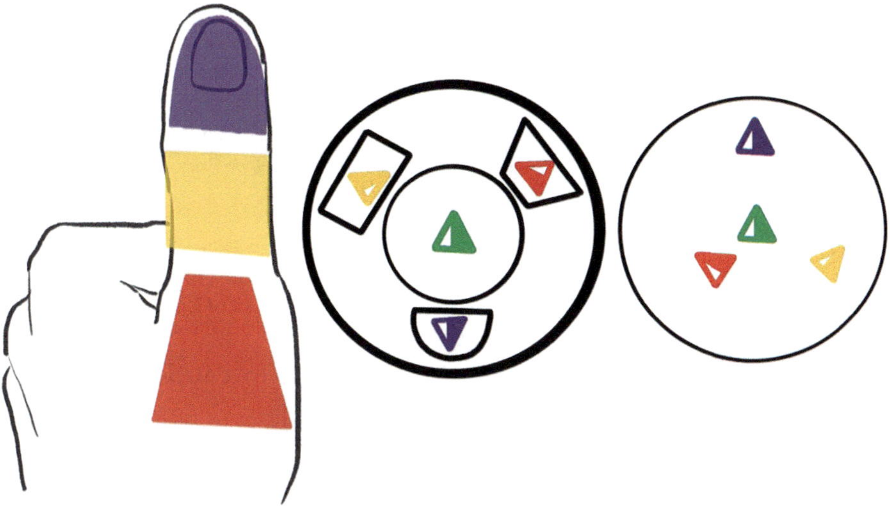

Fig. 6.10 Method for remembering the orientation of the four mirrors of the three-mirror lens

6.3.2 Lincoff's Rules

In May 1971, Dr. Lincoff published an original paper entitled "Finding the Retinal Hole" in the renowned ophthalmology journal *Archives of Ophthalmology*. The study included 1000 patients with RRD. By meticulously recording the shape of retinal detachment and the location of primary breaks, and based on the mechanism of subretinal fluid production and the effect of gravity, a method for localizing breaks was initially proposed.

In 1972, based on these research findings, Lincoff proposed Lincoff's Rules for localizing primary retinal breaks (Fig. 6.11), which remain an important component of the scleral buckling system. With continued clinical experience, one gains a deeper appreciation of their objectivity and accuracy. When applying these principles, the case most easily overlooked by beginners is that of a primary break located superiorly presenting as inferior bullous detachment (Fig. 6.12).

Lincoff's Rules can be applied sequentially in the following scenarios.

1. When the affected eye is suitable for scleral buckling (e.g., young age, limited detachment extent, etc.), but the surgeon has not clearly visualized the break preoperatively using common examination methods such as wide-field fundus photography or indirect ophthalmoscopy.
2. In scenario (1), under the guidance of Lincoff's Rules, use the three-mirror lens combined with changes in the patient's eye position to locate breaks in the peripheral retina, paying particular attention to ora serrata dialysis or small retinal flaps.

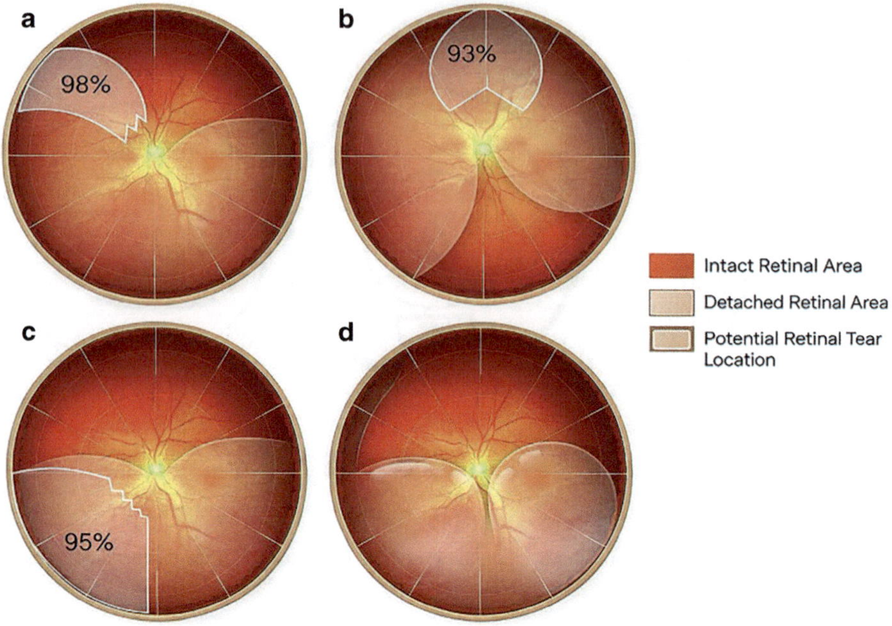

Fig. 6.11 Lincoff's rules for finding primary retinal breaks. (**a**) Temporal superior or nasal detachment: 98% of primary breaks are within 1.5 clock hours of the edge of the highest point. (**b**) Total or superior detachment crossing the 12:00 meridian: 93% of breaks are at the 12:00 position or in a triangular area with the ora serrata as the vertex, and the two sides of the triangular area extend 1.5 clock hours to the left and right of the 12:00 position, respectively. (**c**) Inferior retinal detachment: 95% of breaks are slightly inferior to the highest side of the detachment. (**d**) Inferior and spherical detachment: if the detachment area presents a large blister-like bulge, the break is usually located superiorly

3. If the retinal break remains unfound in scenario (2), after excluding exudative retinal detachment, use a cryoprobe to perform scleral indentation during surgery and examine the peripheral retina with indirect ophthalmoscope, with special attention to possible breaks at the ora serrata.
4. When no definite break is found in scenario (3), or when the refractive media are opaque, apply Lincoff's Rules directly and perform a wide scleral buckle.

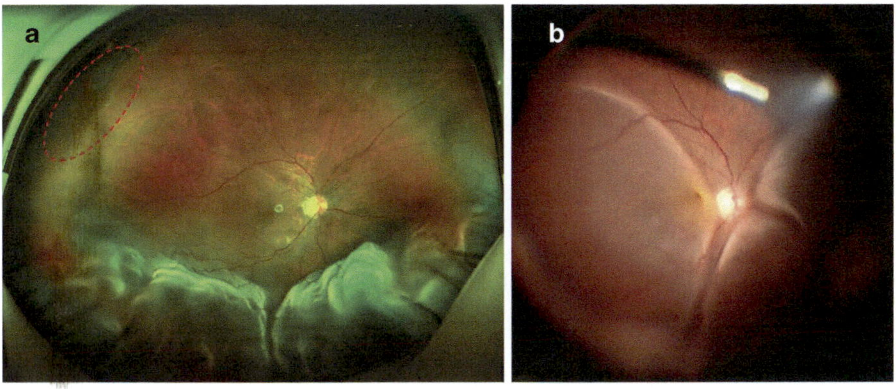

Fig. 6.12 Inferior spherical retinal detachment. (**a**) When the patient undergoes fundus photography in the sitting position, subretinal fluid accumulates inferiorly due to gravity. According to Lincoff's Rules, the primary break should be located within the red dashed line in the superotemporal area. (**b**) When the patient is in the supine position, the configuration of the retinal detachment changes significantly (video snapshot during PPV)

6.4 Basic Steps and Precautions of Scleral Buckling

6.4.1 Understand Different Philosophies of Scleral Buckling

Since the mid-twentieth century, after extensive clinical validation, scleral buckling has developed into a standalone procedure with distinct approaches that differ in some details. Among these, the most representative are the Lincoff school and the Schepens school. The major difference between them is whether subretinal drainage is performed during surgery. Which approach is superior is something every young retina surgeon must ultimately determine based on their own experience and insights.

Interestingly, despite the many differences in specific steps, the safety and efficacy of scleral buckling remain consistently high. The fundamental reason is that all successful procedures adhere to basic principles: ① judicious selection of indications, and ② accurate localization and sealing of the primary breaks.

When learning scleral buckling, we should thoroughly understand the characteristics of different approaches and, in clinical practice, prioritize safety and efficacy as we explore the most suitable surgical strategy for ourselves.

6.4.2 Basic Steps of Scleral Buckling

The key to scleral buckling is preoperative design; the focus during surgery is avoiding complications. Below are the basic steps for scleral buckling without drainage.

1. Incise the conjunctiva to expose the sclera. Subconjunctival or sub-Tenon anesthesia is not necessary. Although it aids analgesia and Tenon's capsule separation, it can cause bulging, hindering accurate conjunctival wound alignment and postoperative healing. After limbal conjunctival incision, use scissors to bluntly separate the intermuscular septum between adjacent rectus muscles, avoiding damage to the extraocular muscle sheaths to reduce bleeding.
2. Sling the extraocular muscles. Slide a strabismus hook backward along the scleral surface under the rectus muscle. The hook tip should always stay close to the sclera to ensure the entire muscle insertion is engaged. After hooking the muscle, pause to wipe away bleeding and confirm complete engagement (Fig. 6.13). Incomplete engagement may cause the scleral implant (especially the encircling band) to pass through the muscle, leading to postoperative dysfunction—this must be strictly avoided.
3. Anterior chamber paracentesis. Use a drainage needle to release aqueous humor and reduce intraocular pressure. Keep the needle tip within the anterior chamber angle to avoid lens damage. Gently squeeze the eyeball to temporarily increase

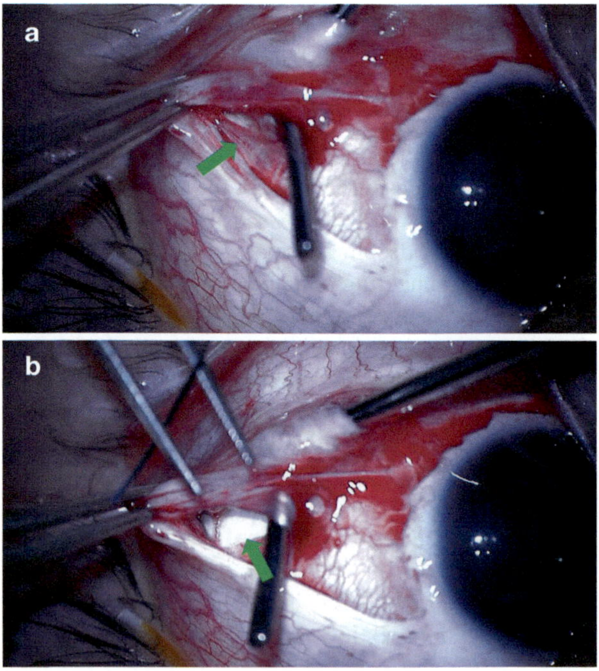

Fig. 6.13 Elevation of the extraocular muscle with a strabismus hook. (**a**) The strabismus hook does not completely engage the extraocular muscle, and the hook splits the muscle fibers (green arrow). (**b**) Withdraw the strabismus hook, then re-elevate the extraocular muscle. Confirm that the muscle has been completely engaged as a whole; no residual fibers remain unengaged. (green arrow)

pressure and promote aqueous outflow (Fig. 6.14). Release >0.2 mL of aqueous humor to facilitate subsequent indentation and buckling. In patients with significant vitreous liquefaction, the anterior chamber may not shallow noticeably, so monitor intraocular pressure closely.

4. Localize the break under indirect ophthalmoscope. This step has a steep learning curve. Intraoperative practice alone is insufficient; beginners should focus on outpatient and ward training. Once mastered, indirect ophthalmoscope provides excellent intraoperative visualization.

   The surgeon wears an additional pair of sterile gloves or a disposable sterile plastic film bag (commonly used at Zhongshan Ophthalmic Center—faster than gloves), then wears the indirect ophthalmoscope and adjusts tightness and focus.

   Focus adjustment steps: ① Extend left hand, close left eye, face palm toward yourself, and adjust the right eyepiece until the light circle is fully cast on your left palm. ② Extend right hand, close right eye, and adjust the left eyepiece until the light circle is fully cast on your right palm. ③ Open both eyes—the complete light circle will appear before you.

   Hold a +20D aspheric lens in the left hand and the cryoprobe handle in the right hand. Press the ocular wall back and forth from the periphery to the equator, carefully searching for breaks in the target area (Fig. 6.15).

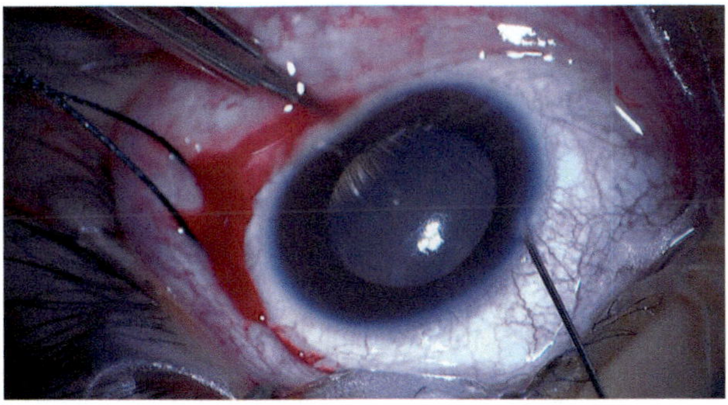

Fig. 6.14 Anterior chamber paracentesis. Attention should be paid to avoiding accidental injury to the iris and lens. By squeezing the eyeball, temporarily increase intraocular pressure to promote aqueous humor outflow

After accurate localization, ask the assistant to mark the break's approximate position on the scleral surface with a cautery or marker pen. This is especially helpful for posterior breaks and long axial lengths, enabling accurate explants placement (Fig. 6.16).

5. Retinal cryopexy: Under indirect ophthalmoscope, step on the cryopexy foot pedal. When the pressed area rapidly changes color—the choroid turns orange-red and the outer retina becomes slightly whitened—stop immediately. The cryoprobe can thaw naturally or be dripped with water to accelerate thawing (Fig. 6.17).

   Cryopexy can be performed simultaneously with break localization. Once the break is accurately localized, cryopexy is not difficult. Do not freeze the RPE layer directly beneath the break; instead, apply moderate freeze to the surrounding RPE at multiple points. The most common beginner mistake is excessive cryopexy. Scleral cryopexy penetrates the entire ocular wall, potentially damaging the sclera, choroid, RPE, and neurosensory retina. Postoperative inflammation leads to scar formation, which seals the break.

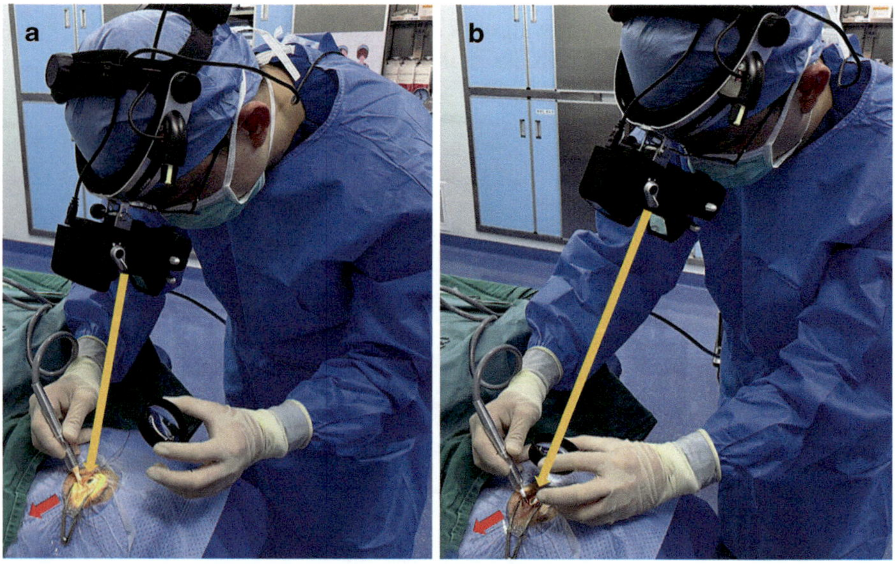

Fig. 6.15 Steps of break localization under indirect ophthalmoscope (**a**) Use the cryoprobe to gently rotate the eyeball toward the intended freezing position (red arrow). The surgeon first observes the elevated peripheral retina through the headlight, keeping the indirect ophthalmoscope light source and the peripheral retina aligned (two points form a line) (yellow arrow). (**b**) Maintain the direction of eyeball rotation (red arrow). The surgeon places the aspheric lens in line with the light source using the left hand, so that three points—indirect ophthalmoscope light source, aspheric lens, and peripheral retina—are aligned (yellow arrow)

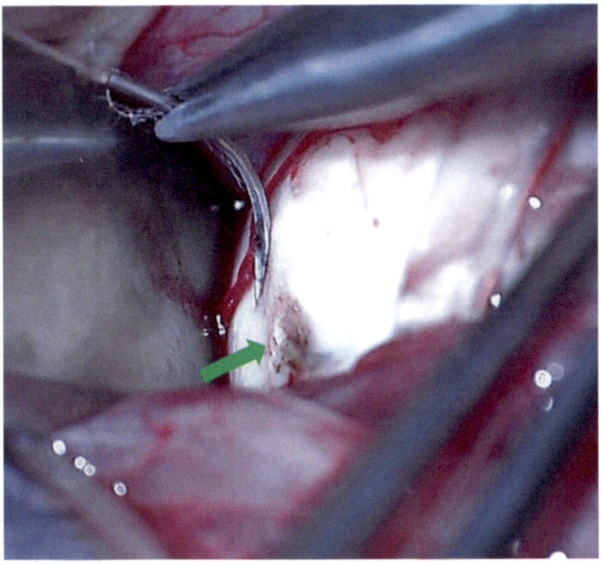

Fig. 6.16 Mark the approximate position of the break on the scleral surface with a cautery (green arrow)

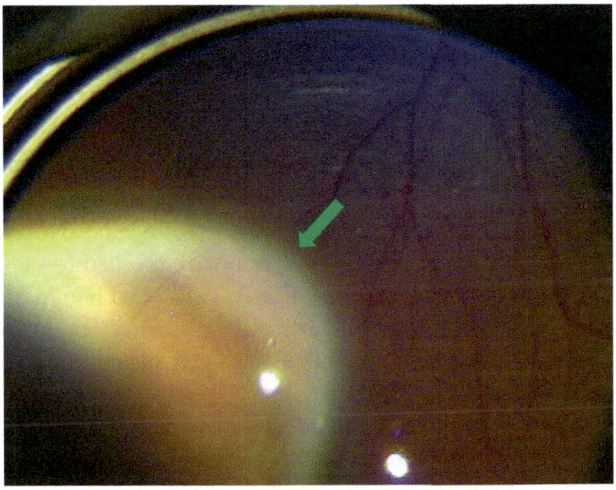

Fig. 6.17 Surgical video screenshot showing slight whitening of the retina under cryotherapy (green arrow)

This inflammatory response is a double-edged sword. Follow the principle: "accurate multiple points, lighter rather than heavier." Excessive cryopexy causes severe inflammation, promoting PVR development, while atrophic changes at the neuroepithelial layer may create new breaks at the cryopexy spot edges, causing recurrent detachment and significantly increasing reoperation difficulty (Fig. 6.18).

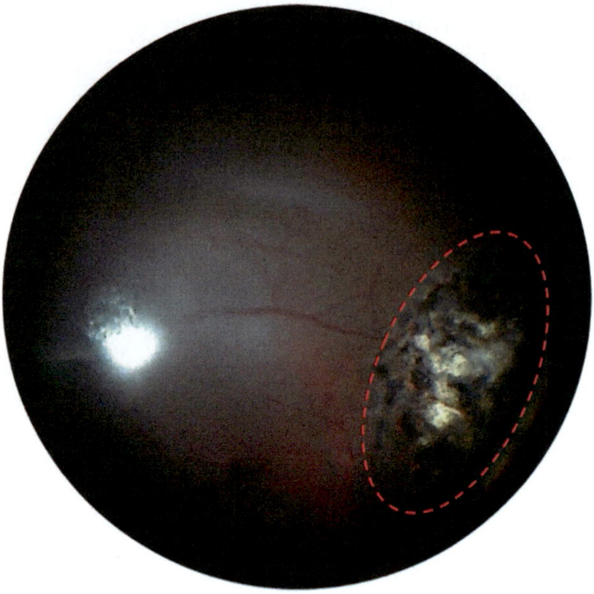

Fig. 6.18 Chorioretinal atrophy caused by excessive cryotherapy (within the red dashed line), eventually leading to recurrent retinal detachment

6. Placement of silicone explants: Explants fixation typically uses 5–0 nylon sutures, which can be pre-placed or directly sutured to the sclera. The anterior suture is generally placed 9–10 mm posterior to the limbus. Beginners should use a caliper to determine suture edges, ensuring good silicone buckle apposition and reducing astigmatism.

   Needle entry point selection is critical. The anterior point should avoid muscle insertions; the posterior point should avoid vortex veins to prevent bleeding. Breaks located under a rectus muscle increase suturing difficulty.

   The assistant uses a retractor to fully expose the sclera. The surgeon holds the corresponding muscle insertion with toothed forceps in the left hand, creating a stable fulcrum to control needle depth and length.

   To prevent scleral tearing at suture entry points, maintain appropriate needle depth and a sufficient needle span, ensuring the scleral tissue has enough toughness to resist suture stress.

   When inserting the needle, hold it in the right hand, gently press the scleral surface, and enter at a 45° angle to reach the scleral lamella. The needle trajectory should be faintly visible on the scleral surface. When placing the posterior suture, carefully identify the vortex vein and strictly avoid its adjacent area (Fig. 6.19).

   During this process, maintain slight, slow wrist rotation to adapt to scleral curvature, ensuring consistent needle depth—avoiding both suture slippage (too shallow) and globe perforation (too deep).

The silicone explant width, suture span, and ligature tightness jointly determine buckle height. The commonly used silicone explant has a 7 mm base width (nicknamed "tire" due to its appearance). #276 (groove on the side) (Fig. 6.20) and #277 (central groove) tires are the most commonly used. Beginners should first master these two styles.

The suture span should be 1–2 mm wider than the silicone explant. For a 7 mm wide tire with a 9 mm suture span, tighten the suture until the two groove margins are roughly apposed (Fig. 6.21). After the first knot, the assistant should fix it with microneedle holders to prevent loosening—otherwise, a definite buckle is difficult to achieve. Figure 6.22 shows shape changes of the eye wall when tightening the encircling band and silicone block.

The buckle arc should sufficiently seal the break and surrounding degenerative area, generally extending ≥1 clock hour beyond each break edge. In practice, especially without drainage, retinal elevation and mobility make clock hour judgment difficult. Beginners may appropriately extend buckling range to avoid missing the break. If the buckling height is insufficient, add sutures to evenly elevate the underlying sclera.

7. Check buckle position and height: Under indirect ophthalmoscope, use a cotton swab or forceps to gently pull the eye toward the observation direction. Observe whether the buckle position is slightly posterior to the break's posterior edge, and adjust as needed. Theoretically, the break's posterior edge should be ≥1 PD and ≤1.5 PD anterior to the buckle crest, but this is difficult to achieve precisely. Beginners should at least confirm that the break's posterior edge lies on the anterior slope of the buckle.

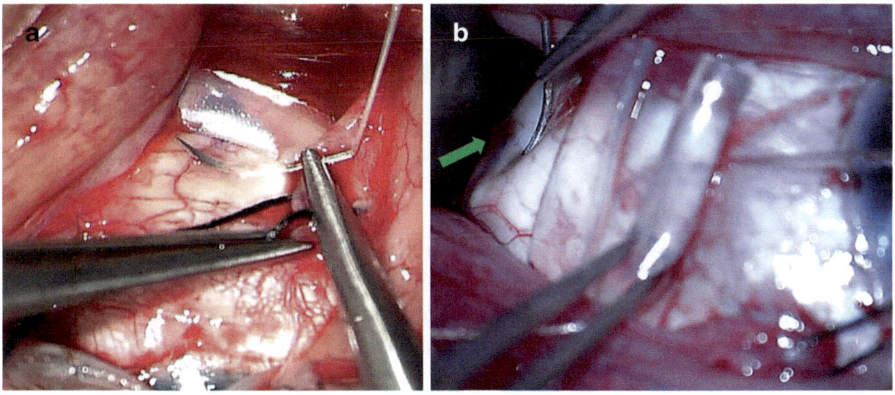

Fig. 6.19 Anterior and posterior edge suture fixation of the silicone explant. (**a**) The needle entry point at the anterior edge should avoid the area around the muscle insertion. The needle entry depth should allow the metal reflection of the advancing needle to be faintly visible, and the span should not be too small—preferably 2–3 mm. (**b**) The needle entry point at the posterior edge should avoid the vortex vein (green arrow) and its surrounding area

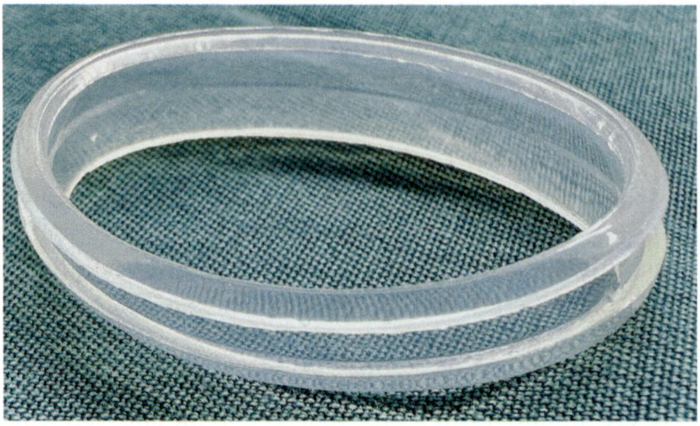

Fig. 6.20 Silicone explant (#276), the width is 7 mm, and the central groove width is 2.5 mm. This groove serves two different functions: (1) When combined with encircling, the encircling band passes through the groove, which helps to fix the band in place. After the encircling band is tightened, the posterior edge of the scleral buckle lies flush with the posterior edge of the silicone explant; (2) When the silicone tire is used alone, tightening the fixation sutures approximates the two sides of the groove, creating a higher scleral buckle. In this configuration, the posterior edge of the buckle lies flush with the midline of the groove

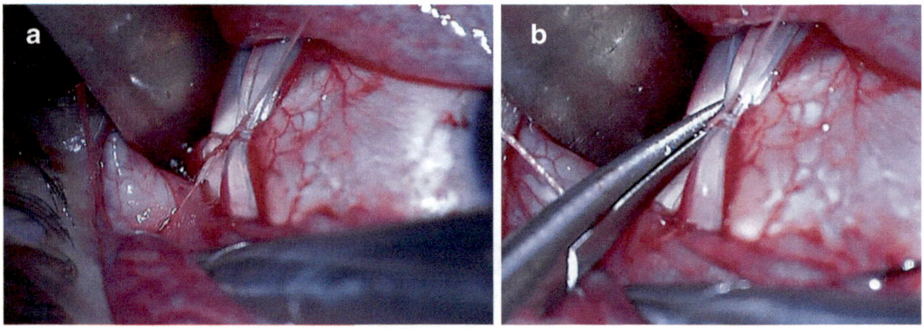

Fig. 6.21 Tightening and fixing the suture. (**a**) Tighten the suture to approximate the two sides of the groove. (**b**) The assistant uses microneedle holder to secure the first knot, preventing slippage

Additionally, continuously monitor intraocular pressure and optic disc perfusion. If optic disc arterial pulsation or cessation of arterial perfusion is observed, perform anterior chamber paracentesis promptly to lower pressure. If pressure is low, inject balanced salt solution or filtered air into the vitreous cavity. Long-acting gas is generally not recommended at this stage.

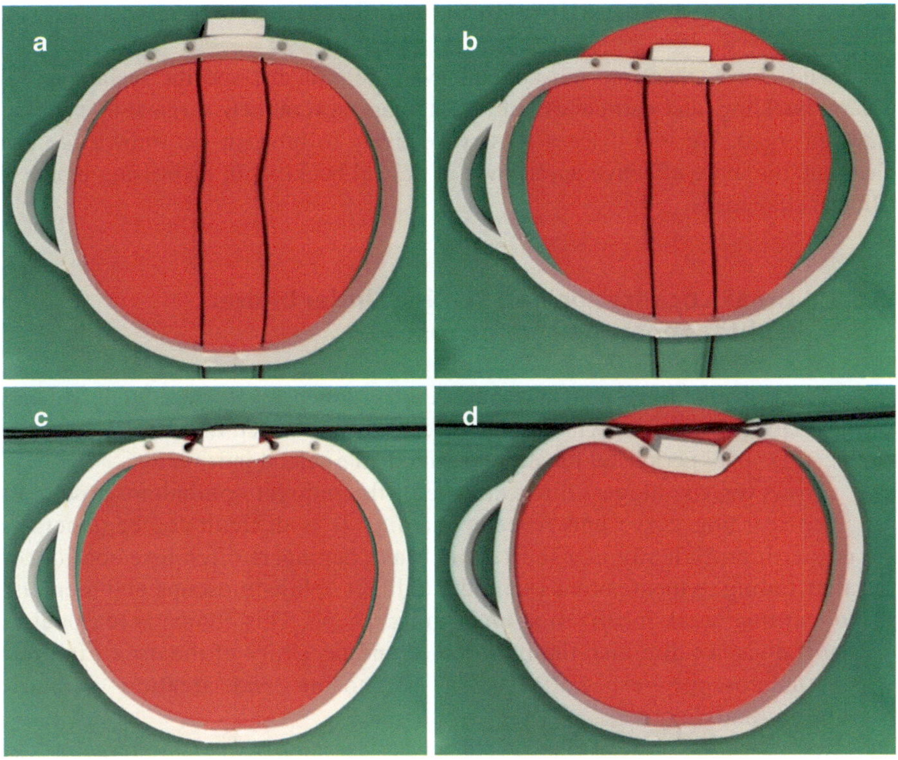

Fig. 6.22 Changes in the shape of ocular wall by silicone explants. (**a**) The ocular wall is nearly circular when the silicone explant is not tightened. (**b**) After tightening the encircling band, the anteroposterior diameter of the vitreous cavity increases, and the anterior chamber becomes slightly shallower. (**c**) When suturing the silicone explant, a small suture span produces a ridge with a low height and gentle slope. (**d**) A larger suture span creates a ridge with greater height and a steeper slope

8. Close the conjunctival incision: Align the conjunctival incision edges and close with interrupted or continuous 8–0 absorbable sutures. If tension is high, place a fixation suture at the limbus to prevent slipping. Wounds heal quickly, typically within 2 weeks, but avoid rough alignment to prevent excessive postoperative edema and scarring. Conjunctival sutures may be removed promptly to reduce ocular foreign body sensation.

6.5 Different Operations in Scleral Buckling

As noted above, there are considerable variations in the specific techniques of scleral buckling, and particularly in recent years, several new surgical approaches have emerged. We will discuss these objectively to broaden our knowledge and facilitate the more effective application of scleral buckling in addressing practical clinical challenges.

6.5.1 Break Localization and Sealing Under Indirect Ophthalmoscope and Microscopes

1. Indirect ophthalmoscope: It provides a three-dimensional, clear fundus image, facilitating dynamic observation of the cryotherapy effect. It offers advantage in locating small peripheral breaks under moderate scleral indentation.

   However, the biggest disadvantage of the indirect ophthalmoscope is its steep learning curve and reverse imaging. It is difficult for beginners to master it proficiently in a short time. Many beginners often lose confidence after failing to locate breaks with the indirect ophthalmoscope and then turn to learning break localization under microscope. This choice is reasonable, but it does not diminish the importance and necessity of the use of indirect ophthalmoscope—especially when diagnosing and treating pediatric vitreoretinal disorders.
2. Microscope: Most steps of are performed under microscope. The surgeon does not need to use an indirect ophthalmoscope for break localization or cryotherapy, ensuring the procedural consistency. This technique is particularly useful in medical institutions that lack access to an indirect ophthalmoscope.

   Because the procedure is performed under the microscope, the highest point of the peripheral retina must be depressed to bring it close to the visual axis. This is difficult to achieve without scleral drainage. Therefore, this technique places high demands on drainage. However, beginners should avoid pursuing maximal efficacy of subretinal drainage at the expense of safety. Additionally, for some small breaks, if the neurosensory retina is not frozen to be white enough, the break may be difficult to visualize clearly. As a result, the total cryoenergy delivered during break localization and cryotherapy may be excessive.

   Mastering the indirect ophthalmoscope requires overcoming a steep learning curve. However, if we approach it as an essential career skill and actively learn it—just as no novice ophthalmologist would give up learning slit-lamp biomicroscopy despite similar difficulty—the lasting and profound sense of fulfillment it brings will be well worth the effort. At the same time, microscopic scleral buckling also offers distinct advantages. Beginners should remain objective and open-minded, trying different techniques in clinical practice to find the approach that best suits you.

6.5.2 Subretinal Fluid Drainage

From the surgeon's perspective, the decision to perform subretinal fluid drainage depends on two major factors: (1) The specific surgical philosophy the surgeon follows; and (2) The clinical balance between its potential advantages and inherent risks. All other secondary considerations revolve around these two fundamental pillars. By carefully examining these factors from both the patient's clinical status and the surgeon's technical perspective, a well-informed final decision can be reached.

(1) Concepts

The Custodis–Lincoff school has demonstrated through long-term practice that scleral buckling can achieve a high success rate without subretinal fluid drainage—even when the retinal break remains unclosed at the end of the procedure. As explained earlier by Bernoulli's equation, the buckling effect around the break promotes retinal reattachment. If the buckle is placed appropriately, subretinal fluid will be gradually absorbed over one or several days after surgery (Fig. 6.23).

Based on the principle of maximizing benefits while minimizing risks—although the probability of choroidal hemorrhage caused by subretinal fluid drainage is low (approximately 10%)—this school emphasizes that it should be avoided whenever possible.

The Schepens school believes that subretinal fluid drainage enables more accurate sealing of the retinal break during surgery, results in more definitive scar formation, and does not require an excessively high buckle to seal the break. Especially in patients with relatively viscous subretinal fluid, drainage promotes complete retinal reattachment. Regarding potential complications, this school believes that the benefits significantly outweigh the risks. As long as proper surgical techniques are followed, the probability of complications such as choroidal hemorrhage remains low—there is no need to "abandon eating for fear of choking."

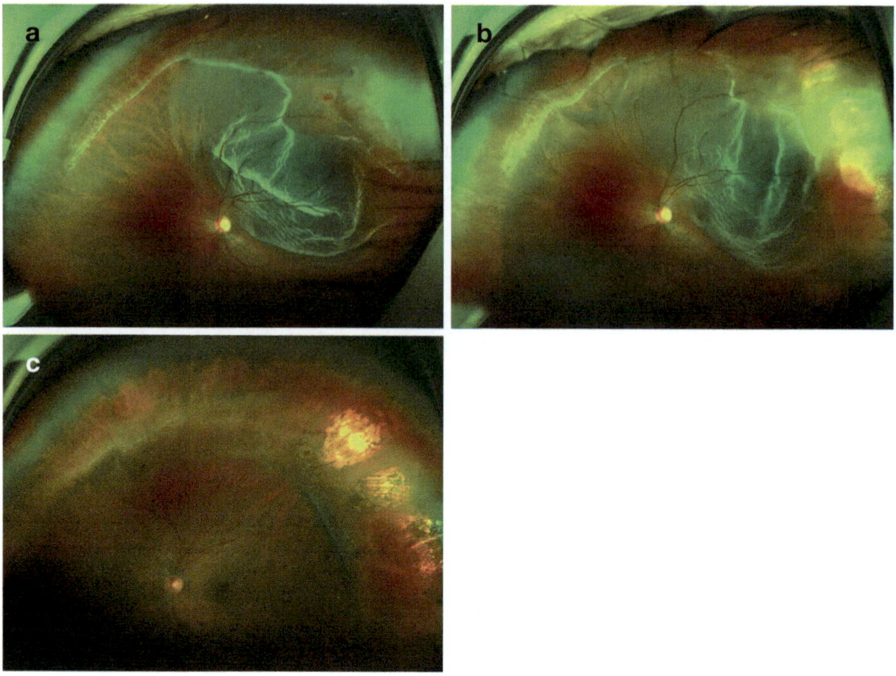

Fig. 6.23 Preoperative and postoperative fundus images of scleral buckling without subretinal fluid drainage. (**a**) Preoperative oval hole and multiple degenerative lesions in the superotemporal area; corrected visual acuity was 0.1. The patient was monocular, so it was ultimately decided not to perform subretinal fluid drainage. (**b**) Twelve hours after scleral buckling, subretinal fluid was partially absorbed; the silicone buckle was faintly visible, and the break was located above the buckle. (**c**) Half a month after surgery, the retina was completely attached, the break was fully apposed to the silicone buckle, and corrected visual acuity was 0.8

(2) Advantages and Disadvantages

1. Advantages of subretinal fluid drainage: (1) Directly reduces the volume of subretinal fluid, thereby enhancing its absorption; (2) Brings the retinal break into closer proximity with the underlying retinal pigment epithelium (RPE), thereby facilitating the effective application of cryotherapy; and (3) Lowers intraocular pressure, which can aid in the precise localization and effective sealing of small peripheral retinal breaks.
2. Disadvantages of subretinal fluid drainage: (1) Significant increase in the risk of choroidal hemorrhage, where small hemorrhages outside the macula generally resolve spontaneously, but severe hemorrhage can result in devastating visual loss and make secondary surgery extremely challenging (Fig. 6.24); (2) High risk associated with the drainage site selection, as drainage from areas with limited subretinal fluid or proximity to high-risk structures like vortex

veins remains hazardous regardless of surgical skill; (3) High incidence of complications secondary to a sudden drop in intraocular pressure, including globe collapse and choroidal detachment; (4) Potential for retinal perforation leading to iatrogenic breaks, though the incidence remains low; and (5) Risk of retinal incarceration or vitreous prolapse, which occurs with very low frequency.

(3) Selection of Draining Location

If the surgeon decides to perform subretinal fluid drainage, a 2-mL syringe needle may be used to puncture the sclera, or a sharp blade may be used for oblique puncture. When subretinal fluid is observed to flow out, a cotton swab or forceps can be used to gently depress the ocular wall to facilitate further fluid egress. If no fluid flows out after puncture, do not manipulate the incision significantly to avoid choroidal hemorrhage. Indirect ophthalmoscopy can be used to reassess the location of subretinal fluid elevation, and an alternative safe drainage site may be selected for puncture.

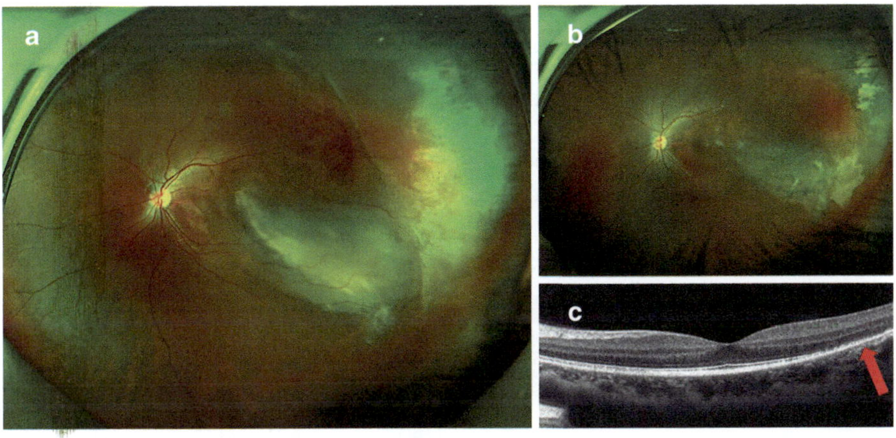

Fig. 6.24 Postoperative fundus images of choroidal hemorrhage during scleral buckling. (**a**) Intraoperative fundus examination revealed subretinal hemorrhage. The patient was immediately instructed to maintain a left lateral decubitus position after surgery. On the first postoperative day, fundus examination showed that the retina was essentially attached, the break was well sealed, and the hemorrhage was predominantly in the temporal area. As the hemorrhage did not significantly involve the macula, the patient's vision recovered well (corrected visual acuity 0.5), although the patient complained of a fixed black scotoma. (**b**) Fundus reexamination six months after surgery showed complete retinal attachment and complete resolution of the subretinal hemorrhage. Because a 6/0 absorbable suture was used to secure the silicone explant, the silicone buckle had completely disappeared after the suture degraded (corrected visual acuity 1.0). (**c**) OCT at six months postoperatively revealed an intact and continuous ellipsoid zone in the macular area, but the ellipsoid zone was absent in the slightly temporal region (red arrow), which was attributed to a toxic reaction caused by the subretinal hemorrhage

Regardless of the drainage method used, the following principles should be followed to select the optimal drainage site: (1) The drainage point must be located within the area of greatest subretinal fluid detachment; (2) Avoid the 3 o'clock and 9 o'clock positions to protect the long posterior ciliary arteries and long ciliary nerves; (3) Avoid the areas surrounding the vortex veins to minimize hemorrhagic risk; (4) The zones one clock hour above and below the medial and lateral rectus muscles are considered the safest for drainage (Fig. 6.25); (5) Maintain an appropriate distance from the limbus, as being too close results in low drainage efficiency while being too far increases the risk of choroidal hemorrhage—a distance of 10–12 mm from the limbus is generally preferable; and (6) Prioritize safety above all, and do not persist with the attempt if significant technical difficulties arise.

6.5.3 Scleral Encircling

For patients with extensive retinal degeneration—particularly adolescents with underlying conditions such as familial exudative vitreoretinopathy (FEVR) or Stickler syndrome—the risk of peripheral vitreous traction and contraction is relatively high. Scleral encircling may be considered in such cases (Fig. 6.26). Alternatively, peripheral retinal laser photocoagulation can be performed preoperatively or postoperatively to seal the degenerative areas and prevent the formation of new breaks.

The following points should be noted during fixation of the encircling band: (1) Ensure that the encircling band passes completely under the rectus muscles;

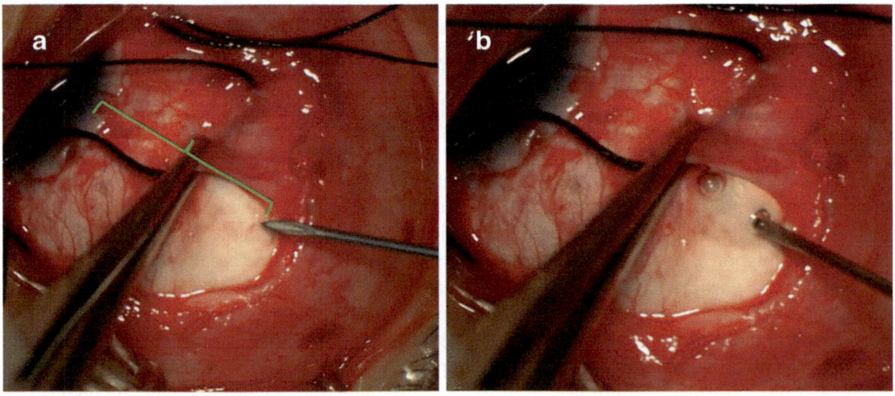

Fig. 6.25 Subretinal fluid drainage. (**a**) Puncture slightly above the lateral rectus muscle using oblique needle insertion; the chord length from the puncture site to the limbus is approximately 12 mm (green line). (**b**) Successful drainage of subretinal fluid: gently depress the scleral wound with the needle to facilitate further fluid egress; no significant bleeding is observed during the procedure

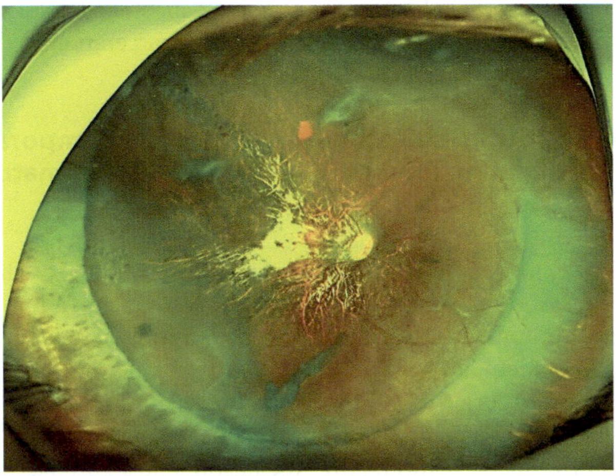

Fig. 6.26 Fundus image after scleral buckling. The patient underwent encircling with scleral buckling for retinal detachment in the right eye over 30 years ago (at age 20). The surgical ridge is well in position. No recurrent retinal detachment was observed during long-term follow-up. Subsequently, his daughter developed the same type of retinal detachment, and genetic testing confirmed that both were diagnosed with Stickler syndrome (COL2A1 gene mutation)

carefully verify that it does not compress any portion of the muscles; (2) Adjust the anteroposterior suture distance according to the position of the silicone explant to ensure that the encircling buckle remains parallel to the limbus; (3) Reasonably adjust the tightness of the encircling band based on the band's position and the axial length of the surgical eye. A mild scleral indentation is preferred; excessive tightening may cause axial elongation, adversely affecting anterior segment perfusion and potentially progressing myopia; (4) If intraocular pressure becomes excessively elevated, perform anterior chamber paracentesis promptly to maintain normal intraocular pressure.

6.5.4 Modified Methods in Scleral Buckling

In recent years, several modified scleral buckling techniques have emerged, including the following: (1) Using a 25G endoilluminator to visualize the break position, assess the degree of cryopexy, and verify the correct placement of the silicone buckle from an internal approach; (2) Using a 25G light fiber combined with an external scleral cryoprobe to localize and seal the break; (3) Internal buckling: incising the sclera beneath the break and injecting viscoelastic material into the subscleral space to create a temporary buckling ridge under the break (this method typically requires internal illumination). These modified techniques have enriched the scope of scleral buckling. However, because they involve entry into the vitreous cavity, attention must be paid to incision maintenance during surgery to prevent complications such as wound leakage and vitreous incarceration.

6.5.5 Modified Suturing Technique to Produce Temporary Scleral Buckling Effect for Noncomplex Rhegmatogenous Retinal Detachment

The modified buckling technique was proposed by the author (Zhang) in 2024. It uses both nonabsorbable and absorbable sutures to create a temporary scleral buckling effect for noncomplex rhegmatogenous retinal detachment. This technique provides an adequate buckling effect while inducing minimal permanent refractive changes. Figure 6.27 shows the main steps of this technique.

This technique offers a distinct advantage: it does not cause significant changes in axial length or refractive power. After the absorbable suture has been absorbed, the shape of the eyeball remains essentially unchanged (Fig. 6.28), and the risk of inducing or exacerbating anisometropia is relatively low. However, its long-term efficacy, safety, and optimal indications require further validation.

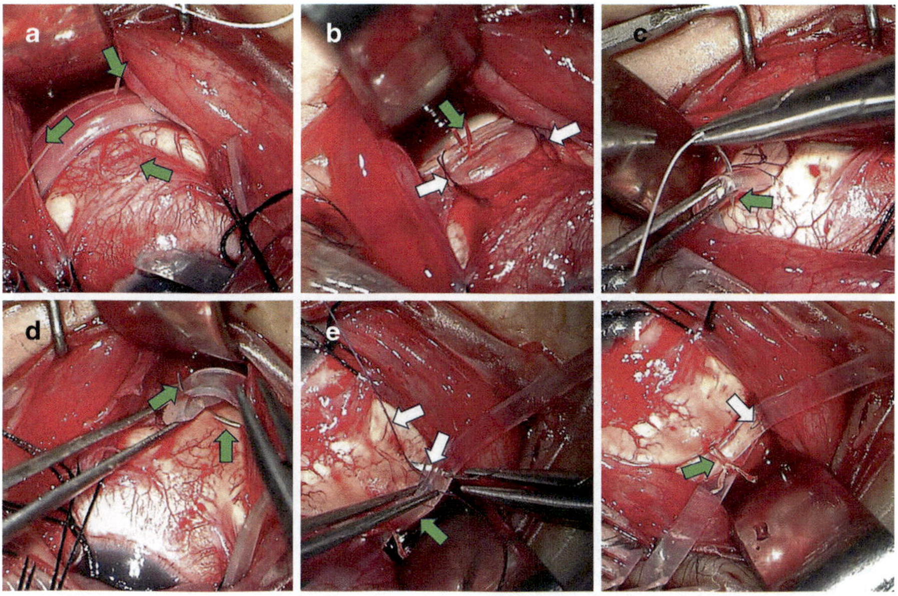

Fig. 6.27 Key steps of the technique using a combination of nonabsorbable and absorbable sutures to produce a temporary buckling effect. (**a**) The segmental silicone tire is fixed to the sclera with a 5-0 nonabsorbable suture (green arrow). (**b**) After the 5-0 nonabsorbable suture is tied (green arrow), 6-0 absorbable sutures are added to tighten the silicone tire and create a scleral ridge (white arrow). (**c**) One end of the silicone tire is fixed to the sclera with a 5-0 nonabsorbable suture (green arrow). (**d**) The other end of the silicone tire is fixed to the sclera with a 5-0 nonabsorbable suture (green arrow). (**e**) A silicone sleeve (green arrow) is used to hold the two ends of the encircling band, which are then tightened with a 6-0 absorbable suture. (**f**) After a 5-0 nonabsorbable suture is tied to secure the band in place (green arrow), the silicone sleeve is removed. The 6-0 absorbable suture then becomes the only element tightening the two ends of the band

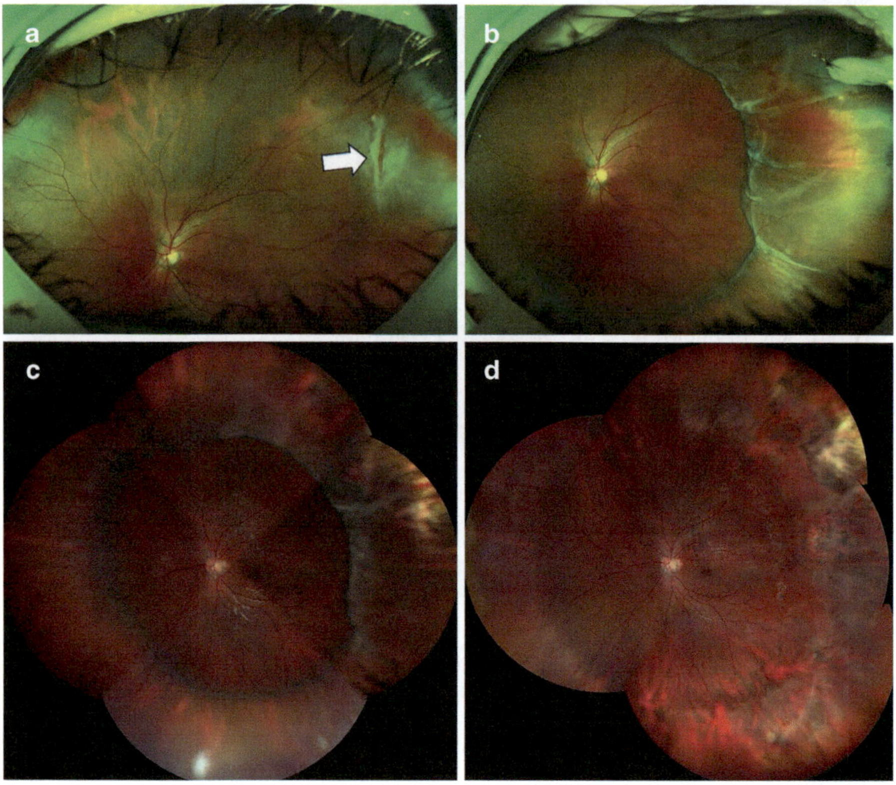

Fig. 6.28 Typical case who underwent the suturing technique with both segmental silicone tire and encircling band. (**a**) Before surgery, a retinal tear (white arrow) and superficial macula-off retinal detachment were observed, with an axial length 26.97 mm. (**b**) One day after the surgery, retinal reattached, with an obvious scleral ridge. (**c**) One month after surgery, the ridge was still present and in situ. (**d**) Three months after surgery, the retina remains attached, the scleral ridge is basically resolved, axial length 26.99 mm, corrected visual acuity 1.0

6.6 Postoperative Complications and Management of Scleral Buckling

Aside from choroidal hemorrhage, scleral buckling is generally safe when proper surgical techniques are followed; however, several postoperative issues still warrant close attention.

6.6.1 Persistent Subretinal Fluid

Subretinal fluid may persist for an extended period in certain patients, particularly in cases involving: (1) Adolescents; (2) Chronic retinal detachment; and (3) Situations where no drainage or insufficient drainage of subretinal fluid was performed. When persistent subretinal fluid is encountered, the peripheral retina must be carefully examined to confirm that the primary break is completely apposed to the buckle. If the break is well sealed and no additional breaks are identified, the subretinal fluid will typically resolve over time. Although this absorption process may be quite slow, the patient's visual acuity generally remains stable—as the trapped subretinal fluid can provide a relatively stable environment for neurosensory retinal metabolism—and no further intervention is required.

6.6.2 Recurrent Retinal Detachment

First, observe whether the primary break is well sealed, then determine the presence of missed or new breaks, and finally formulate a secondary surgical plan based on the clinical findings. Lincoff's Rules can be used to assess whether missed or new breaks are present.

If the primary break is located superiorly (between the 8:00 and 4:00 o'clock positions), intravitreal gas injection may be considered. Inject a small volume of filtered air or an inert gas (e.g., 0.2 mL of C_3F_8), combined with appropriate head positioning, to allow the gas bubble to seal the break and promote retinal apposition. This method is particularly suitable for "fish-mouth" breaks that remain unclosed.

If the buckle is improperly positioned, revision surgery may be performed to adjust the position of the silicone explant. However, due to the significant postoperative inflammatory response, attention should be paid to intraoperative analgesia and hemostasis (Fig. 6.29). If new breaks occur or PVR develops, an internal approach may be required to achieve retinal reattachment.

6.6.3 Elevated Intraocular Pressure

Most cases are temporary and spontaneously resolve. However, a few cases may be pathological, generally due to the following causes: (1) Anterior chamber shallowing caused by the explant (e.g., anterior displacement of the ciliary body); (2) Obstruction of the choroidal venous outflow pathway for aqueous humor; (3) Preexisting undiagnosed glaucoma, which may be exacerbated postoperatively; and (4) Pupillary block from various factors (e.g., extensive posterior iris synechiae). Persistent intraocular pressure elevation can lead to irreversible visual damage. If intraocular pressure remains uncontrolled despite appropriate measures such as mydriatics, anti-inflammatory agents, and ocular hypotensive medications, the patient should be promptly referred to the glaucoma service for further management.

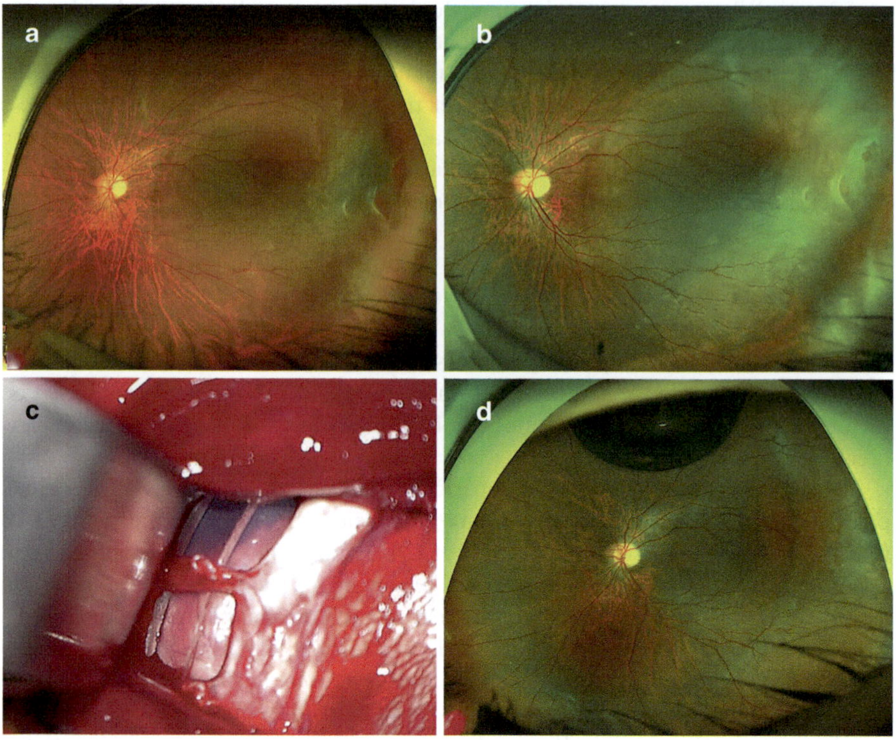

Fig. 6.29 Preoperative and postoperative images of secondary silicone explant adjustment. (**a**) Primary retinal break located in the temporal area of the left eye. (**b**) Fundus examination on the first day after scleral buckling surgery shows that the retina remains detached and the scleral buckle is malpositioned. (**c**) During revision surgery, after incising the conjunctiva, suture slippage is noted, and the groove of the silicone explant is not aligned. Re-suturing is performed, and approximately 0.5 mL of filtered air is injected. The patient is instructed to maintain a right lateral decubitus position for one day. (**d**) Fundus examination on the first postoperative day shows that the break is well sealed and the silicone buckle is properly positioned

6.6.4 Anterior Segment Ischemia

The incidence of this complication is extremely low. To prevent it, the rectus muscles should be handled with care during surgery, and the encircling band should not be excessively tightened. The main manifestations include a severe ischemic inflammatory response in the anterior chamber, such as corneal edema, anterior chamber flare, fibrous exudation, and even iris neovascularization, along with acute intraocular pressure elevation. Mild cases may be managed with systemic and topical glucocorticoids; however, the prognosis for severe cases is often poor. In such instances, the scleral explants should be removed promptly, and symptomatic treatment should be administered.

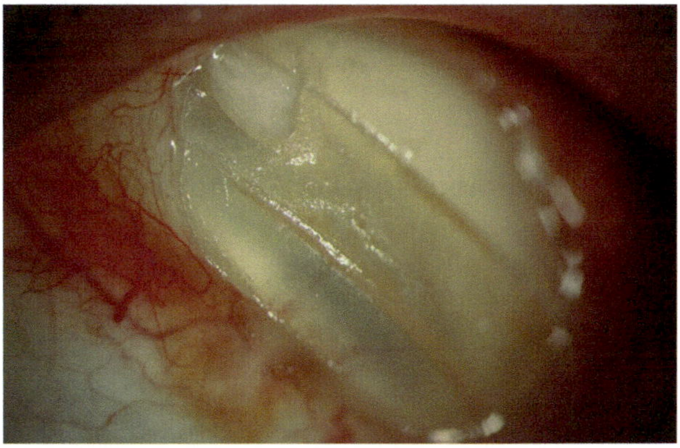

Fig. 6.30 Extrusion of the silicone tire and encircling band

6.6.5 Explant Displacement and Extrusion

If the explant penetrates the conjunctiva and becomes exposed (Fig. 6.30), the patient may complain of significant foreign body sensation, and some cases may present with concurrent ocular surface infection. Prompt removal of the implant is necessary. However, due to severe scarring and bleeding during removal, careful sharp dissection is required to maintain a clear surgical field and avoid damaging the extraocular muscles or the ocular wall.

6.6.6 Extraocular Muscle Dysfunction

This complication may manifest as abnormal ocular motility, strabismus, or diplopia; while these findings are typically transient, they may become permanent in a small number of cases. Possible causes include: (1) Severe iatrogenic injury to the extraocular muscles during surgery; (2) Extensive adhesions forming between the extraocular muscles, Tenon's capsule, and the sclera; and (3) Splitting or compression of the extraocular muscles by the explant. During surgery, meticulous attention must be paid to protecting the extraocular muscles, maintaining a clear surgical field, and strictly avoiding muscle damage during sharp dissection.

6.6.7 Refractive Changes

Postoperative refractive changes are a frequently criticized complication of scleral buckling, most commonly presenting as myopia progression. Some patients may develop irregular astigmatism. For patients with poor baseline visual acuity, such changes often do not cause significant discomfort. However, for patients with good baseline visual acuity, the resulting anisometropia may cause significant discomfort, affecting work and daily life. Preoperatively, the spherical refractive power of both eyes should be examined to determine whether scleral buckling will exacerbate the interocular refractive difference. Additionally, the external scleral explant should not be placed too anteriorly, and the encircling band should not be excessively tightened.

6.6.8 Common Issues of Retinal Detachment

Complications such as choroidal detachment, epiretinal membrane, macular edema, and PVR may occur. These should be managed with either observation or secondary surgery, depending on the cause and severity of the condition—this will not be elaborated further here.

6.7 Summary

"As a stone sharpens a blade, turning bluntness into sharpness." This chapter has provided a comprehensive overview of scleral buckling, covering its current status, foundational principles, indications, and key surgical maneuvers. We have navigated through the diverse schools of thought and the management of potential complications, all with the goal of helping the novice surgeon broaden both the depth and breadth of their professional knowledge. By mastering these fundamental techniques, you are not merely learning a procedure; you are sharpening your clinical intuition to identify the most effective surgical strategy for each unique patient. The true charm—and the persistent perplexity—of scleral buckling lies in its unpredictability. Despite our best planning and execution, the outcomes often surprise us, reminding us of the limits of our control.

Even today, no surgeon can assert with absolute certainty that the retina will be perfectly reattached by the first postoperative day. Furthermore, the biological mystery remains: no one can fully explain the subtle, invisible forces that compel the detached neurosensory retina and the retinal pigment epithelium to "embrace" each other so tightly once again. As you refine your skills, let this blend of scientific rigor and clinical wonder guide your growth in this intricate art.

Surgical Intervention of Rhegmatogenous Retinal Detachment: Part 2 (Pars Plana Vitrectomy)

7

For the treatment of rhegmatogenous retinal detachment (RRD), pars plana vitrectomy (PPV) has become the mainstream approach worldwide. In a narrow sense, PPV is often referred to as ab interno surgery, primarily to emphasize its fundamentally different approach from scleral buckling. Compared with scleral buckling, PPV follows a relatively fixed operative pattern. Intraocular illumination provides full, clear visualization of the vitreoretinal lesions. The coordinated use of various intraocular instruments enables direct and precise relief of vitreous traction on the retina, allowing complete closure of retinal breaks during the procedure. These advantages largely account for its widespread acceptance among retinal surgeons. This chapter will focus on introducing conventional surgical techniques for RRD treatment and will incorporate complex scenarios to explore the precautions and surgical skills essential for PPV.

7.1 Patient Selection for Vitrectomy

The vitreous of the human eye occupies most of the volume of the intraocular contents. Vitrectomy involves removing nearly all of this tissue, which is a fundamental difference from many other surgical subspecialties. The vitreous plays an important physiological role in the eye. We should not regard it as an insignificant "silent bystander", the decision to proceed with vitrectomy must be approached prudently.

"Und wenn du lange in einen Abgrund blickst, blickt der Abgrund auch in dich hinein (When you gaze long into an abyss, the abyss also gazes into you)." This metaphor is likely fitting here. If we treat the vitreous hastily, it may soon trouble us in return. In RRD surgery, extensive residual vitreous can lead to serious complications. Therefore, when considering whether to perform vitrectomy, we should first consider the purpose of vitreous removal, then the difficulty of the procedure, and finally the potential benefits and risks.

Z. Zhang, U. Spandau, *Vitreoretinal Surgery*,
https://doi.org/10.1007/978-3-032-25271-5_7

In the following RRD patients, PPV may be the preferred approach: (1) Extensive bullous retinal detachment; (2) Older age accompanied by posterior vitreous detachment (PVD) or significant vitreous liquefaction; (3) Obvious vitreoretinal traction; (4) Multiple retinal breaks involving different quadrants; (5) Pseudophakic eyes; (6) Presence of significant proliferative changes (PVR ≥ C1) (see Sect. 11.2 of Chap. 11 for grading); (7) Severe pre- and subretinal proliferative retinopathy; (8) Giant retinal tears (GRTs); (9) Macular hole retinal detachment (MH-RD); and (10) Coexistence of clinically significant vitreous hemorrhage.

The above relative indications generally align with one of the following three major principles: (1) The overall surgical difficulty and potential risk associated with achieving an adequate vitrectomy are relatively low; (2) The pathological changes within the vitreous are sufficiently severe to render its pathological impact greater than its physiological value; and (3) Vitrectomy stands as an unavoidable clinical measure for the effective management of complex retinal pathologies.

7.2 Why You Should Be Familiar with the Underlying Logic of Parameters Settings on Vitrectomy Machine

Using 23G and 25G vitrectomy platforms as examples, the main parameters and precautions are set as follows (Table 7.1). The surgeon should adjust them dynamically based on the specific intraoperative conditions.

Beginners must master the parameter settings for infusion, endoillumination, and vitrectomy, and deeply understand the underlying physical principles and design logic in order to adapt flexibly to special situations.

Table 7.1 Common parameter settings and precautions for vitrectomy

Item	Parameter	Details
Intravitreal perfusion	20~30 mmHg	(1) For children and patients with diabetic retinopathy, hypertension, and glaucoma, the perfusion pressure must be strictly controlled, and attention must be paid to the perfusion of the optic disc blood vessels throughout the process (2) Notice the hanging height of the liquid bottle and prevent additional intraocular pressure due to hanging too high (3) First, empty the air in the entire perfusion line before connecting to the infusion trocar (4) Prevent excessive curling and folding of the perfusion line
Vacuum	0~500 mmHg	(1) The vacuum level is typically set to increase linearly with foot-pedal depression depth (2) Maintaining a large vacuum difference makes it easier for beginners to adjust precisely through the pedaling depth

(continued)

Table 7.1 (continued)

Item	Parameter	Details
Cutting rate	5000~2500 cpm	(1) Under constant vacuum, vitrectomy with higher speed is safer to remove the peripheral vitreous (2) Under constant vacuum, vitrectomy with a relatively lower speed is more effective to remove the vitreous; the surgeon can adjust the vacuum level to shave the central vitreous but must be careful to avoid iatrogenic retinal breaks (3) Beginners can fix the speed at 5000 cpm. At this time, they only need to pay attention to controlling the vacuum, which will make things simpler for beginners
Endoilluminator	30%~40%	(1) Pay attention to the bulb life. The maximum illumination brightness of a newly replaced bulb is relatively high (when set to 100%). At this time, do not increase the illumination brightness at will to avoid retinal phototoxicity (2) Avoid direct exposure to the macular for a long time (3) If the bulb is aging, the parameters can be appropriately increased, but not arbitrarily increased to a higher level. The surgeon can first shine the light on himself to test the brightness. If there is a glare like the direct exposure of a car's high beam, the brightness must be reduced
Diathermy	10%~20%	(1) Should be prepared at all times, because if bleeding occurs during surgery, it must be stopped in time (2) The diathermy pen is a fragile accessory, so it can be checked before use and must be equipped with sufficient supplies (3) Always begin with the lowest energy setting

7.3 Fundamental Steps and Key Precautions

For noncomplext RRD surgery, as long as the surgeon strictly adheres to standard surgical protocols, the surgical success rate will be satisfactory. Anesthesia and trocar insertion techniques have been described in detail in previous chapters; therefore, this section will focus only on other basic steps.

7.3.1 Cutting Central Vitreous

First, insert the cutter and endoilluminator into the vitreous cavity. Hold the intraocular instruments firmly with both hands to avoid iatrogenic damage. Adjust the microscope (first focus, then magnification). The surgeon can simultaneously assess whether the vitreous adheres tightly to the underlying retina (i.e., whether a Weiss ring is present), thereby roughly predicting the difficulty and planning the following steps (e.g., whether to prepare triamcinolone acetonide for vitreous staining). First, insert the cutter and endoilluminator into the vitreous cavity.

7.3.2 Confirming or Creating Posterior Vitreous Detachment

In younger patients or those with high myopia, posterior vitreous detachment (PVD) is often deceptive. Triamcinolone acetonide (TA) can be used to repeatedly confirm the presence of PVD and to identify any residual vitreous.

7.3.3 Relieving Traction on Primary Retinal Breaks

After removing the central vitreous, the vitreous around the retinal breaks should be removed with the cutter while maintaining a high cutting rate and low vacuum. The vitreous between the anterior edge of the breaks and the ora serrata must be removed as completely as possible, as it is the most direct factor in the formation of retinal tears. This maneuver helps restore retinal mobility. If the breaks are located peripherally, the procedure must be performed under scleral indentation with bimanual instrument exchange; otherwise, lens injury is very likely (Fig. 7.1).

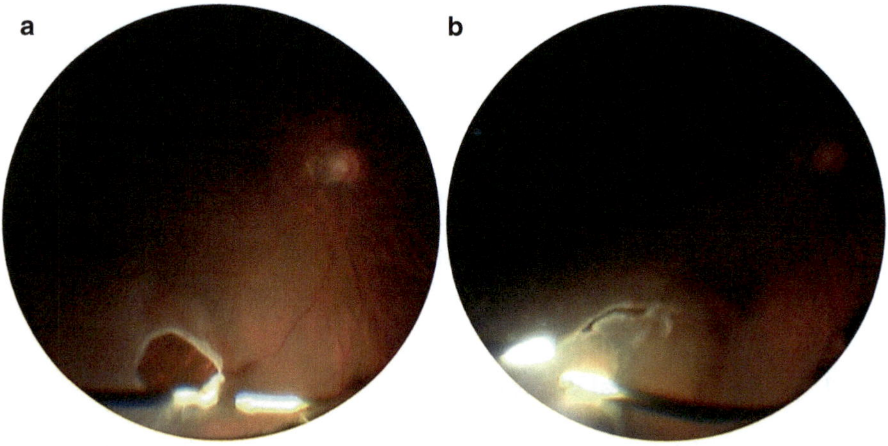

Fig. 7.1 Relieving vitreous traction on retinal flaps. (**a**) Without scleral indentation, the peripheral vitreous on the anterior flap of the tear could not be well visualized. (**b**) Under scleral indentation, the peripheral vitreous was well exposed to the surgeon

7.3.4 Examination of the Peripheral Retina (Generally Performed Simultaneously with Step 5)

We must apply a "zero-tolerance" principle to peripheral retinal abnormalities in order to maximize the long-term postoperative success rate. We recommend performing a 360° peripheral inspection with scleral indentation. For beginners, scleral indentation must be applied to 100% of retinal detachment cases.

"Snatching defeat from the jaws of victory." Why must we be so persistent? Because in vitrectomy, the tolerance for missed retinal degenerative areas or breaks is extremely low.

7.3.5 Removing Peripheral Vitreous

While exploring the peripheral retina, the "skirt" of peripheral vitreous can be removed simultaneously. This maximizes the restoration of retinal mobility and helps prevent traction and breaks caused by postoperative vitreous contraction (Fig. 7.2).

All efforts are not in vain; hardships temper one into success. The inferior vitreous deserves special attention: if not adequately removed, RPE cells dispersed into the vitreous cavity can accumulate there under gravity, eventually becoming a nidus for proliferation.

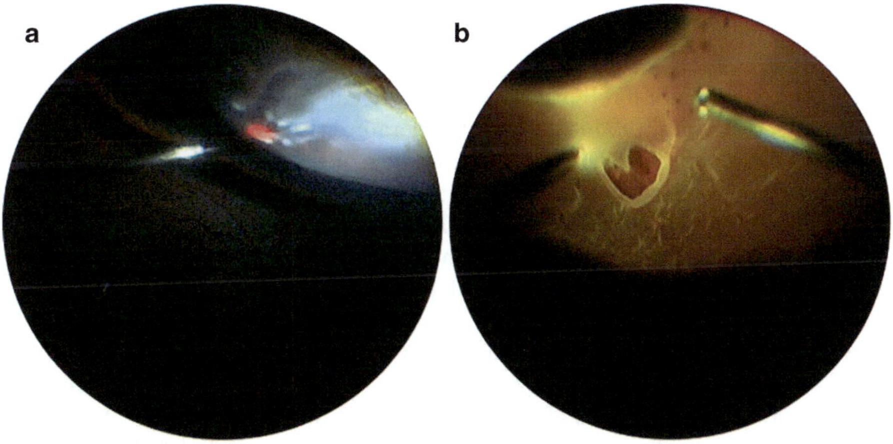

Fig. 7.2 Exploring peripheral retina under scleral indentation. (**a**) Identifying small inferior breaks and applying laser photocoagulation to the peripheral break. (**b**) Discovering multiple inferior RPE cell deposits

7.3.6 Reattaching the Retina

Since a detached retina cannot reattach spontaneously, external forces are required to reattach it. For beginners, this is the step where complications are most likely to occur during the entire procedure. The two most commonly used methods for retinal reattachment are fluid/air exchange and heavy liquid tamponading.

Before performing retinal reattachment, do not rush. First, patiently remove the vitreous and maximize retinal mobility. Strictly speaking, the retina is not "blown" back by air or "pressed" back by heavy liquid; these methods only "squeeze" subretinal fluid out through the breaks. Good retinal mobility is an important prerequisite.

With a wide-field surgical lens, retinal reattachment can generally be achieved through fluid/air exchange. A small amount of residual subretinal fluid at the posterior pole can be completely absorbed within a short period. In most cases, there is no need to inject heavy liquid or create a hole for subretinal draining. Beginners are prone to hesitation at this stage. As long as the retina is well attached with the underlying RPE, we can proceed to the next step without overdoing it.

7.3.7 Sealing Retinal Breaks

(1) Laser and Cryotherapy

Retinal laser photocoagulation is typically used to close breaks due to its precision and mild inflammatory response. Cryotherapy in PPV is rarely used today, but it remains highly effective—especially for small peripheral breaks that are difficult to fully expose.

(2) Role of Laser

Laser photocoagulation relies on the photothermal effect. When the target tissue absorbs intense light, the local tissue temperature rises sharply, denaturing proteins and inducing scar formation. Excessive laser energy causes photovaporization, leading to the evaporation of intracellular and extracellular water and potentially resulting in iatrogenic small retinal breaks. This should be avoided whenever possible. If it occurs, laser energy must be reduced immediately, and a small number of laser spots should be placed around the small breaks to seal them.

Substances in fundus tissues that absorb laser energy include: (1) Melanin, present in retinal pigment epithelium (RPE) cells and the choroid, which primarily absorbs wavelengths between 400 and 700 nm; (2) Lutein, concentrated in the macula, which protects photoreceptor cells by filtering short-wavelength light; and (3) Hemoglobin, whose laser absorption characteristics depend primarily on its oxygen saturation levels.

For laser closure of retinal breaks, two methods are generally employed: (1) The spot array method, in which laser spots are arranged in an orderly pattern around the break, spaced 0.5–1 spot diameter apart, and typically consisting of 3–5 consecutive rows (Fig. 7.3); and (2) The continuous method, in which laser spots are interconnected to form a linear chain that encircles the entire break, generally requiring only two rows. Beginners should strive for neatly placed laser spots, though absolute perfection is not required; this is akin to handwriting, where whether one uses regular script or cursive, the result is acceptable as long as the placement is accurate and the intention is clear.

Since hemoglobin absorbs laser energy, laser can also serve a hemostatic function. After fluid/air exchange, if a small amount of bleeding occurs at the break edge, laser photocoagulation can be used to achieve rapid hemostasis without electrocautery.

The time for a laser spot to mature is generally 5 days (which explains why PPV with filtered air tamponade has a high success rate for retinal detachment with superior breaks). As the laser spots mature, their diameters expand to approximately 1.5 times their original size.

(3) Laser Parameter Settings

Laser parameters for retinal photocoagulation primarily involve three adjustable settings: (1) Laser power, where starting at 100 mW is appropriate, with subsequent titration based on the clinical appearance of the laser spots; (2) Duration, with a standard range of 150–200 ms being appropriate; and (3) Interval, with 150–200 ms being appropriate. Beginners may benefit from setting a longer interval to allow

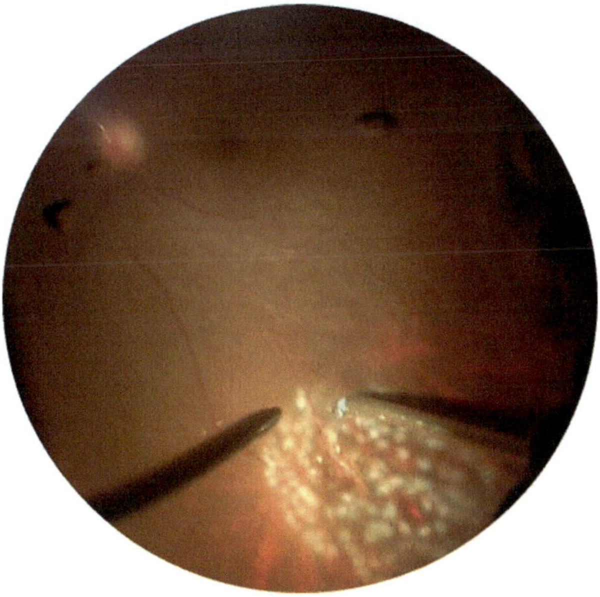

Fig. 7.3 Laser photocoagulation to seal retinal breaks

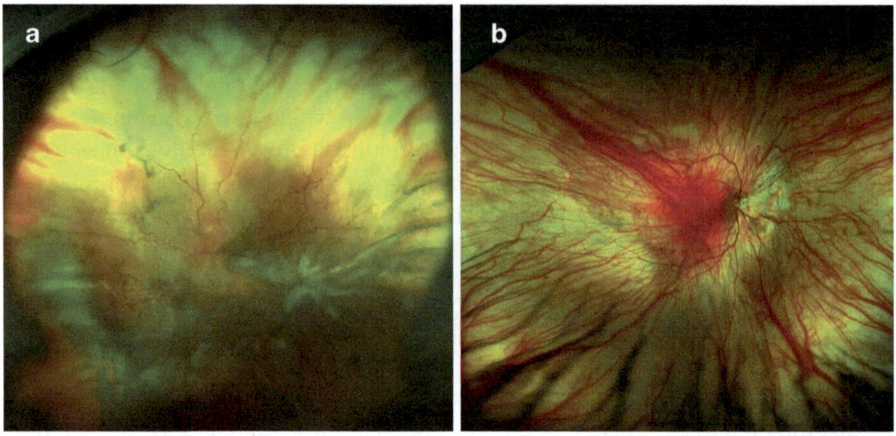

Fig. 7.4 Fundus of a patient with ocular albinism, in which the effect of retinal laser photocoagulation is often poor. (**a**) Retinal detachment with fixed folds in the left eye; no breaks were found. (**b**) Fundus photograph of the right eye

sufficient time for intraoperative reflection and judgment, thereby minimizing the risk of accidental tissue injury—particularly to the macula—caused by surgical anxiety.

The closure of retinal breaks relies primarily on the absorption of laser energy by melanin in the RPE layer. In cases of chronic retinal detachment with tissue edema, laser energy and duration may need to be appropriately increased to produce reliable laser spots. Additionally, in individuals with lighter RPE pigmentation—such as Caucasians and patients with ocular albinism (Fig. 7.4)—laser energy should also be increased accordingly.

7.3.8 Intraocular Tamponade Agents

Select the most suitable intraocular tamponade agents based on the location and size of the retinal breaks, as well as the severity of retinal detachment. Beginners often tend to use silicone oil, which is understandable. However, given the higher incidence of silicone oil-related complications and the need for secondary removal, the use of silicone oil should be gradually reduced. Filtered air also has a definite effect on superior breaks, but it is not particularly recommended for beginners because its volume dissipates quickly.

7.3.9 Adjusting Intraocular Pressure

. After injecting an intraocular tamponade agent, IOP must be carefully monitored, as fluctuations are common—for instance, hypertension is frequently associated with silicone oil, while hypotony is often seen with gas tamponade. IOP can be assessed using two practical methods: (1) Observing optic nerve head perfusion using a light guide fiber to ensure adequate vascular flow; and (2) Gently palpating the sclera with the pulp of the index finger to gauge firmness. If uncertain, the surgeon may palpate the patient's nose or forehead through the surgical drape for comparison; a scleral firmness similar to that of the nasal tip typically suggests a normal IOP range.

7.3.10 Closing Scleral Incisions and Advising the Patient to Maintain a Face-Down Position

To determine whether there is leakage from the scleral incisions, beginners are advised not to overlook the importance of suturing, even for self-sealing incisions. Suture if necessary; sutures can be removed one week postoperatively. In addition, it is important to check for incarceration of uveal tissue or vitreous at the incision sites. A cutter may be used to remove tissue exposed outside the incision. When suturing scleral incisions, the depth of needle insertion must be strictly controlled to avoid full-thickness penetration of the eyewall; otherwise, bacteria may be introduced into the vitreous cavity during postoperative suture removal, potentially causing infection.

Finally, if silicone oil or gas tamponade is used, the patient and their family should be instructed to maintain a face-down position postoperatively. Although some studies suggest that strict face-down positioning may not be necessary for detachments caused by superior breaks, the face-down position remains the most universal and easiest for patients to follow. For highly compliant patients, however, they can be individually instructed.

7.4 Details of Air/Fluid Exchange

7.4.1 Advantages and Disadvantages

The most direct benefit of air/fluid exchange to drain off subretinal fluid is that it maximally reduces the use of heavy liquid, which facilitates laser photocoagulation or cryotherapycryopexy. Additionally after air/fluid, the peripheral retina can be directly visualized without scleral indentation. However, in cases where clarity is poor, scleral indentation should be combined to achieve a thorough 360° inspection and treatment of peripheral abnormalities.

7.4.2 Key Points and Difficulties

For beginners, air/fluid exchange generally does not present great difficulty. The key points are adequate exposure of the breaks and proper use of the flute needle. The main difficulties include the following two aspects.

1. Decreased clarity of the surgical field. Due to the mixture of fluid and air, the refractive interface within the vitreous cavity is temporarily disrupted. However, as the proportion of gas increases, the blurring will resolve in a short time. This process is similar to an airplane passing through clouds during take-off and landing (Fig. 7.5). As long as surgical norms are strictly followed, the procedure is relatively safe, and the surgeon need not be overly nervous. For beginners, it is not recommended to aspirate subretinal fluid directly with a cutter, as this may accidentally engage the edge of the break, potentially enlarging the retinal break (Fig. 7.6). This is especially concerning when the break is located at the posterior pole, where such accidental aspiration may involve the macula and result in irreversible visual impairment.
2. Unskilled drainage technique. Either active drainage with a cutter or passive drainage with a flute needle may be used. However, due to the negative pressure at the instrument tip and the decreased clarity of the surgical field after air/fluid exchange, certain complications are more likely to occur, primarily including: (1) the tip easily aspirating the edge of the break, causing enlargement of the break; (2) the tip contacting the underlying RPE and choroid, leading to bleeding (Fig. 7.7); and (3) failure to adjust the eye position adequately to drain sufficient subretinal fluid.

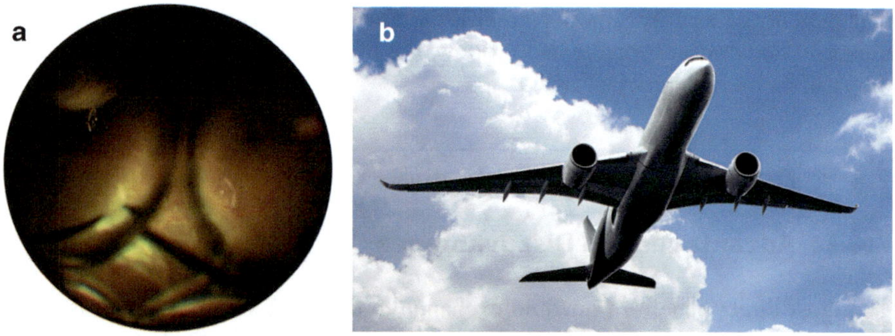

Fig. 7.5 Air/fluid exchange can temporarily reduce fundus visibility. (**a**) The entry of air bubbles reduces visibility in the vitreous cavity. (**b**) Schematic diagram of an airplane passing through clouds

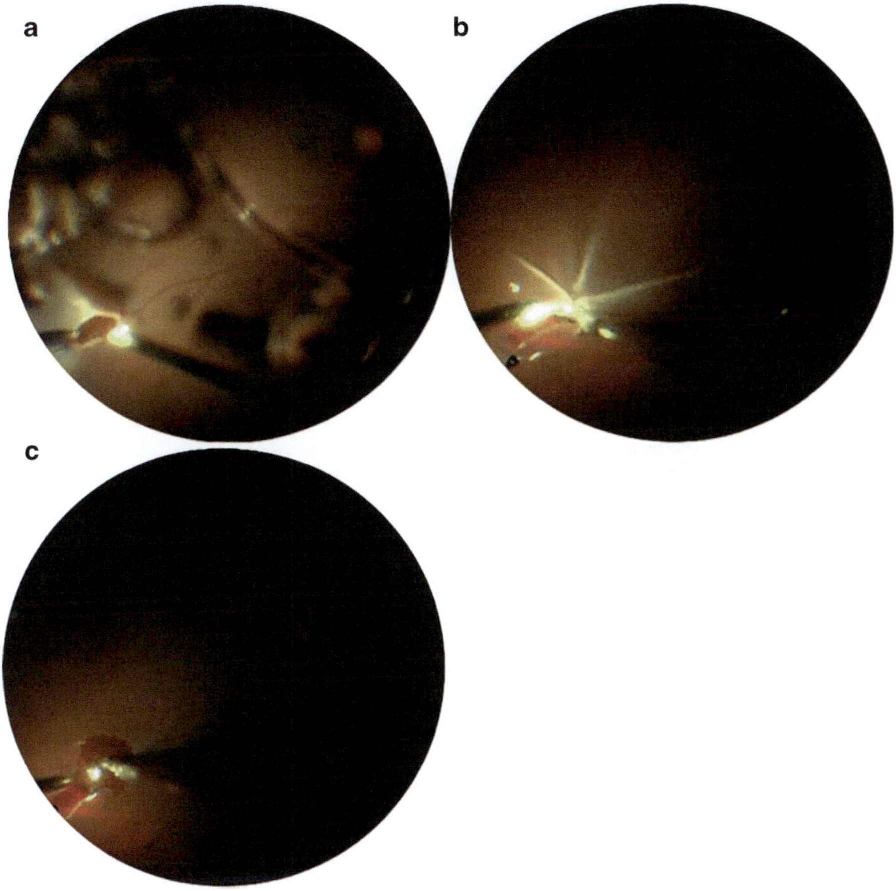

Fig. 7.6 Drainage of subretinal fluid with a cutter during air/fluid exchange. (**a**) Using a cutter to drain subretinal fluid from the primary break. (**b**) The retina at the posterior edge of the primary break is accidentally aspirated by the cutter. (**c**) The range of the retinal break is significantly enlarged

7.4.3 Application of Flute Needle

(1) Passive Aspiration

When using a flute needle to drain subretinal fluid via passive aspiration, the following two physical principles are primarily involved.

1. Siphon effect. When gas perfusion is turned on, the gas in the vitreous cavity exerts continuous downward pressure on the retina and the underlying fluid. At this time, the pressure at the inner opening of the flute needle (from the subretinal fluid) is higher than the atmospheric pressure at its outer opening. This pressure difference drives the fluid upward along the tube and out of the eye.

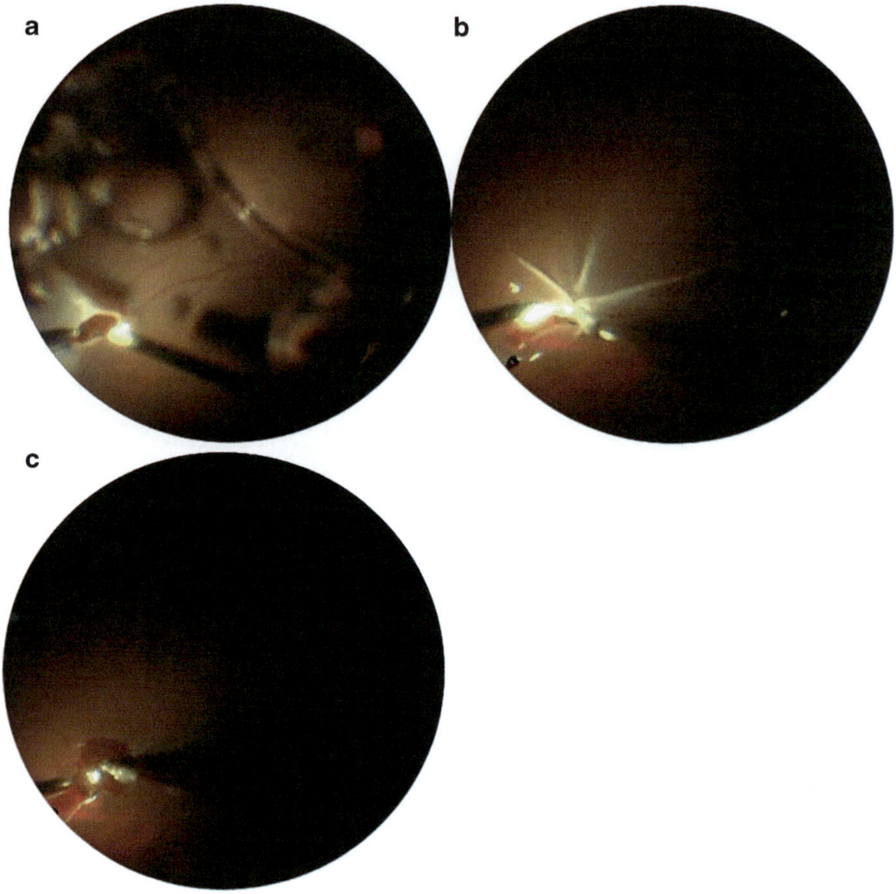

Fig. 7.7 Bleeding caused by the tip of the flute needle touching blood vessels when draining subretinal fluid

2. Capillary effect. This refers to the phenomenon in which liquid flows into a narrow tube or small gap without external force, driven by the adhesion between the liquid and the object, as well as the surface tension generated by cohesion among liquid molecules. This effect allows liquid to rise against gravity. When the tip of the flute needle contacts subretinal fluid, capillary action draws a small amount of fluid into the needle. Once this initial contact is established, the siphon effect (pressure gradient) takes over to evacuate the fluid from the eye.

Therefore, when using a flute needle to drain subretinal fluid through a relatively peripheral break, in order to ensure unobstructed and thorough drainage—in addition to using a sufficiently high gas perfusion pressure (usually 30–50 mmHg)—the tip should be kept within the fluid at all times (but not too deep, to avoid injuring the RPE layer), and the surgeon should strive to drain sufficient fluid "in one go."

(2) Active Aspiration

In addition to using a cutter, a flute needle can also be used for active aspiration of subretinal fluid. The proximal vacuum connector of the cutter can be unscrewed, and the flute needle can be connected to the vacuum. This method is efficient, but care must be taken to avoid accidental aspiration of the retina, which may enlarge the break.

7.4.4 Cooperation of Patient's Head Position and Eye Position

One of the great advantages of using a wide-angle lens in PPV is that, during air/fluid exchange, sufficient subretinal fluid can be drained by adjusting the patient's head and eye position without the need for heavy liquid tamponade. This is also an important reason for the significant reduction in the use of heavy liquid.

How to better adjust the patient's head position to assist subretinal fluid drainage can be accomplished through the following steps.

1. Determine the position of the break. If there are multiple breaks, select the retinal break closest to the posterior pole for drainage.
2. Adjust head position. Based on the position of the break to be drained, ask the patient to move their head toward the break's clock-hour position (or gently assist them). For example, if the break is located at the 6 o'clock position, ask the patient to tuck their chin or adjust the eye position downward using the upper two trocars as fulcrums (Fig. 7.8).
3. Adjust eye position. Using the upper two trocars as fulcrums, hold the light fiber and flute needle with each hand and gently push the eyeball toward the break's clock-hour position. This further helps drainage of the subretinal fluid.

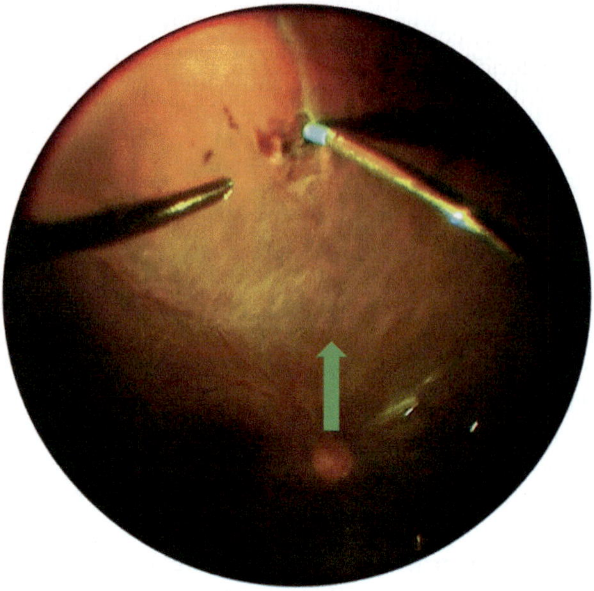

Fig. 7.8 The retinal break is located at the 6 o'clock position. The head and eye are directed downward (green arrow) to bring the break to the lowest position, thereby facilitating adequate aspiration of subretinal fluid

7.5 Systematic Approach to Prevent Inadvertent Perfusion in Eyes with Extensive Choroidal Detachment, Suprachoroidal Fluid, and Hypotony During Pars Plana Vitrectomy

Approximately 10% of RRD cases are complicated by extensive choroidal detachment. High-risk factors include older age, high myopia, long axial length, aphakia, pseudophakia, and low intraocular pressure. In these cases, surgical difficulty increases significantly, presenting an inevitable challenge for junior surgeons.

RRD with choroidal detachment is generally accompanied by suprachoroidal effusion and hypotony (Fig. 7.9). Anatomically, suprachoroidal effusion makes trocar insertion difficult. At the same time, hypotony renders the ocular wall soft, leading to difficulty positioning the inner opening of the trocar within the vitreous cavity. Moreover, when the inner opening of the trocar is surrounded by uveal tissue, fluid or gas infusion into the vitreous cavity becomes even more challenging (Fig. 7.10).

When dealing with these challenges, we must address three mutually reinforcing unfavorable factors: (1) Choroidal detachment; (2) Suprachoroidal effusion; and (3) Hypotony. These three factors are intricately interrelated and often form a vicious cycle. All appropriate surgical maneuvers must be centered on breaking this cycle, as the key to resolving these issues lies in the effective restoration and maintenance of stable intraocular pressure.

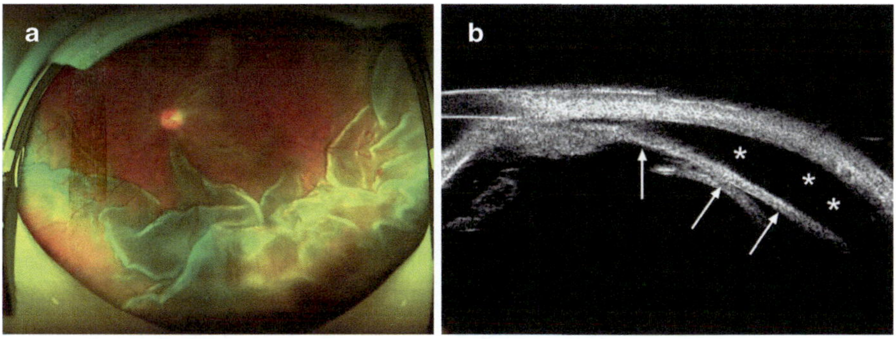

Fig. 7.9 Choroidal detachment and suprachoroidal effusion. (**a**) Wide-field fundus photography shows retinal detachment and choroidal detachment. (**b**) UBM shows suprachoroidal effusion (white asterisk) and ciliary epithelial detachment (white arrow)

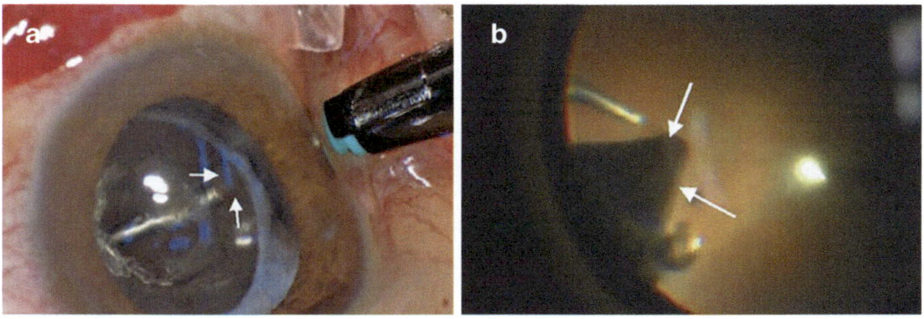

Fig. 7.10 The inner opening of the trocar is surrounded by the uveal tissue. (**a**) When inserting the trocar, the inner opening of the trocar is partially surrounded by the dark brown uveal tissue (white arrow). (**b**) The inner opening of the trocar is completely surrounded by the uvea (white arrow)

How can intraocular pressure be improved and maintained? The author (Zhang) has developed a step-by-step surgical approach that has been proven to be safe and efficient. It does not require additional scleral incisions for drainage of suprachoroidal effusion (please refer to the website for detailed demonstration: https://link.springer.com/article/10.1007/s12325-018-0801-2). This approach is briefly presented here for reference (Fig. 7.11).

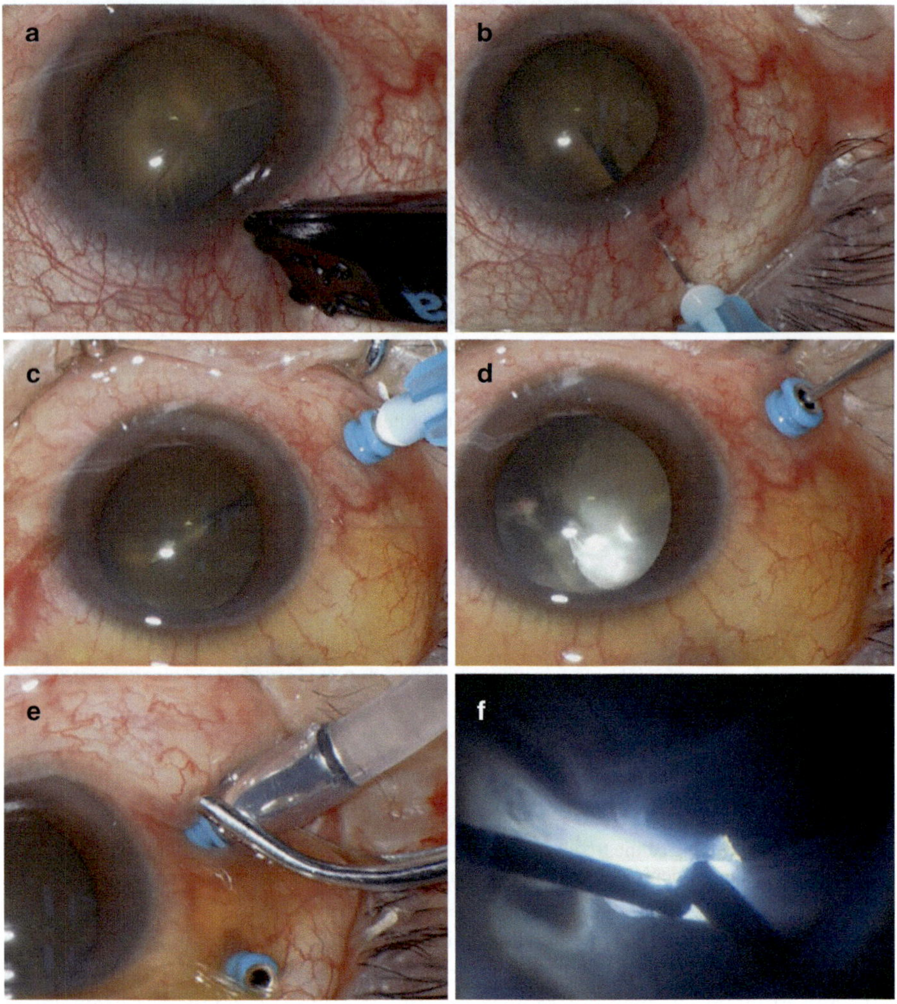

Fig. 7.11 Step-by-step surgical management of choroidal detachment complicated with suprachoroidal effusion (**a**) Measure the point 4 mm behind the limbus. (**b**) Injecting balanced salt solution 4 mm behind the limbus (transconjunctival intravitreal injection) to increase IOP. (**c**) Orange-yellow suprachoroidal fluid is observed overflowing passively into the subconjunctival space through the injection site. After inserting the inferotemporal trocar-cannula, a fine needle is used to continue injecting fluid into the vitreous cavity. (**d**) Inserting an endoillumination light pipe into the inferotemporal region to inspect whether the inner opening of the infusion cannula has been successfully created and to observe any surrounding condensed intraocular tissues. (**e**) The assistant uses curved forceps to create a centripetal indentation of the inferotemporal infusion cannula. (**f**) With endoillumination, using a vitrectomy probe to carefully peel off the uveal tissue covering the inner opening of the infusion cannula and to remove the peripheral dense vitreous. After confirming that the inner opening of the infusion cannula has completely entered the vitreous cavity, the fluid infusion is turned on

7.6 Etiology and Surgical Treatment of Giant Retinal Tear

7.6.1 Pathological Basis

Giant retinal tear (GRT) refers to a special type of retinal break spanning more than 3 clock hours (one quadrant). Although some breaks in rhegmatogenous retinal detachment may also exceed 3 clock hours, most of them present as U-shaped tears. Strictly speaking, such cases should not be classified as GRT but rather as typical retinal tears, because their pathological basis is quite different from that of GRT.

Its pathological basis is that the posterior vitreous has undergone extensive liquefaction, while the adhesion between the peripheral vitreous and the retina remains relatively tight. The shrinkage of the peripheral vitreous generates a broad area of centripetal traction, whereas the posterior vitreous cannot provide stable support for the corresponding retinal area. This imbalance of forces leads to extensive tearing of the peripheral retina (Fig. 7.12).

7.6.2 Surgical Principles

The use of heavy liquid has significantly reduced the treatment difficulty of GRT, but beginners must still understand its pathological basis and formulate a rational surgical strategy. The following four key points should be emphasized.

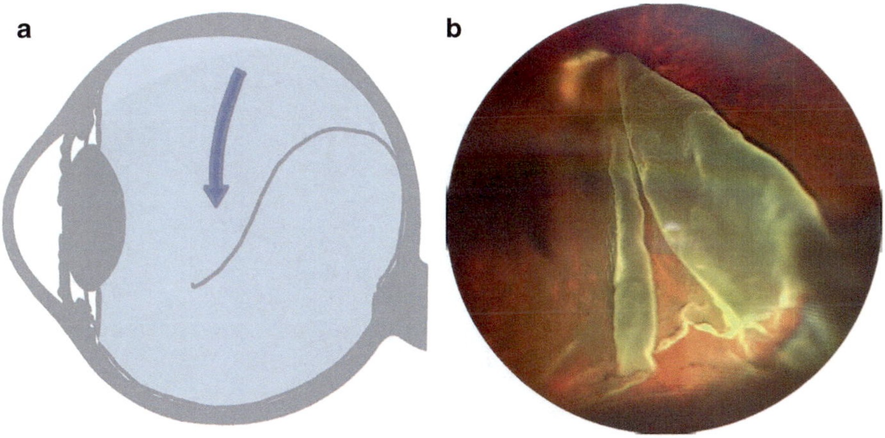

Fig. 7.12 Schematic diagram of giant retinal tear. (**a**) Liquefaction of the posterior pole and shrinkage of the peripheral vitreous cause extensive traction on the peripheral part. (**b**) Fundus image of a giant retinal tear

1. Low difficulty in removing posterior vitreous. Due to extensive liquefaction of the posterior vitreous, PVD may already be present preoperatively, and inducing PVD is relatively easy. However, because patients with GRT are generally young, TA is recommended to confirm that no residual vitreous at the posterior pole.
2. High difficulty in removing peripheral vitreous. The peripheral vitreous is dense and exerts significant traction on the anterior edge of the break. Complete removal is challenging, and residual vitreous as well as iatrogenic breaks are common risks. Even with a wide-angle lens, 360° vitrectomy must be performed with the aid of scleral indentation.
3. Relieving the edge of the break is the key to the operation. The pathological basis of GRT is an imbalance of vitreous forces, and this imbalance is most severe at the edge of the break. The vitreous here is the densest and most tightly adherent (Fig. 7.13). Therefore, it must be completely removed to achieve full retinal reattachment. However, because this area is located peripherally, exposure is difficult. Good assistant cooperation and the use of high-speed, low-negative-pressure vitrectomy are essential to avoid iatrogenic breaks.
4. Repositioning the retinal flap is the challenge. If heavy liquid is drained via air/fluid exchange, the pressure gradient decreases from the periphery to the posterior pole, making the posterior edge of the GRT prone to curling and slippage. If silicone oil is then injected, the surgical difficulty increases greatly and the postoperative outcome is significantly compromised (Fig. 7.14). Therefore, if silicone oil tamponade is selected, oil/fluid exchange technique is still recommended.

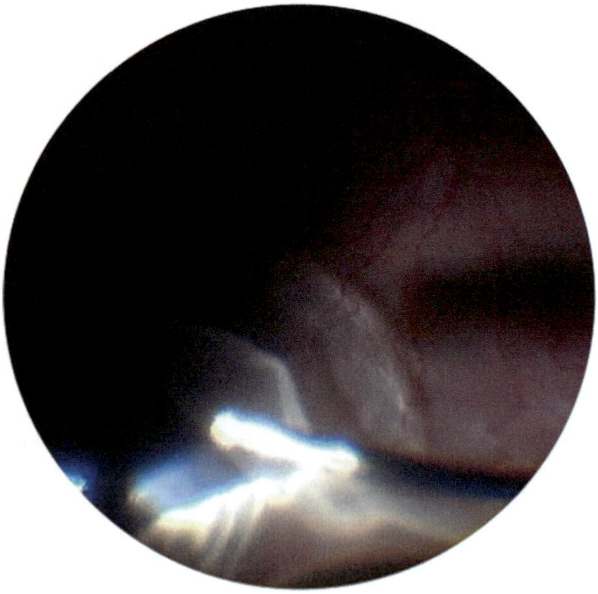

Fig. 7.13 Removing dense vitreous at the corner of the GRT under scleral indentation

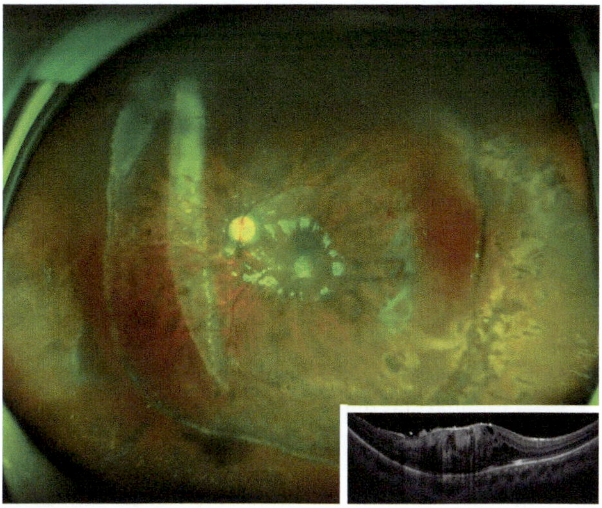

Fig. 7.14 After surgery for GRT, the retinal flap curls and slips, and OCT also indicates epimacular membrane and edema (inside the white border)

7.6.3 Surgical Strategies

Due to the rapid onset and progression of GRT, once the macula becomes involved, visual acuity drops sharply to hand motions. Many patients seek medical attention promptly. The surgical strategy for GRT is primarily determined by the severity of PVR, with grade C1 serving as the cutoff.

(1) PVR < C1 (See Sect. 11.2 of Chap. 11 for Grading)

For GRT without obvious PVR, the surgical principles are essentially the same as described above, with the main difference being the choice of tamponade agents.

The author (Zhang) often use PPV with short-term tamponade of heavy liquid to treat GRT without obvious PVR, with satisfactory surgical outcomes (Fig. 7.15). The surgical strategy primarily involves the following key objectives: (1) Relieving peripheral vitreous traction to ensure retinal stability; (2) Preventing heavy liquid from inadvertently entering the subretinal space during injection; and (3) Maintaining strict postoperative positioning and administering comprehensive anti-inflammatory treatment. Especially for superior GRT, the head should be slightly tilted back after surgery (Fig. 7.16). 7–10 days after the primary surgery, remove the heavy water. If the retina is well reattached, there is no need to tamponade with gas or silicone oil. Please refer to the website for detailed demonstration of the surgical approach: https://link.springer.com/article/10.1007/s10792-017-0613-4.

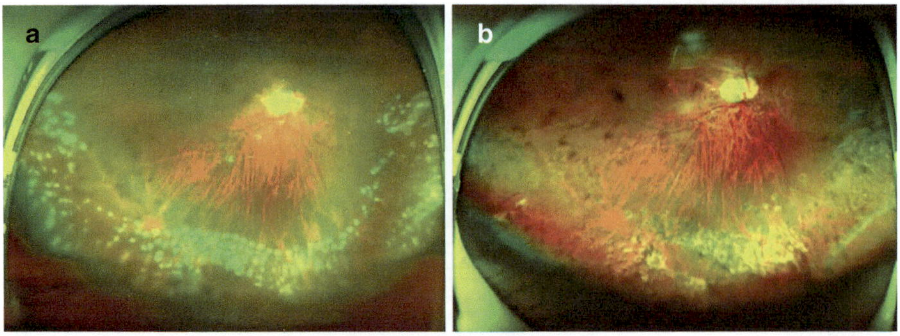

Fig. 7.15 Postoperative fundus images of giant retinal tear. (**a**) Fundus photography on the first day after heavy liquid tamponade. (**b**) Fundus photography 1 month after heavy liquid removal

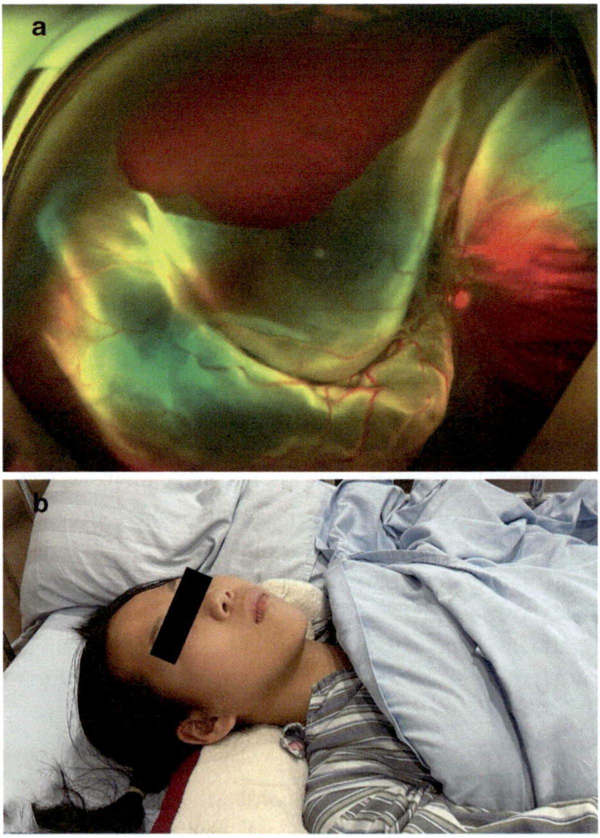

Fig. 7.16 Preoperative fundus image and postoperative head positioning for GRT. (**a**) Preoperatively, a retinal tear spanning approximately 120°. (**b**) After heavy liquid tamponade, the patient is instructed to maintain a supine position with the head slightly tilted back, as the break is located in the superior retina

(2) PVR ≥ C1

Silicone oil tamponade is generally selected, and the surgical principles are the same as described above. The main surgical challenge is to prevent curling and slippage of the posterior edge of the tear. Air/fluid exchange is generally not recommended; instead, oil/fluid exchange is preferred, as it better prevents curling and slippage of the posterior edge. Some patients may additionally undergo scleral encircling.

Although it is relatively challenging for beginners to finish a GRT surgery, the complications are preventable and controllable. As long as the pathological basis is well understood and the principles of heavy liquid use are followed, good outcomes can usually be achieved.

7.7 Surgical Treatment of Retinal Detachment Secondary to or Concomitant with Macular Hole

Retinal detachment complicated by macular hole (MH-RD) is a complex form of RRD. Retinal detachment with the macular hole as the primary break occurs predominantly in patients with high myopia. Some macular holes are secondary, mainly appearing in patients with RRD who have marked vitreous liquefaction, high retinal elevation, and a relatively long disease duration.

If the retinal detachment is extensive and highly elevated, or if the macular hole is small in diameter, OCT may sometimes fail to detect a clear macular hole. Preoperative examination should be carefully performed, especially when scleral buckling is planned, to thoroughly rule out the presence of a macular hole.

MH-RD is characterized primarily by the following two features: (1) The detachment is centered on the macula, with the superior retina typically remaining attached or exhibiting less detachment compared to the inferior retina; and (2) The detachment pattern does not follow Lincoff's rules, potentially manifesting as a shallow macular detachment or being complicated by concomitant choroidal detachment, where the inferior detachment shows symmetrical elevation on both sides without a distinct lateral slope (Fig. 7.17).

For MH-RD secondary to high myopia, the three most significant surgical challenges are: (1) Long axial length, which complicates maneuvers at the posterior pole due to the increased working distance; (2) Residual vitreous cortex that is easily overlooked, necessitating careful staining and removal; and (3) Tight adhesion of the peripheral vitreous, which makes thorough vitrectomy challenging and increases the risk of iatrogenic retinal breaks.

To address these issues, the following surgical strategies may be adopted:

Complete removal of posterior vitreous. Double staining with TA and indocyanine green (ICG) can be used. TA stains only the vitreous, whereas ICG stains the internal limiting membrane (ILM). If the ILM cannot be stained by ICG, it indicates that the ILM is still covered by residual vitreous. Intraocular forceps can be used to lift a flap from the stained area and expand the peeling range, which often allows simultaneous peeling of the ILM and residual vitreous.

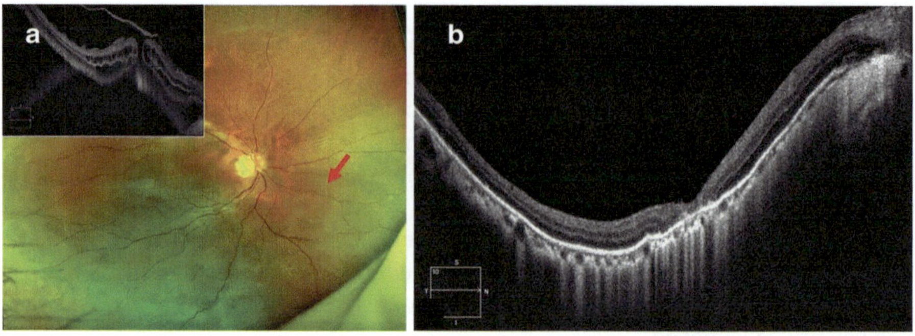

Fig. 7.17 High myopia with MH-RD (**a**) Shallow detachment of the macula and inferior retina. No obvious break is visible in the macula on fundus photography, but OCT reveals a small macular hole. Due to its small diameter, a retinotomy was created at the site indicated by the red arrow during surgery to drain subretinal fluid. (**b**) Postoperative OCT confirms retinal reattachment and closure of the macular hole

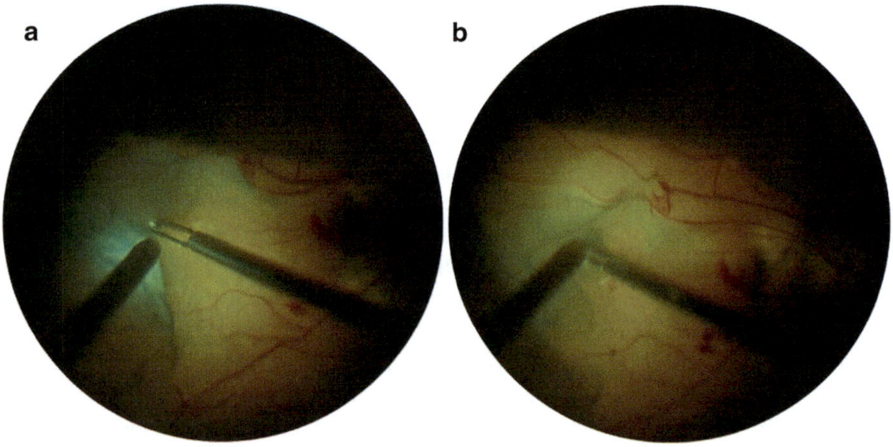

Fig. 7.18 ILM peeling for high myopia with MH-RD. (**a**) Flap creation using the "end-grasping" technique. (**b**) Expanding the peeling range from the edge of the ILM flap

Strategic peeling of the ILM. Flap lifting is the key, and surgery under heavy liquid tamponade is generally not recommended. Because the posterior retina elevated with edema, the forceps can easily reach the retinal plane without causing iatrogenic breaks. The surgeon lifts the flap with the distal end of the forceps near the vascular arcade. Due to the high mobility of the underlying retina, the surgeon may appropriately increase the grasping force. Once the flap is successfully lifted, the peeling range can be easily expanded. The key to the procedure is "end-grasping" of the ILM with the forceps (Fig. 7.18).

"Persistently" removing peripheral vitreous: Under TA staining, identify the edge of the peripheral vitreous. Use a vitrectomy probe (with high cutting rate and low vacuum) to begin the shaving. Iatrogenic breaks in the inferior quadrant should be avoided as much as possible, because silicone oil tamponade provides poor sealing effect for inferior breaks.

Selecting the appropriate subretinal fluid drainage method: Fluid/air exchange is generally preferred. If the macular hole is large, drainage can be performed directly through the hole. However, if the hole is small, direct drainage may be difficult and could enlarge the hole. In such cases, a drainage retinotomy can be created in the mid-peripheral detached retina. The retinotomy should preferably be located in the superior quadrant; if the superior retina is not detached, choose a location where silicone oil can effectively tamponade postoperatively.

Adequate drainage of subretinal fluid around the macular hole: Before injecting silicone oil, subretinal fluid in the macular area should be completely drained off, leaving the hole in a "dry" state. Silicone oil should then be injected quickly to cover the macular hole, preventing reaccumulation of fluid at the posterior pole. This strategy can improve the success rate and help avoid recurrent detachment of the hole.

Preventing pupillary block: Some patients are prone to pupillary block after surgery, and even silicone oil migration into the anterior chamber. Close observation and timely treatment are required. In pseudophakic eyes, an inferior Ando iridectomy can be created during surgery for.

If the macular hole remains in a flat-open state after surgery, the probability of retinal re-detachment following silicone oil removal increases. For patients with a large macular hole (Fig. 7.19), an inverted ILM flap can be used to cover the macular hole (Fig. 7.20).

Finally, it should be noted that if the retina is completely reattached after surgery but the macular hole is not closed (flat-open state), some patients will have symptoms of central scotoma. However, this should not be considered a surgical failure, and explanations should be provided to the patient before and after surgery.

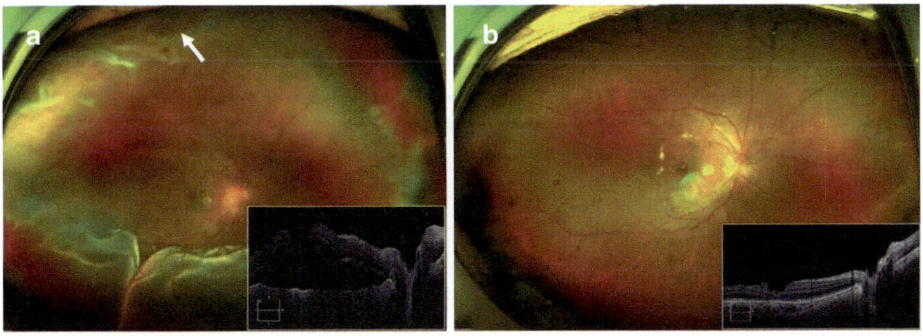

Fig. 7.19 Preoperative and postoperative fundus images of MH-RD. (**a**) Preoperatively, retinal detachment is visible, with the primary retinal break located in the superior peripheral area (white arrow), and OCT shows a macular hole. (**b**) In the postoperative silicone oil tamponade state, the retina is flat and the hole is closed

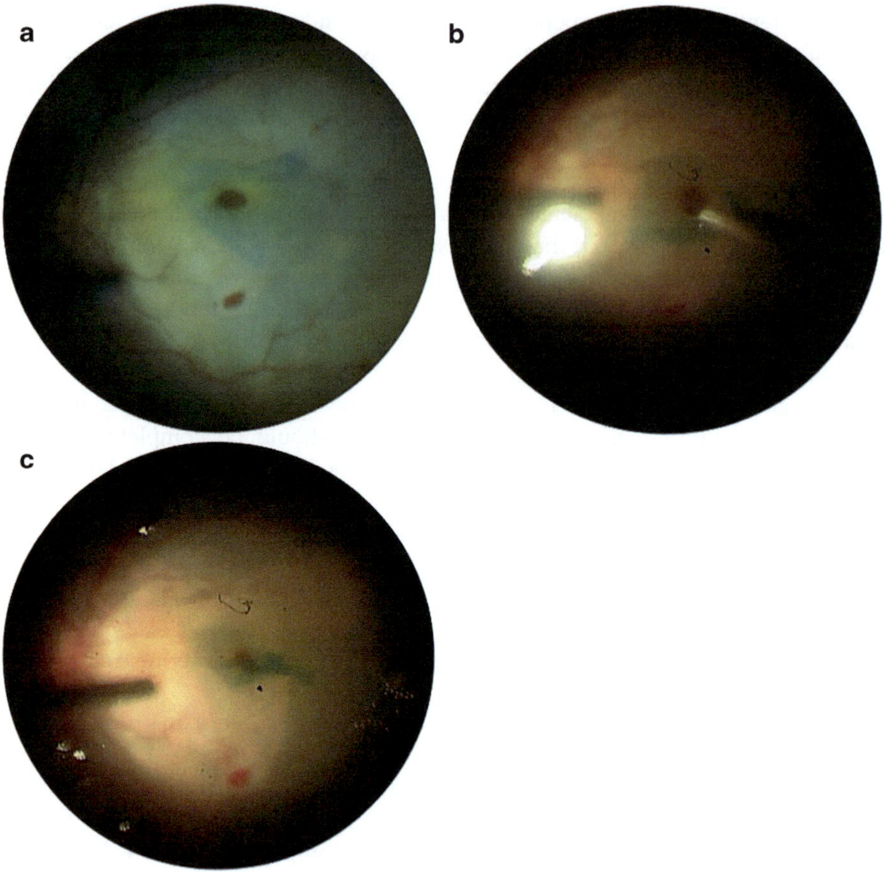

Fig. 7.20 Inverted ILM flap to cover MH in MH-RD. (**a**) After ILM staining, first lift a flap from a position far from the macula to create a wide-based and large ILM flap. (**b**) Before draining subretinal fluid from the macular hole through air/fluid exchange, gently flatten the ILM flap to its original position to avoid damage and aspiration by the flute needle. (**c**) When the macular hole is completely "dry," use intraocular forceps to cover the macular hole with the ILM flap, followed by immediate silicone oil injection

7.8 How to Modify the Surgical Approach When Primary Break(s) Cannot Be Found

Approximately 5% of patients with RRD, especially young pseudophakic patients, have no identifiable primary retinal break either preoperatively or intraoperatively. In such cases, exudative causes should first be ruled out, and a surgical strategy should be formulated based on the vitreous status. The following steps can be taken:

Rule out macular hole. If PVR is severe or the posterior pole detachment is high, a macular hole may be masked.

Infer break location using Lincoff's rule. As long as a primary break exists, the morphology of retinal detachment will follow Lincoff's rule, which can be used to estimate the approximate break location.

Formulate a surgical plan based on vitreous status. Scleral buckling should not be overlooked. If the vitreous is relatively clear and the patient is young, the break location can be inferred using Lincoff's rule, and scleral buckling can be attempted first. This approach has inherent advantages, particularly for inferior retinal detachment, and can often avoid internal surgery.

Select a good position to create a retinal break for subretinal fluid drainage. An incision should be made at a slightly superior and posterior location within the detached area for drainage. The tip of a flute needle can be used to aspirate intermittently and repeatedly to create a small break. Subretinal fluid can then be drained via air/fluid exchange. Laser photocoagulation should be applied to the peripheral retina, as there may be tiny breaks.

If the retinal mobility is good, long-acting gas tamponade is sufficient, and silicone oil can be used in a few cases. If the inferior retinal mobility is poor, auxiliary scleral buckling can be performed.

7.9 Additional Steps to Ensure Possibly Higher Long-Term Reattachment Rate

Although the long-term (>6 months) anatomical success rate of noncomplex RRD has exceeded 90%, maximizing the long-term prognosis is still the constant goal of all retina surgeons. We mainly try to improve the long-term healing rate of RRD through two methods:

7.9.1 360° Laser Encircling

There remains considerable controversy regarding the necessity and effectiveness of this technique. After closing all primary breaks, if the ora serrata is visible under a wide-angle lens, two to three rows of laser photocoagulation may be applied to the peripheral retina near the ora serrata without scleral indentation. This may benefit patients with high myopia, weak ora serrata, or multiple peripheral degenerative areas (Fig. 7.21).

7.9.2 Scleral Buckling

In fact, the use of adjunctive scleral buckling for routine RRD is gradually decreasing. However, it still plays a positive role in retinal detachment with multiple primary breaks in the inferior quadrant. Numerous clinical studies have shown that adjunctive scleral buckling can improve the surgical success rate of RRD, and therefore beginners should not overlook its importance (Fig. 7.22). Adjunctive scleral buckling may be performed either before or after PPV. If gas tamponade is planned postoperatively, it is recommended to perform buckling before; if silicone oil tamponade is planned, buckling should be performed after.

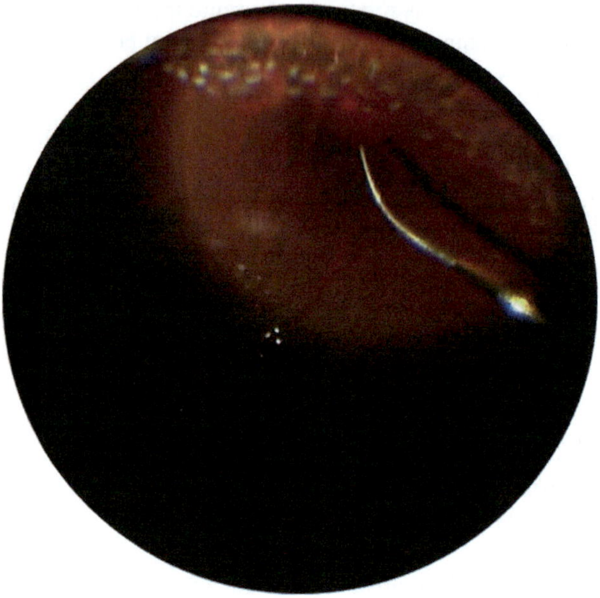

Fig. 7.21 Laser encircling. Beginners performing 360° laser encircling should pay attention to the following details: (1) Protect the lens; (2) Strictly control the total amount of laser. (3) Avoid creating laser-induced breaks

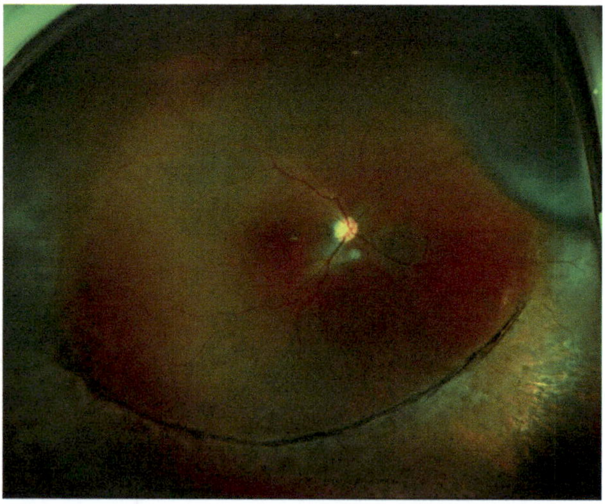

Fig. 7.22 Postoperative fundus photograph of a patient with retinal detachment due to inferior breaks. PPV with silicone oil tamponade and scleral encircling was performed to improve surgical success

7.10 Surgical Complications and the Management

Surgery-related complications (e.g., elevated IOP, cataract, PVR) are consistent with those of PPV and intraocular tamponade agents. Their prevention and management are discussed in the relevant chapters and will not be repeated here.

7.11 Summary

"True caution is watching for the smallest flaw; true wisdom is mastering the grand scheme." Mastering PPV for the treatment of RRD is a definitive milestone for every retina surgeon. This procedure serves as an exceptional training ground for beginners, as it demands a delicate balance between microscopic precision and global intraocular awareness. While meticulous attention to the smallest detail—such as identifying subtle peripheral breaks or ensuring the complete removal of vitreous base—is crucial to prevent recurrence, one must never lose sight of the "grand scheme."

The learning curve of RRD surgery is steep, often oscillating between the technical rigor of maneuvers and the psychological pressure of managing unexpected intraoperative changes. However, by formulating a cohesive and logical surgical plan grounded in the underlying physics of the eye, a surgeon can transcend mere technical repetition. This strategic depth allows even a novice to navigate the complexities of the procedure with composure and foresight, transforming a series of challenging steps into a controlled, goal-oriented journey toward anatomical and functional restoration.

8 Surgical Management of Diabetic Retinopathy

Preventing and managing proliferative diabetic retinopathy (PDR) remains a complex and demanding challenge. Among all treatment modalities, surgery is the most technically demanding, particularly for novice surgeons. However, the advent of minimally invasive vitreoretinal surgery (MIVS) and the intraocular application of anti-vascular endothelial growth factor (anti-VEGF) agents have revolutionized PDR management. These advancements have significantly reduced surgical complexity by protecting healthy retinal tissue from iatrogenic trauma and minimizing the risk of intraoperative hemorrhage.

While surgical outcomes are inherently tied to disease severity, three other critical factors are paramount: first, precise perioperative assessment, which draws heavily on clinical experience; second, proficient surgical skills, cultivated through rigorous and consistent training; and third, reliable equipment, which serves as the foundation for optimizing surgical expertise. Although MIVS has significantly advanced PDR surgery, the rapidly evolving concepts and techniques can be overwhelming for beginners. This chapter provides a comprehensive guide, starting with the anatomical pathology of PDR and focusing on strategic surgical planning and essential operative techniques.

8.1 Underlying Logic for Surgeons to Better Understand Surgical Techniques

Successful surgical management of PDR requires exceptional spatial awareness to accurately identify lesions across different layers and understand their interrelationships. This expertise begins with a comprehensive mastery of the pathological anatomy of PDR.

The pathological anatomy of PDR primarily manifests in two dimensions: (1) the extent of fibrovascular proliferation and (2) the status of the vitreous. Together, these factors dictate the surgical complexity. When approaching complex PDR cases, beginners should prioritize a thorough assessment of these two key elements (Fig. 8.1).

Z. Zhang, U. Spandau, *Vitreoretinal Surgery*,
https://doi.org/10.1007/978-3-032-25271-5_8

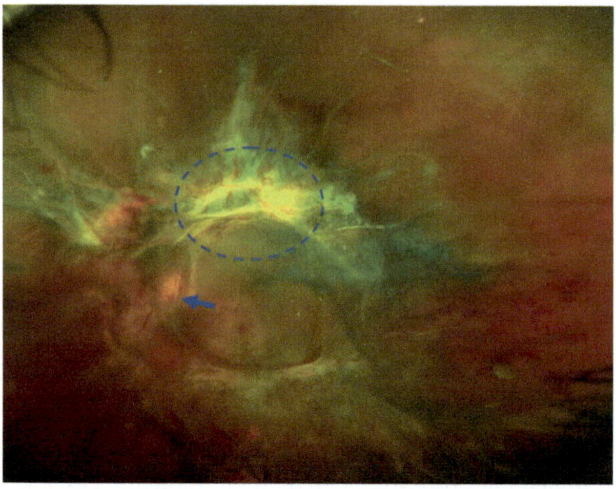

Fig. 8.1 Representative fundus image showing classic features of severe PDR. Surgeons can assess case complexity by evaluating the extent of retinal proliferation and the vitreous status: (1) residual posterior hyaloid adherent near the optic disc (blue arrow) indicates the absence of a complete posterior vitreous detachment (PVD); and (2) a prominent, dense fibrovascular membrane (FVM) firmly attached to the superior vascular arcade (within the blue dashed line) signifies severe retinal proliferation. The primary surgical objective is to induce PVD to relieve the tangential and anteroposterior traction exerted by the membrane. The critical challenges involve preventing iatrogenic retinal breaks and managing intraoperative hemorrhage

8.1.1 Retinal Proliferative Changes

Ischemic lesions in PDR primarily affect the mid-peripheral retina beyond the vascular arcades and the area nasal to the optic disc. Subsequent neovascularization typically emerges posterior to these ischemic zones, manifesting as fibrovascular tissue along the superior/inferior vascular arcades and the nasal aspect of the optic disc.

Neovascular tissue originating from retinal venules penetrates the internal limiting membrane (ILM) and proliferates into the vitreous cavity. In advanced cases, this forms planar fibrovascular membranes across the posterior pole. These membranes become intertwined with the posterior hyaloid, establishing dense vitreoretinal adhesions. Furthermore, the friable walls of these neovascular vessels are prone to spontaneous rupture, leading to localized hemorrhage.

While retinal proliferation itself exerts minimal traction, subsequent vitreous organization and contraction disrupt the delicate balance of vitreoretinal interface. Extensive and forceful vitreous traction can lead to tractional retinal detachment (TRD). Conversely, if partial or complete PVD occurs, it may trigger vitreous hemorrhage (VH) due to the avulsion of fragile vessels. In severe cases, these two conditions often coexist, significantly compounding the surgical complexity.

From the perspective of the vitreoretinal interface, the core surgical challenge lies in the precise identification and systematic relief of traction sites, while simultaneously preserving retinal integrity to minimize iatrogenic breaks and vascular trauma.

8.1.2 Vitreous Status

If retinal ischemia is the 'seed' of PDR, the vitreous serves as the 'fertile soil.' Pathophysiologically, the vitreous provides a scaffold for fibrovascular proliferation originating from the inner retina. Molecularly, it acts as a reservoir for

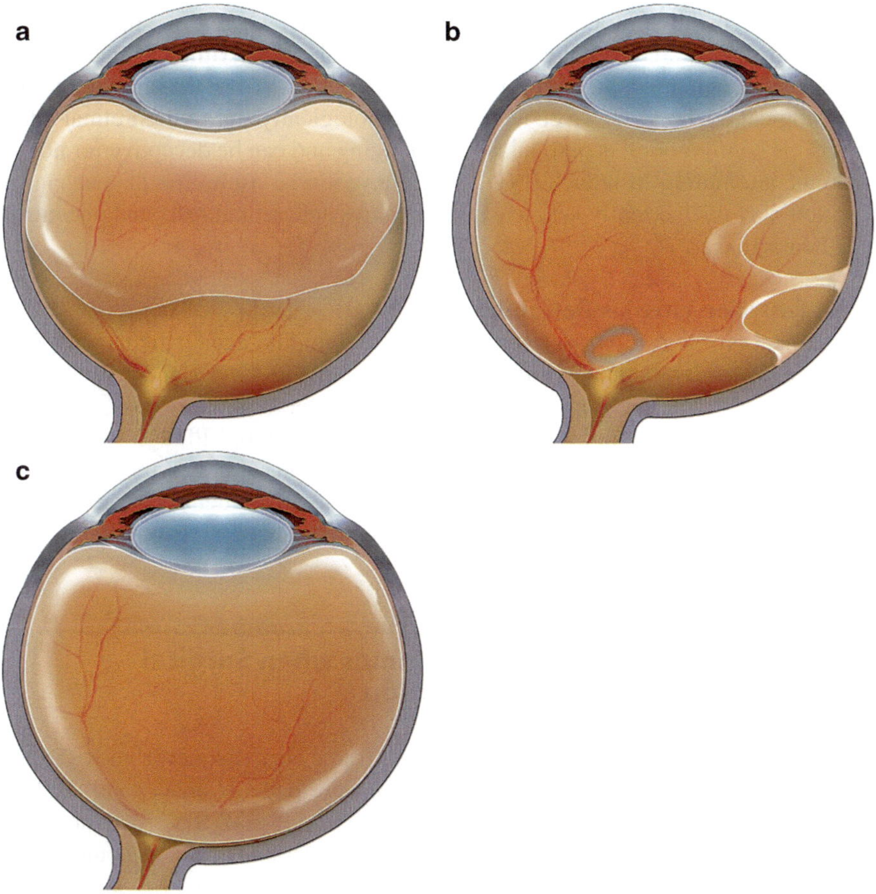

Fig. 8.2 Three types of vitreous status in PDR patients. (**a**) Complete posterior vitreous detachment. (**b**) Partial posterior vitreous detachment. (**c**) No posterior vitreous detachment

pro-angiogenic factors while also serving as a critical conduit for the distribution of anti-VEGF agents.

The vitreous status in PDR patients can be categorized into three types (Fig. 8.2):

(1) Complete Posterior Vitreous Detachment (Complete PVD)
This presentation typically manifests as diffuse vitreous hemorrhage (VH) that obscures the fundus, requiring B-scan for diagnosis. Intraoperatively, the posterior pole appears remarkably free of prominent fibrovascular membranes. The hemorrhage usually stems from tractional avulsion of retinal vessels during PVD or the spontaneous rupture of fragile neovascular tissue. This 'hemorrhagic-type' PDR is relatively straightforward to manage, making it an ideal starting point for novice surgeons. Nevertheless, preoperative dynamic B-scan is mandatory to evaluate the PVD status and exclude occult retinal tractions.

(2) Partial Posterior Vitreous Detachment (Partial PVD)
Partial PVD typically initiates in the peripheral vitreous, whereas the posterior pole remains firmly incarcerated by fibrovascular membranes. Although the vitreous body is often contracted, the proliferative tissue extending from the inner retina acts as 'biological anchors' or 'rivets,' creating pathologically tight vitreoretinal adhesions. This configuration is particularly challenging and can be deceptive for novice surgeons: attempting to induce PVD using conventional aspiration or mechanical elevation may inadvertently lead to extensive iatrogenic retinal tears and uncontrollable hemorrhage.

(3) No Posterior Vitreous Detachment (No PVD)
This clinical profile is most prevalent in young and middle-aged patients with PDR who have not undergone panretinal photocoagulation (PRP) or standardized medical management. In such cases, fibrovascular proliferation is diffuse, extending from the posterior pole to the periphery. This 'adherent-type' PDR is exceedingly demanding for novice surgeons, as its management necessitates the mastery of advanced, multifaceted maneuvers. Precise preoperative identification is paramount, and it is strongly recommended that inexperienced surgeons defer these complex cases to more seasoned specialists.

8.2 How to Better Analyze Dilemmas when Surgical Intervention Is the Only Option

Surgery for PDR requires a unique assessment framework distinct from RRD protocols. Preoperative counseling is essential to ensure patients understand the high risks involved, such as intraoperative bleeding that may stall the procedure, poor visual outcomes or deterioration, and recurrent postoperative vitreous hemorrhage.

PDR surgery involves three critical dilemmas for the surgeon:

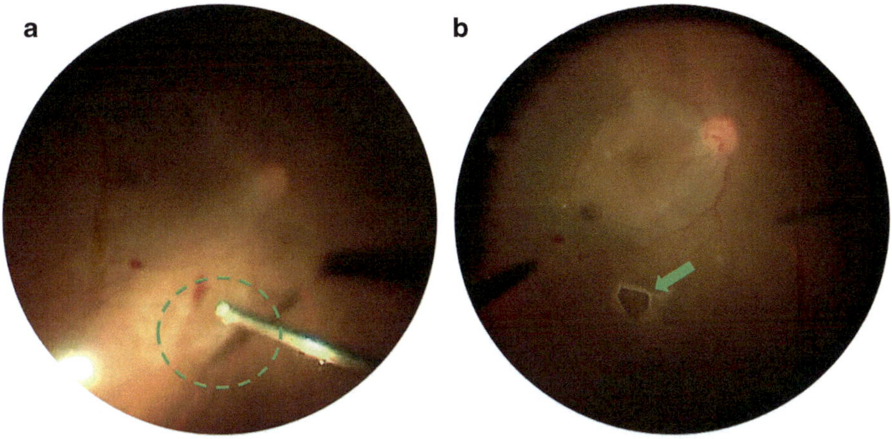

Fig. 8.3 Iatrogenic retinal break in PDR surgery. (**a**) Gently lifting the posterior vitreous with a vitrectomy probe. (**b**) Iatrogenic tear induced by the vitrectomy probe (green arrow)

8.2.1 Significant Discrepancy Between Preoperative and Intraoperative Findings

Preoperative assessment of PDR is often hindered by VH, which limits fundus visibility. However, even a transparent vitreous can mask complications such as tight vitreoretinal adhesions or occult subretinal proliferation, both of which are difficult to detect before the procedure begins.

8.2.2 A Fine Line Between Treatment and Harm

The primary objective of PDR surgery is the maximum relief of vitreoretinal traction; however, maneuvers such as peeling off proliferative membranes can inadvertently induce retinal tears and hemorrhage (Fig. 8.3). Consequently, achieving the optimal balance between "persistent proceeding" and "judicious cessation" serves as a critical test of a surgeon's clinical judgment.

8.2.3 Coordination of Interventional Strategies

PDR predominantly affects middle-aged and elderly populations, and diabetes itself serves as a significant risk factor for cataract progression. Consequently, patients often present with varying degrees of lens opacity, which markedly complicates vitreoretinal procedures. While combined phaco-vitrectomy addresses both issues, it also increases intraoperative complexity and exacerbates postoperative inflammation. For novice surgeons, determining the optimal timing for cataract extraction is a critical decision.

Furthermore, while preoperative anti-VEGF agents reduce vascular activity, they may also trigger fibrovascular membrane contraction, potentially inducing or aggravating tractional retinal detachment. Mastering the interval between anti-VEGF injection and pars plana vitrectomy (PPV) is therefore a vital skill for beginners.

Finally, managing persistent postoperative VH remains a significant challenge. Beginners must learn to strategically choose between conservative observation, further intravitreal injections, or intravitreal irrigation based on the clinical presentation.

8.3 When to Use Anti-VEGF

Chronic hyperglycemia is the primary driver of PDR, influencing clinical outcomes throughout the therapeutic process. The biochemical alterations increase blood viscosity and induce a pro-inflammatory state. This cascade eventually leads to the loss of capillary contractility, compromised vascular integrity, and aberrant endothelial cell proliferation, culminating in microcirculatory dysfunction and regional retinal ischemia.

Retinal ischemia triggers the pathological expression of multiple cytokines, with VEGF being the most significant and well-characterized mediator. Elevated VEGF levels compromise retinal health through four primary mechanisms: (1) inducing capillary inflammation and leukostasis, (2) increasing vascular permeability, (3) stimulating pathological angiogenesis, and (4) promoting cellular apoptosis.

Intravitreal anti-VEGF therapy directly counteracts these mechanisms. Preoperatively, its primary objective is to attenuate vascular activity, thereby minimizing intraoperative and postoperative hemorrhage, shortening procedural duration, reducing the risk of iatrogenic tears, and facilitating the dissection of fibrovascular membranes—ultimately enhancing surgical success rates.

However, the most critical risk associated with preoperative anti-VEGF administration is tractional retinal detachment (TRD) secondary to fibrovascular membrane contraction. Known in the literature as "crunch syndrome" (Fig. 8.4), this phenomenon has an incidence of approximately 10%. If the macula is involved, visual prognosis is severely guarded, and surgical dissection becomes markedly more complex. High-risk factors include extensive proliferative changes, significant preretinal fibrosis, and pre-existing TRD. Studies indicate that crunch syndrome typically manifests 1–6 weeks post-injection, with an average onset of 13 days.

Crunch syndrome warrants particular vigilance due to limited patient awareness of diabetic retinopathy and substantial regional disparities in medical resources. For clinicians, anti-VEGF intervention—regardless of the severity of proliferative changes—demands meticulous preoperative assessment and standardized follow-up protocols. Common clinical challenges include:

1. Patient Non-compliance: Improved visual acuity following injection may lead to complacency, causing patients to miss follow-up appointments and resulting in rapid, unmonitored disease progression.

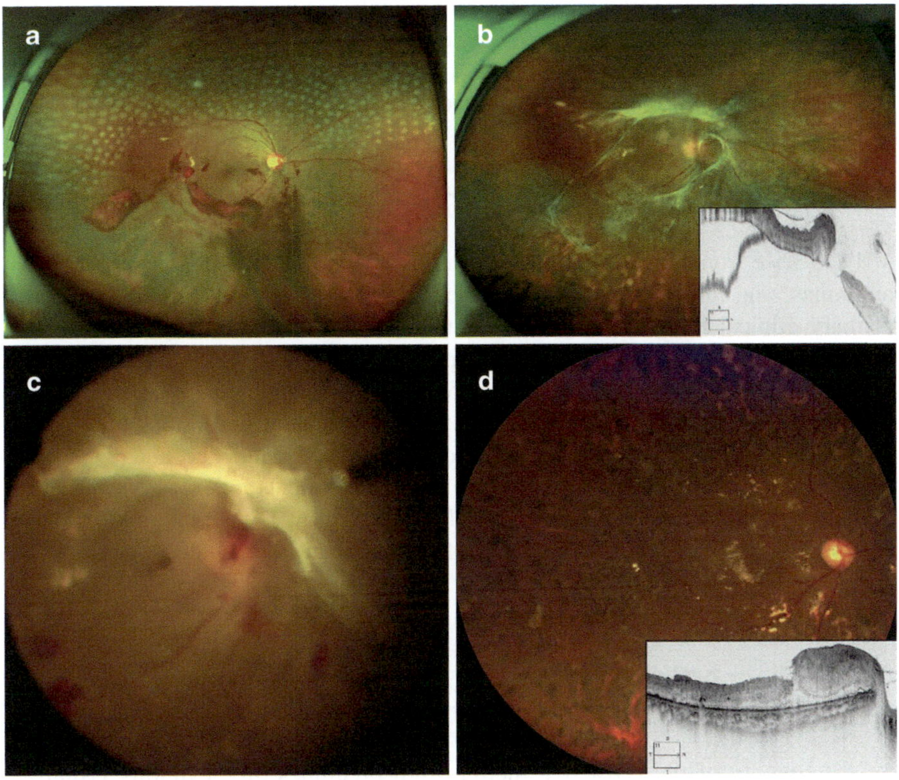

Fig. 8.4 Crunch syndrome. (**a**) Baseline: status post-laser photocoagulation; BCVA 0.5. minimal VH without obvious PVD. (**b**) 3 weeks post-anti-VEGF: BCVA dropped to HM. Fundus imaging shows RD; OCT reveals an associated macular hole (black border). (**c**) Intraoperative: dense fibrovascular membranes adherent to the optic disc and vascular arcades. (**d**) Postoperative: the retina reattached, OCT confirmed that the macular hole was nearly closed (black border), BCVA improved to 0.1

2. Delayed Laser Intervention: Overreliance on anti-VEGF therapy can defer essential laser photocoagulation, leading to advanced retinal proliferation by the time symptomatic visual impairment occurs.
3. Systemic Comorbidities: Patients with poorly controlled systemic factors (e.g., hypertension or hyperglycemia) may experience a paradoxical exacerbation of retinal proliferation after injection while focusing on managing their underlying diseases.

Currently, a definitive consensus on the optimal timing for PPV following anti-VEGF injection is lacking. While vitrectomy 7 days post-injection is a common and scientifically sound practice, it should not be applied as an absolute rule; instead, a multi-factorial clinical judgment is required. Evidence suggests that patients undergoing surgery 5–10 days post-injection achieve superior visual outcomes and fewer intraoperative complications compared to those treated within 1–3 days.

In summary, a surgical interval of approximately one week post-injection remains a safe and effective protocol. However, in cases of pre-existing retinal detachment or extensive preretinal fibrosis, intensive fundus monitoring is mandatory, and earlier surgical intervention may be indicated to preempt progressive traction.

8.4 Surgical Treatment of Vitreous Hemorrhage

VH can arise from various fundus pathologies, including retinal tears, retinal hemangiomas, and retinal vein occlusion; however, VH secondary to PDR remains a primary clinical focus. Notably, the first human vitrectomy was performed on a diabetic patient with long-standing VH, marking a milestone in ophthalmic surgery.

Historically, VH served as a catalyst for the advancement and popularization of PPV. This was driven by two key factors: (1) the potential for dramatic postoperative visual recovery, which bolsters surgeon and patient confidence, and (2) the relative simplicity of certain cases that require fewer instruments and steps. Nevertheless, modern comprehensive assessment of VH now necessitates the integration of two critical independent factors: the status of prior retinal laser photocoagulation and the adjunctive use of anti-VEGF.

8.4.1 Diagnostic Evaluation and Etiology of Vitreous Hemorrhage

Severe opacity of the refractive media often precludes direct fundus visualization. In such cases, ocular B-scan ultrasonography—particularly dynamic B-scan—is indispensable for evaluating the posterior segment and providing a critical reference for surgical planning. Furthermore, a dilated fundus examination of the contralateral eye is essential, as the pathological status of the fellow eye frequently mirrors the extent of retinal involvement in the affected eye.

The onset of VH is typically multifactorial. Key triggering factors include: (1) highly active neovascularization, (2) vascular wall rupture, (3) posterior pole vitreoretinal traction, (4) vitreous contraction, (5) posterior vitreous detachment (PVD) (Fig. 8.5), and (6) acute hypertensive episodes. It is crucial to recognize that these factors often coexist and interact synergistically, necessitating a comprehensive clinical assessment.

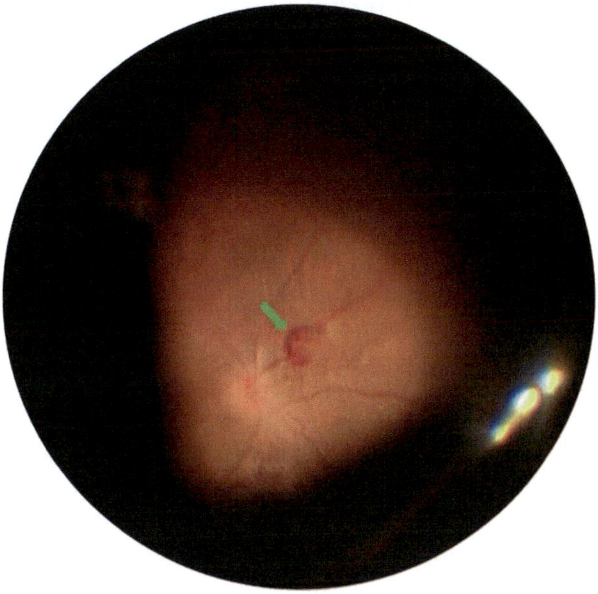

Fig. 8.5 Posterior pole vein rupture caused by posterior vitreous detachment, leading to extensive vitreous hemorrhage

8.4.2 Timing of Surgery for Vitreous Hemorrhage

Perspectives on the timing of surgical intervention for VH have evolved significantly. The observation period for non-clearing VH is shortening, a trend primarily driven by advancements in anti-VEGF therapy and the high safety profile of minimally invasive vitrectomy. Early intervention is increasingly favored to expedite visual recovery and allow for definitive management of the underlying retinopathy.

In cases of mild VH, where blood settles inferiorly and leaves the macula and superior retina visible, laser photocoagulation (PRP) should be prioritized. This intervention reduces intraocular VEGF expression in a manner comparable to anti-VEGF injections but with a more sustained effect. Provided there is no evidence of tractional retinal detachment, timely laser therapy establishes a critical foundation for stabilizing the disease.

However, prompt vitrectomy is indicated in specific high-risk scenarios, including: (1) neovascularization of the iris (NVI), (2) long-standing diabetes with a history of inadequate management, (3) refractory ocular hypertension secondary to VH (e.g., ghost cell or hemolytic glaucoma), and (4) patients with Type 1 diabetes.

For patients with well-controlled systemic parameters and high treatment compliance, early surgery is a reasonable strategy. This approach facilitates the immediate clearance of opacities, enables complete intraoperative PRP, and allows for the dissection of any fibrovascular membranes. Nevertheless, surgeons—particularly novices—must remain vigilant. Even in seemingly "routine" cases, meticulous vitreous resection and comprehensive endolaser are essential to optimize long-term outcomes and prevent postoperative complications.

8.4.3 Surgical Techniques and Intraoperative Precautions

When preoperative B-scan ultrasonography indicates mild posterior pole proliferation, the procedure is generally straightforward. The surgical approach typically follows these structured steps:

(1) Central Vitrectomy and Media Clearing

Upon inserting the endo-illuminator and vitrectome, if the metallic tip is visible through the media, vitrectomy may proceed directly using a wide-angle viewing system. However, in cases of dense VH where the visual axis is completely obscured, the anterior vitreous must first be resected under direct microscopic visualization. This initial clearance creates a safe workspace. Throughout this stage, meticulous care is required to avoid iatrogenic lens injury and to maintain a safe distance from the underlying retina (Fig. 8.6).

If the optic disc and retinal vasculature are clearly visible at this stage, it typically indicates a highly liquefied vitreous with complete PVD, generally leading to a straightforward procedure. Conversely, if the posterior pole remains obscured, extreme caution is mandatory to prevent iatrogenic retinal injury from the vitrectome.

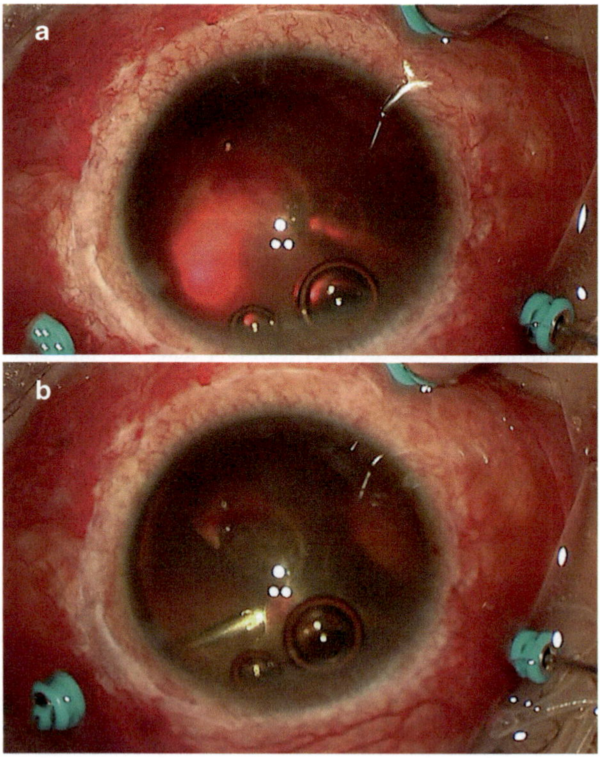

Fig. 8.6 Anterior vitrectomy under direct microscopic visualization. (**a**) To prevent blood from entering the anterior chamber, first inject viscoelastic agent into the anterior chamber to fill the entire space, under microscopic transillumination, the vitrectome resects the retrolental vitreous on the same side. (**b**) The vitrectome is switched to the opposite side to clear the remaining peripheral vitreous, markedly restoring visualization of the posterior segment

(2) Vitrectomy Starting from the Superior Vitreous Cavity

Surgeons should remain vigilant to the possible presence of a mobile, detached retina below. During advancing the vitrectomy, even a minor error can result in irreversible, extensive retinal loss. As a general principle, vitrectomy should be first performed in the superior vitreous cavity (between the 10 o'clock and 2 o'clock positions). In the event of an iatrogenic retinal tear, superior breaks are typically more manageable than those located elsewhere.

(3) "Finding the Beacons in the Mist"

The optic disc and retinal vasculature serve as essential "beacons" during VH surgery. Identifying these landmarks clarifies the surgical field and provides reliable anatomical reference points. This principle is fundamental across all VH cases—whether secondary to RRD, polypoidal choroidal vasculopathy (PCV), or PDR—and must be prioritized consistently.

The surgeon should search for vascular clues through clear gaps in the vitreous. The vascular architecture serves as a diagnostic guide: a standard anatomical course suggests attachment, while a displaced or anteriorly shifted vascular pattern is a hallmark of retinal detachment (Fig. 8.7).

(4) Inducing Posterior Vitreous Detachment (PVD)

The presence or absence of PVD in cases of VH can be highly deceptive; novice surgeons must remain vigilant to prevent from misjudgments. If a complete PVD

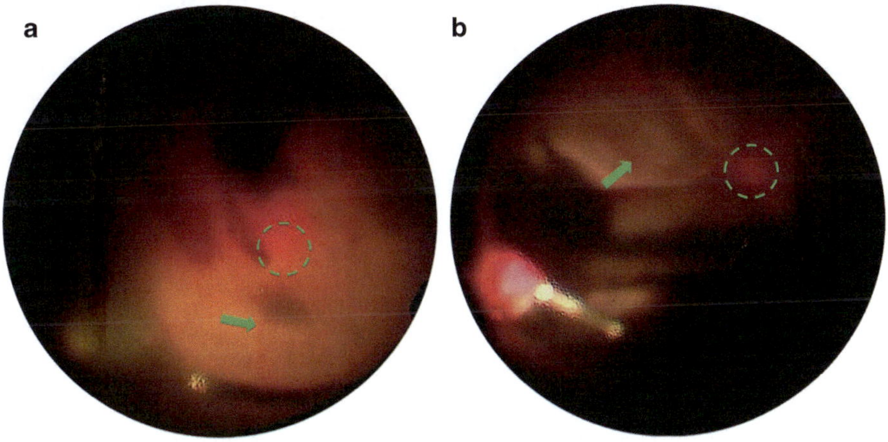

Fig. 8.7 Landmark identification and surgical safety. (**a**) Partial clearing reveals the optic disc (green dashed line) and retinal vessels (green arrows) at a standard depth. (**b**) Overlying clots obscure the disc (green dashed line), and vessels (green arrows) appear displaced toward the surgeon. In this case, the aspiration function of the vitrectome should be used first to create a safe distance between the vitreous and retina before resecting the vitreous

exists, the posterior pole is typically clear of dense adhesions; any residual blood can usually be aspirated using a flute needle or the vitrectome. Conversely, if hemorrhage remains firmly adherent to the posterior pole, it signifies tight vitreoretinal adhesion. In such instances, TA should be injected to visualize the vitreous interface, then use the vitrectome's suction to cautiously induce a PVD (Fig. 8.8).

(5) Posterior Vitreous Resection

Once the PVD is induced, the posterior hyaloid interface becomes easier to identify. While extending the PVD, carefully monitor for tight vitreoretinal or vitreovascular adhesions. Avoid aggressive aspiration in these areas to minimize the risk of bleeding or iatrogenic retinal breaks.

(6) Peripheral Shaving and Scleral Indentation

After the posterior pole is cleared, perform scleral indentation to check the peripheral retina for pre-existing or iatrogenic tears (Fig. 8.9). Residual vitreous in the periphery is a primary risk factor for postoperative tractional detachment; however, the shaving process itself must be meticulous to prevent new tears. In the event of a retinal break, shave off the surrounding vitreous, control any bleeding, and apply endolaser treatment to seal the site.

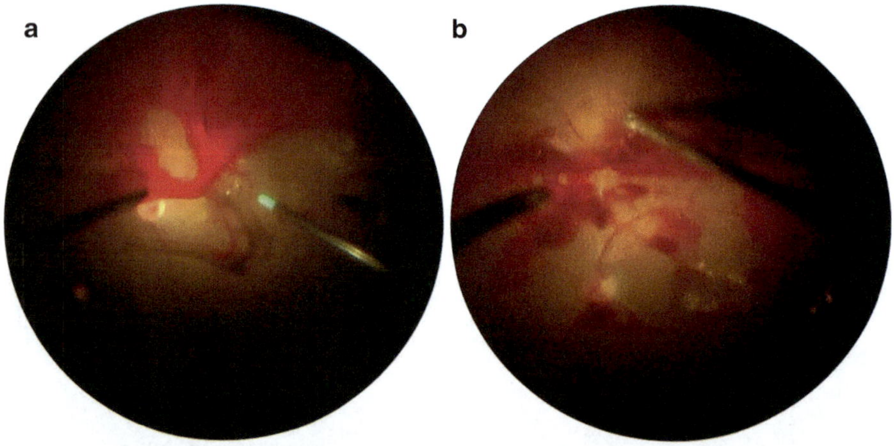

Fig. 8.8 Evaluating PVD using the "blowing and aspiration tests." (**a**) Blowing the hemorrhagic area with a flute needle reveals that blood can be completely cleared from the retinal surface, indicating complete vitreous resection. Blood is easily cleared from the retinal surface with a flute needle, indicating a complete PVD and adequate vitreous removal. (**b**) Blood accumulates in stubborn patches that resist aspiration, confirming that it is "trapped" beneath the posterior hyaloid. This finding indicates that an intact posterior vitreous cortex is still adherent to the retinal surface

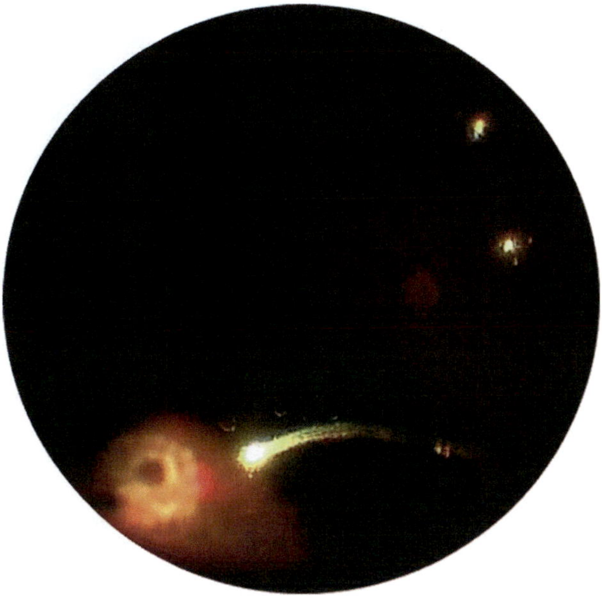

Fig. 8.9 Scleral indentation and peripheral repair. Identification of a peripheral retinal tear via scleral indentation, followed by thorough vitreous base shaving and laser retinopexy to seal the lesion

(7) Comprehensive Pan-retinal Photocoagulation (PRP)

Once PDR is confirmed as the etiology of the vitreous hemorrhage, extensive PRP is indicated. The integration of wide-angle viewing systems has significantly streamlined intraoperative laser delivery. It is generally recommended to extend from the vascular arcades to the post-equatorial region, reaching just posterior to the ora serrata. Laser parameters must be adjusted dynamically. Given that laser scars typically expand by approximately 50% during the postoperative healing phase, adequate spacing between spots must be maintained (Fig. 8.10). While a symmetrical arrangement of laser spots is aesthetically ideal, clinical efficacy depends primarily on the total coverage area rather than the alignment pattern. Excessive energy levels should be avoided to minimize the risk of iatrogenic, laser-induced retinal breaks. Furthermore, focal photocoagulation can be applied to target localized vascular leakage. For patients with prior incomplete laser treatment, supplementary peripheral PRP should be performed under scleral indentation to ensure comprehensive coverage in a single surgical session ("single-stage completion").

Novice surgeons must strictly avoid iatrogenic macular injury. When initiating laser therapy, the following safety protocol is essential: (1) verify the operative eye once more; (2) identify the macular boundaries, noting that macular edema may obscure the foveal reflex and prolonged intraoperative manipulation can diminish fundus visibility; and (3) first delineate the macula by placing an initial row of protective laser spots around its periphery.

(8) Choosing the Optimal Tamponade

If retinal proliferation is mild, balanced salt solution (BSS) can be used. For some patients, filtered air or inert gas may be selected based on specific conditions; silicone oil tamponade is generally unnecessary.

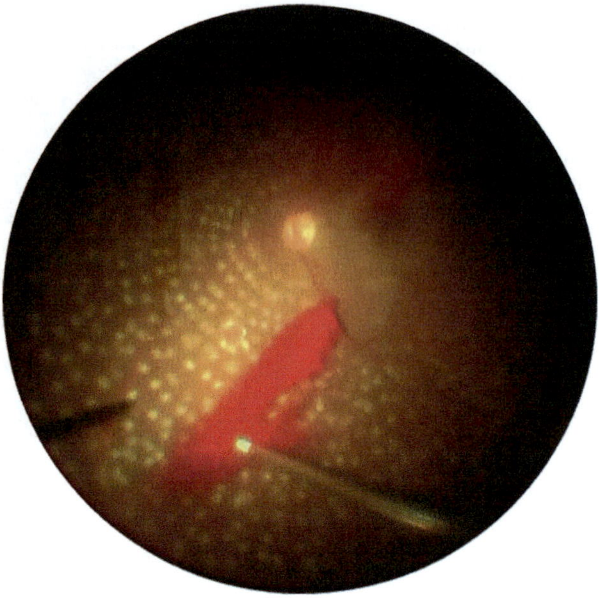

Fig. 8.10 Pan-retinal photocoagulation. Minor bleeding sites are manageable after most areas have been treated with laser; completing the PRP first helps stabilize the overall fundus environment

(9) Postoperative Anti-Inflammatory Therapy
PDR and extensive intraoperative laser treatment often predispose patients to severe postoperative inflammation. In such cases, enhanced local anti-inflammatory regimens are necessary. Additionally, mydriatic eye drops should be prescribed to maintain pupillary activity and reduce the risk of inflammatory complications like pupil seclusion.

8.4.4 Management of Postoperative Recurrent Hemorrhage

Recurrent VH occurs in approximately 30% of patients postoperatively. While it causes patient anxiety, thorough preoperative counseling can mitigate this pressure.

Most cases resolve spontaneously within 2–3 weeks, especially in an “aqueous eye” (post-vitrectomy without tamponade) where blood dilutes rapidly. Starting one week post-surgery, B-scan ultrasonography should be used to monitor blood volume and retinal status. If the retina is visible and the initial PRP is adequate, observation is typically sufficient. However, surgeons must monitor for elevated IOP, corneal staining, and iris neovascularization.

About 10% of patients require a repeat vitrectomy. While generally less complex, the surgery carries risks of sudden hypotony, globe collapse, and choroidal hemorrhage during port creation. Using valved trocars enhances safety. Intraoperatively, the focus should be on identifying bleeding sites and applying supplementary laser therapy; electrocoagulation is not generally recommended as the first option to manage the bleeding sites.

8.5 Techniques for Relieving Vitreoretinal Traction

Tractional retinal detachment in PDR is frequently accompanied by varying degrees of VH. However, due to vitreous contraction and dense adhesions, the VH is often localized rather than diffuse. For novice surgeons, the primary challenge lies in the meticulous relief of vitreoretinal traction.

If scleral buckling is likened to "the delicate crafting of a work of art," PDR surgery is akin to "the strategic encirclement and neutralization of a formidable army." It demands not only technical proficiency but also strategic planning, perseverance, and clinical courage.

To master these complexities, beginners must move beyond basic skills and integrate their technical expertise with a deep understanding of intraocular instrument mechanics. This synergy is essential to fully leverage the advantages of modern micro-incisional vitrectomy.

The procedure typically begins with the identification of the posterior hyaloid interface. When a PVD is present in the mid-periphery, a clear gap often exists between the hyaloid and the underlying retina. The surgeon should first utilize the vitrectome to incise this mid-peripheral interface, thereby creating a "safe surgical channel" for instruments to access the posterior pole (Fig. 8.11).

The next phase involves the relief of fibrovascular membrane traction. Regardless of whether a single-handed or bimanual approach is used, the surgeon typically employs three fundamental, interrelated techniques for membrane dissection. These maneuvers must be strategically integrated based on the specific morphology and severity of the lesion to achieve optimal clinical outcomes.

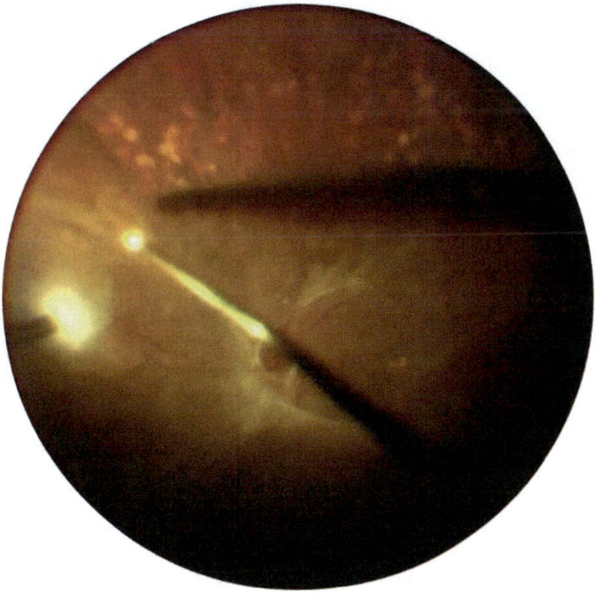

Fig. 8.11 Incision of the mid-peripheral posterior hyaloid

8.5.1 Segmentation Technique

As the most common approach, segmentation follows a "divide and conquer" strategy. Using a small-gauge vitrectome in high-cut-rate, low-vacuum mode, surgeons can partition expansive fibrovascular membranes into smaller segments across the fundus.

This technique is ideal for resecting bridging membranes with an underlying sub-membranous space (Fig. 8.12). While accessible for beginners, the primary challenge is the precise depth perception required to avoid iatrogenic retinal injury, tears, or hemorrhage while "conquering" each segment.

Following segmentation, the remaining membrane fragments can be meticulously debulked using the vitrectome.

8.5.2 Delamination Technique

For membranes with diffuse, moss-like adhesions and no clear surgical plane for segmentation, delamination is required to cautiously peel the membrane from the underlying retina (Fig. 8.13).

In a single-handed approach, intraocular forceps are typically used to expand the delamination from the area of least resistance. When membranes are present at the optic disc, peeling can be initiated peripapillarly (Fig. 8.14), using the endo-illuminator tip for gentle blunt separation of firmer adhesions. If adhesions are

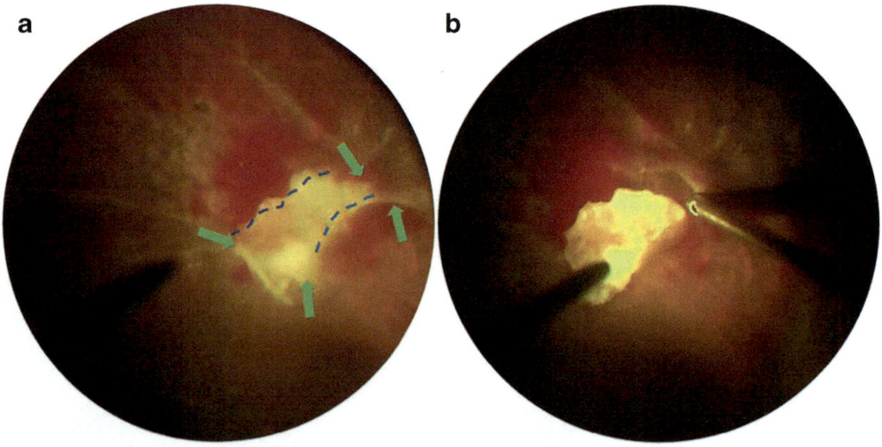

Fig. 8.12 Segmentation of bridging proliferative membranes. (**a**) The fibrovascular membrane spans between two vessels, with dense adhesions at the vascular walls (green arrows). These focal points act as "bridge piers" and are prone to tearing; thus, forceful peeling must be avoided. A sub-membranous space exists between the membrane and the underlying retina (blue dashed area), forming a "bridge" configuration. (**b**) Using a 25G vitrectome, the bridging membrane is incised at its point of maximum elevation to safely expose the underlying retina

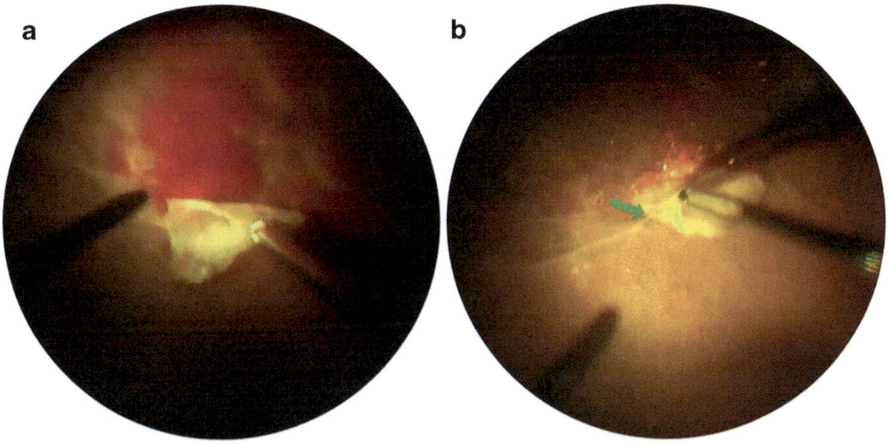

Fig. 8.13 Delamination technique. (**a**) The fibrovascular membrane is gently elevated using a vitrectome to evaluate the extent and tenacity of vitreoretinal adhesions, ensuring a controlled dissection. (**b**) Using intraocular forceps, delamination is initiated from the area of least resistance (the "loose edge"). Focal, striated adhesions between the membrane and retinal vasculature become visible (green arrows)

Fig. 8.14 Peeling the proliferative membrane near the optic disc with intraocular forceps

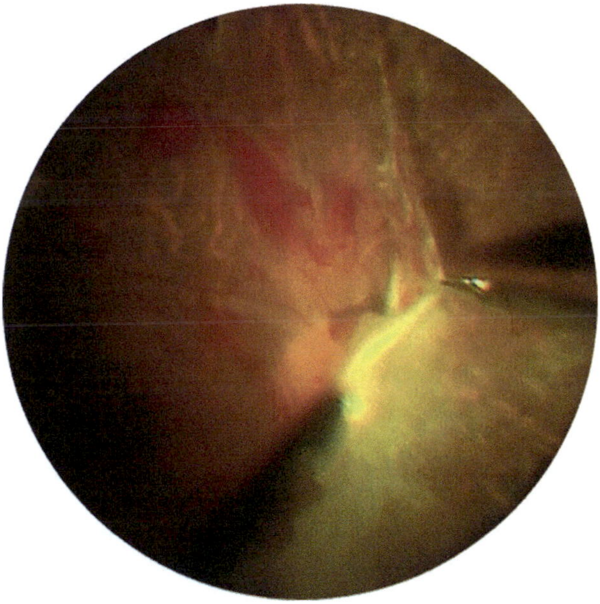

extremely tenacious, forced peeling must be avoided; the surgeon should instead seek alternative surgical planes. If a plane cannot be established, dissection should not be forced to prevent iatrogenic injury.

The bimanual technique is particularly effective for complex delamination. Utilizing a chandelier illumination system, the surgeon uses one hand to tension the membrane edge with intraocular forceps, while the other hand employs a vitrectome or intraocular scissors to release vitreoretinal adhesions. The primary advantage is the enhanced flexibility in identifying surgical planes; intraocular scissors can facilitate sharp dissection to create or expand these planes where blunt separation fails. However, this approach has a steep learning curve; improper execution can compromise efficiency and increase the risk of iatrogenic retinal injury.

8.5.3 En Bloc Technique

The "En bloc" technique (derived from the French for "as a whole") is a strategic approach akin to a "surgical strike." Its primary objective is to release adhesions between the posterior pole membrane and the retina with minimal manipulation. This method uniquely leverages the anteroposterior traction—the very force that causes TRD—as a functional "third hand." This inherent tension tautens the membrane, mimicking the effect of intraocular forceps in bimanual surgery and facilitating precise dissection.

In clinical practice, all three techniques—segmentation, delamination, and en bloc—share a common core principle: identify all vitreoretinal adhesion sites and establish surgical planes to address the primary pathology. The goal is to "utilize the membrane's own force against itself" as an operational platform. When resecting membranes, surgeons must minimize both the extent and intensity of traction applied to the underlying retina. Novice surgeons should adhere to these tenets: proceed with deliberate caution, allow sufficient time for diagnostic judgment, minimize redundant maneuvers, and maintain complications within a manageable threshold.

8.6 Vital Dyes and Intraocular Tamponade Agents

8.6.1 Staining Agents

(1) Staining Agents

Surgeons utilize various chromodissection agents to enhance the visualization of the vitreous and proliferative membranes. TA is commonly used, particularly when managing non-liquefied vitreous with firm retinal adhesions or when PVD status is ambiguous. TA effectively delineates the residual vitreous interface, enabling

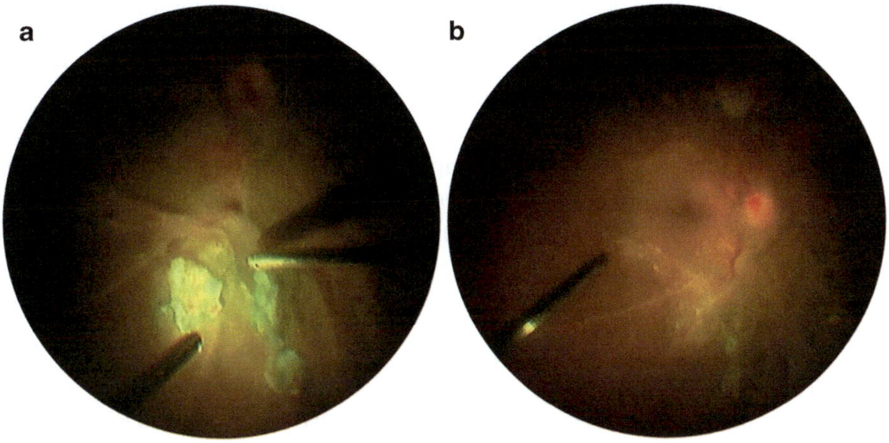

Fig. 8.15 ICG staining aids in identifying proliferative membranes. (**a**) After ICG injection, the membrane edge becomes visible; trim it using a vitrectome, (**b**) Most of the proliferative membrane has been removed

precise resection. Other available agents for staining pathological tissues include trypan blue, brilliant blue G (BBG), and indocyanine green (ICG).

(2) Common Application Methods

ICG is commonly used in China for its strong affinity for the ILM. Although it stains vitreous and proliferative tissues weakly, the resulting color contrast highlights the underlying retinal surface, helping surgeons identify the precise margins and course of fibrovascular membranes (Fig. 8.15).

The use of these staining agents remains controversial due to potential retinal toxicity, which may manifest as localized visual field defects. However, it is generally accepted that such adverse effects are preventable by strictly controlling the dosage and exposure duration. Several clinical strategies are available to mitigate risk:

1. Immediate dilution: When using standard concentrations (e.g., 5 mg/mL ICG), the agent should be aspirated and diluted with the vitrectome immediately after injection. This ensures sufficient rapid staining while preventing the prolonged retention of high-concentration dye within the vitreous cavity.
2. Pre-injection dilution: The agent can be diluted with balanced salt solution (BSS)—for instance, a tenfold dilution of 5 mg/mL ICG to 0.5 mg/mL. If

adequate staining is achieved upon injection, immediate aspiration follows. If visualization is insufficient, the endo-illuminator should be withdrawn, allowing the agent to dwell for 30–60 seconds before aspiration and washout. This approach balances minimal toxicity with enhanced visualization.

3. Hyperbaric delivery: Diluting the dye with a 5% glucose solution (which is relatively hyperbaric/higher density compared to BSS) allows the agent to settle directly onto the posterior pole. This prevents unwanted diffusion throughout the vitreous cavity and focuses the staining on the target tissue.

8.6.2 Tamponades

(1) Intraoperative Tamponades

Perfluorocarbon liquid (PFCL) is a vital intraoperative tool for stabilizing the posterior pole and protecting the macula from mechanical traction. Acting as a "third hand," PFCL enables surgeons to resect peripheral vitreous and dissect proliferative membranes with greater safety and efficiency. Despite these advantages, novice surgeons should exercise caution when using PFCL for retinal flattening. In cases involving rigid, contracted retina, PFCL can become sequestered within retinal folds or migrate into the subretinal space through occult micro-tears. Therefore, PFCL should be reserved as a last resort if air/fluid exchange fails to achieve adequate reattachment. During administration, a gentle injection technique is essential to prevent "fish-egg" droplet formation, IOP spikes, or iatrogenic retinal damage.

Viscoelastic agents may also assist with adhesions, though their use should be limited due to uncertain safety profiles and difficulty in detecting residual material in the vitreous cavity.

(2) Postoperative Tamponades

For uncomplicated vitreous hemorrhage (VH) where the retina is flat and laser photocoagulation is secure, balanced salt solution (BSS) may be used for primary tamponade, or filtered air for short-term support. In cases of moderate retinal proliferation, provided the membranes are completely removed and retinal hemorrhage is minimal, inert gas is an appropriate tamponade choice (Fig. 8.16).

Silicone oil is indicated for severe PDR with high vascular activity due to its hemostatic properties and its role in preventing iris neovascularization by blocking the anterior migration of VEGF. For elderly patients, oil removal is generally recommended at 3–6 months. Delayed removal often leads to advanced cataracts with harder nuclei and poor pupillary dilation, complicating future surgery for novice surgeons. In these challenging scenarios, the risk of serious complications like corneal endothelial decompensation is significantly elevated.

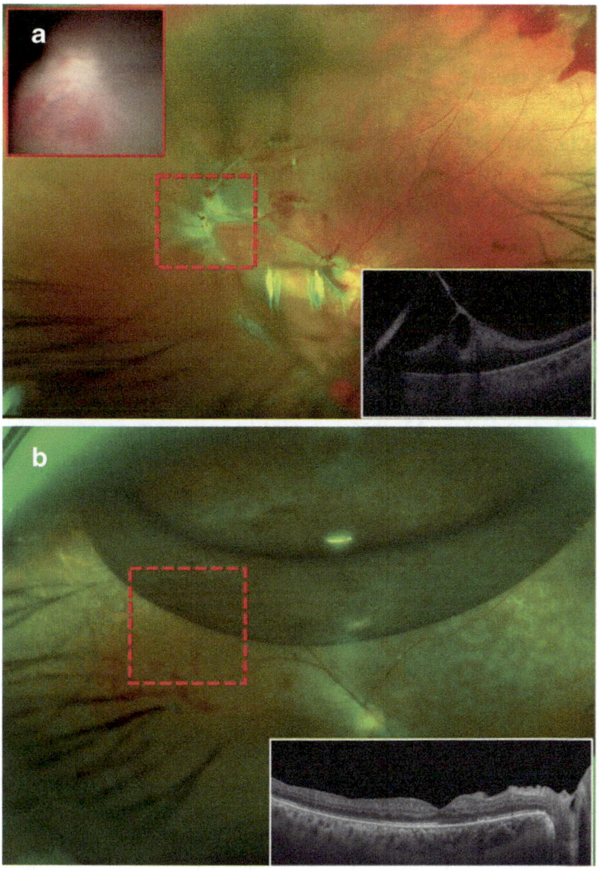

Fig. 8.16 Management of severe PDR with TRD. (**a**) Preoperative fundus showing superotemporal TRD (red dashed line) and tight posterior hyaloid adhesion on OCT (white box). Post-membrane excision, residual retinal folds remained (red box). (**b**) Three weeks postoperatively, the folds resolved spontaneously, and the retina is now fully attached (red dashed line). BCVA improved from 0.02 to 0.6, with nearly normal macular anatomy

8.7 How to Get Rid of Intraoperative Dilemmas

8.7.1 Corneal Edema

Corneal edema is common in PDR patients during surgery. If it occurs early in the procedure, it significantly impairs intraocular visualization. The following measures can be taken to reduce the incidence and severity of corneal edema:

1. Limit Preoperative chemical exposure: Control the duration of povidone-iodine contact with the conjunctival sac (ideally ≤1 min) to reduce epithelial toxicity.
2. Maintain epithelial hydration: Intraoperatively, apply viscoelastic sodium to shield the corneal surface, or irrigate with BSS to ensure the epithelium remains adequately hydrated.
3. Optimize fluid dynamics: Maintain a stable infusion pressure, ideally between 20–25 mmHg. Avoid premature PFCL injection or air/fluid exchange, as sudden IOP fluctuations can trigger corneal decompensation.
4. If necessary, scrape off the edematous corneal epithelium with a blade.

8.7.2 Lens Opacity

Beyond avoiding iatrogenic trauma, utilizing valved trocars is essential to minimize IOP fluctuations. Ensure the infusion cannula is angled toward the center of the vitreous cavity. This prevents localized turbulent flow from directly impacting the posterior lens surface. Although BSS contains glucose, a significant gradient between the infusion fluid and the patient's elevated systemic glucose levels can trigger acute osmotic lens opacification. Therefore, preoperative blood glucose must be stabilized within a therapeutic range. Avoid premature air-fluid exchange or PFCL injection, as these maneuvers can induce sudden IOP shifts that compromise corneal and lens clarity.

Furthermore, combined cataract surgery with PPV is not recommended in PDR cases. Combining these procedures acutely increases surgical complexity and elevates the risk of postoperative inflammatory complications.

8.7.3 Pupillary Constriction

Due to diabetes-related reductions in iris elasticity, some PDR patients exhibit inadequate mydriasis or progressive intraoperative miosis, which can compromise the visualization of surgical maneuvers. Fortunately, the integration of wide-angle viewing systems has made this issue less limiting by providing a broader field of view despite a smaller pupillary aperture.

In patients with stable systemic blood pressure, intrameal epinephrine can be administered to enhance pupillary dilation. A common clinical preparation involves diluting 0.1% epinephrine in a 10-mL BSS-filled syringe (aspirating a volume approximately equal to a small air bubble). Generally, the use of iris retractors is discouraged in PDR cases, as the fragile, inelastic iris tissue is highly susceptible to iatrogenic tears and hemorrhage.

8.7.4 Iatrogenic Retinal Tears

Iatrogenic retinal tears represent a significant complication in PDR surgery, often arising from a combination of complex factors. Despite the implementation of various surgical techniques, the manipulation required for proliferative membrane management may result in iatrogenic tears. While such incidents can occur during surgery, focus remains on prevention through refined maneuvers.

In the event that an iatrogenic retinal tear is identified, the vitreous surrounding the break should be resected thoroughly, and any adhering proliferative membranes should be removed. When managed appropriately, these tears can be utilized effectively during the procedure as conduits for draining subretinal fluid during air/fluid exchange. Following successful reattachment of the retina, laser photocoagulation is employed to seal the tear. With timely and precise intervention, these events typically do not lead to severe long-term complications.

8.7.5 Intraoperative Bleeding

Intraoperative bleeding in PDR surgery can originate from multiple sources, including neovascularization, the optic disc, retinal vasculature, the iris, scleral ports, or the choroid. As in conventional vitrectomy, the most critical preventive strategy is the judicious adjustment and maintenance of infusion pressure.

Hemorrhage is most frequently encountered during the resection or delamination of proliferative membranes with firm vascular adhesions (Fig. 8.17). Once active bleeding is identified, immediate intervention is mandatory. Due to the increased blood viscosity characteristic of PDR patients, large-volume hemorrhage becomes difficult to aspirate and can severely obscure the surgical field, hindering further maneuvers. The following techniques should be employed to achieve effective hemostasis:

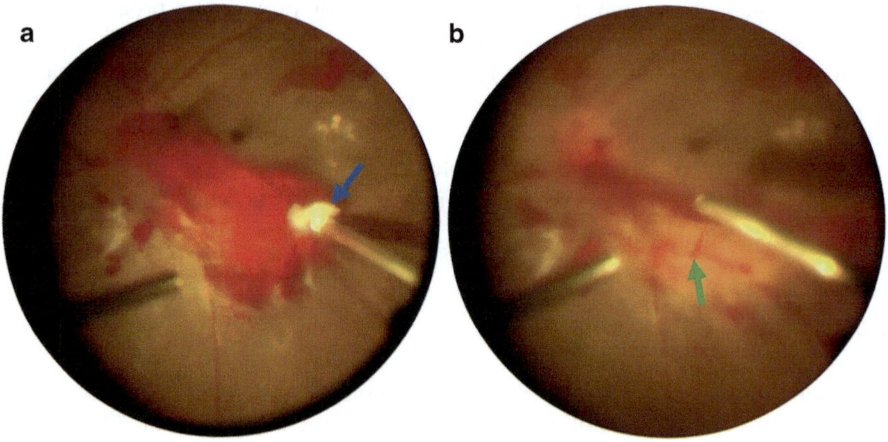

Fig. 8.17 Retinal bleeding during proliferative membrane resection. (**a**) Severe bleeding occurs when resecting a proliferative membrane tightly adherent to the retina (blue arrow) with a vitrectome. (**b**) After aspirating the blood clot with a vitrectome, an active bleeding site is identified (green arrow)

(1) Temporarily Increasing Infusion Pressure

The duration must be strictly controlled ($\leq$3 min) to avoid severely impairing retinal perfusion. After bleeding is controlled, the infusion pressure can be gradually reduced to the normal range in a stepwise manner.

(2) Intraocular Instrument Compression Hemostasis

Use the tip of a flute needle or vitrectomy cutter to gently press the bleeding site for at least 1 min. Avoid ineffective compression due to hand tremors.

(3) Timely Air/Fluid Exchange

Bleeding dissolves quickly in BSS, impairing surgical field visibility. Air/fluid exchange can be performed to allow hemostatic manipulation under gas tamponade.

(4) Electrocoagulation

Precision is essential: the intensity should be controlled within a reasonable range to avoid iatrogenic tears.

(5) Laser Photocoagulation

This is a safe and effective method that beginners should master. The tip of the laser fiber does not need to contact the bleeding site; the laser beam can accurately target the bleeding point, using thermal effects to induce coagulation and hemostasis.

(6) "Luring the Snake Out of Its Hole"

To thoroughly address all bleeding sites intraoperatively, after initial hemostasis, temporarily reduce the infusion pressure to 15–20 mmHg and wait briefly. Carefully observe for active bleeding; if detected, use laser photocoagulation for precise sealing.

8.8 Postoperative Complications and the Management

Beyond the complications inherent to vitrectomy and intraocular tamponades, PDR patients are predisposed to specific postoperative challenges.

8.8.1 Elevated Intraocular Pressure

Postoperative ocular hypertension can manifest in early or late stages. Management should be guided by the severity of the IOP elevation and anterior segment findings, specifically anterior chamber depth and inflammatory status. Approximately one-third of patients experience transient IOP elevation. Notably, corneal edema may result in overestimated readings via non-contact tonometry (NCT); therefore, clinical symptoms such as headache and ocular pain must be assessed. Observation is typically sufficient for IOP 30 mmHg, 1–2 types of topical hypotensive agents should be initiated, with systemic medications added if necessary. If the elevation is secondary to pupillary block, it often progresses rapidly. Management includes immediate intensive anti-inflammatory and mydriatic therapy, strict adherence to a prone position, and prompt surgical intervention if conservative measures fail.

Delayed IOP elevation is frequently caused by silicone oil emulsification. In rare instances, it may be secondary to neovascular glaucoma (NVG) or progressive retinal proliferation. Treatment must be tailored to the underlying etiology.

Middle-to-late postoperative IOP elevation is often caused by silicone oil emulsification; in rare cases, it is secondary to iris neovascularization or worsening retinal proliferation. Management should be tailored to the specific cause.

8.8.2 Uveal Reaction and Inflammation

Significant postoperative uveal reactions are common in PDR patients, driven by a systemic pro-inflammatory state and extensive intraoperative manipulation. Manifestations include pupillary exudative membranes, keratic precipitates (KPs), aqueous flare, and cells. Compared to standard vitrectomy, PDR cases require intensified postoperative anti-inflammatory regimens. If indicated, systemic corticosteroids may be administered under rigorous blood glucose monitoring. Cycloplegic therapy is essential: atropine ointment is preferred during the initial postoperative week, followed by a transition to tropicamide eye drops.

8.8.3 Lens Opacity

If no iatrogenic damage occurs, post-inflammatory lens opacity often resolves. Late-onset cataracts are common and require experienced surgeons, with pre-operative stabilization of retinal proliferation and mandatory post-operative monitoring for macular edema and neovascularization.

8.8.4 Iris Neovascularization and Secondary Glaucoma

Neovascularization of the iris (NVI) typically manifests several weeks postoperatively. Key risk factors include aphakia, pseudophakia, and combined anterior-posterior segment procedures (e.g., phaco-vitrectomy) (Fig. 8.18). To mitigate the risk of NVI, surgeons should prioritize the following strategies: (1) Ensure the judicious use of perioperative anti-VEGF agents and the administration of comprehensive, confluent PRP; (2) Minimize intraoperative manipulation of the anterior segment to reduce the release of pro-angiogenic inflammatory mediators; (3) Verify that the PRP is sufficiently extensive to eliminate retinal ischemia, which is the primary driver of VEGF production. If the elevated IOP remains refractory despite aggressive pharmacological intervention, a timely referral to a glaucoma specialist is mandatory for the management of potential neovascular glaucoma (NVG).

8.8.5 Anterior Hyaloidal Fibrovascular Proliferation

Anterior hyaloidal fibrovascular proliferation (AHFP) is a distinct manifestation of proliferative vitreoretinopathy (PVR) following PDR surgery, predominantly affecting young male patients with Type 1 diabetes. It is characterized by fibrovascular

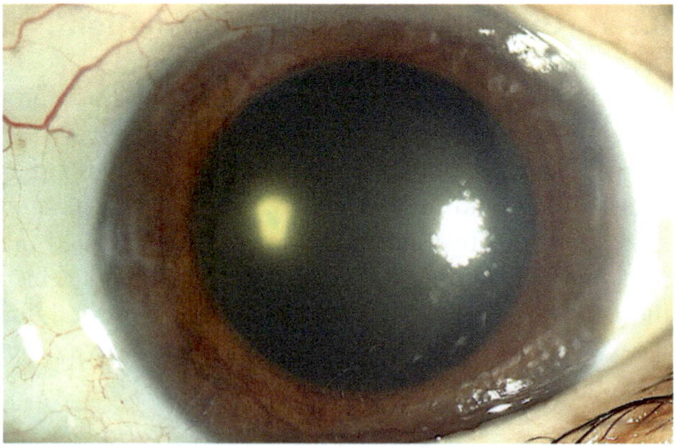

Fig. 8.18 Postoperative iris neovascularization. Neovascularization of the iris observed one month following phaco-vitrectomy for PDR

membranes that originate from the peripheral retina and extend anteriorly toward the ciliary epithelium, the posterior lens capsule, and the posterior iris surface. Clinically, patients present with rapid, severe vision loss, accompanied by significant anterior segment inflammation and hyphema. Due to its aggressive nature, AHFP is challenging to treat and carries a poor visual prognosis.

Prevention during the primary surgery is critical. Two key strategies are essential to mitigate this risk: (1) Performing extensive, confluent PRP that reaches the posterior edge of the ora serrata; (2) Executing a thorough peripheral vitreous shaving under scleral indentation to remove the scaffold for future proliferation.

8.8.6 Intraocular Fibrin Syndrome

This complication is rare but notoriously difficult to manage, often carrying a poor visual prognosis. It is characterized by extensive intraocular fibrin exudation and deposition, which can lead to pupillary membrane occlusion, tractional retinal detachment, and secondary neovascularization (Fig. 8.19). Key risk factors include: (1) Combined anterior-posterior segment surgery (e.g., phaco-vitrectomy); (2) Excessive or high-intensity laser photocoagulation, which triggers a massive inflammatory response.

8.8.7 Vitreous Hemorrhage

Early postoperative vitreous hemorrhage may arise from minor leakage from retinal vessels, residual fibrovascular membranes left after surgery, or postoperative dispersion of residual blood from the peripheral vitreous into the vitreous cavity. Close observation, mainly using B-scan ultrasonography, is recommended, and surgical intervention is generally unnecessary in the short term. Some patients may benefit from repeat intravitreal anti-VEGF injection. If the hemorrhage does not clear after 1–2 months of observation, or if retinal detachment or elevated IOP develops, second surgery may be performed, with caution to avoid complications associated with a vitrectomized eye. The bleeding source should be treated concurrently, and silicone oil tamponade should be considered when indicated.

Mid-to-late postoperative vitreous hemorrhage may result from recurrent retinal fibrovascular proliferation. Neovascularization of the iris and angle may also lead to vitreous hemorrhage. Management should be individualized according to the underlying cause.

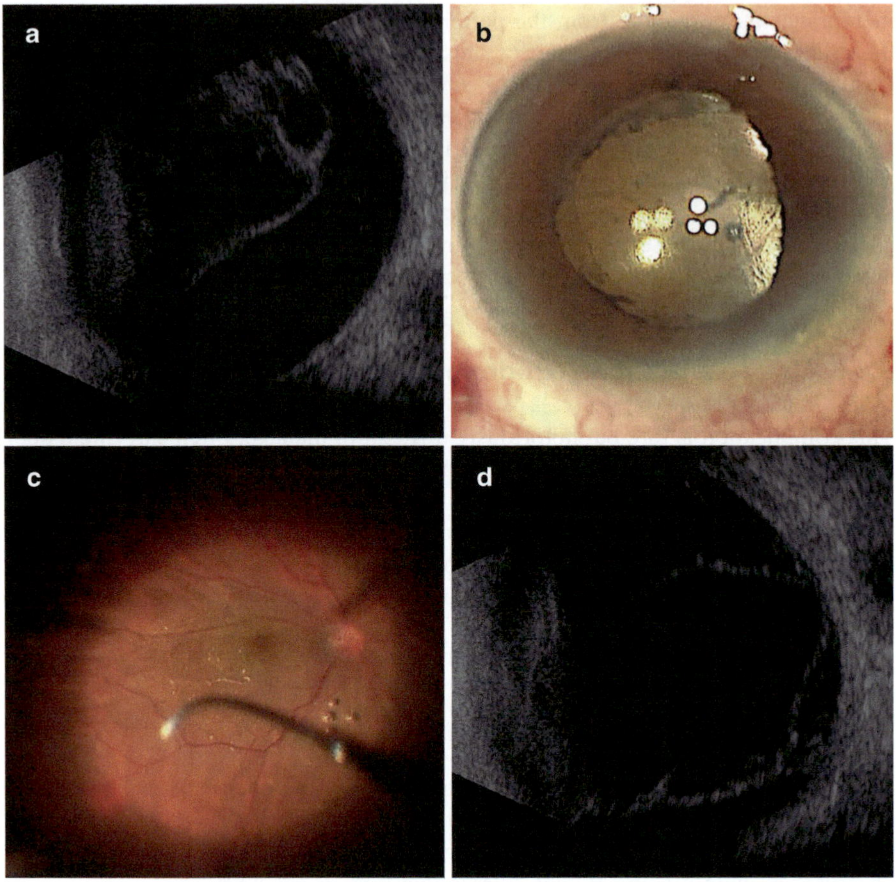

Fig. 8.19 Postoperative fibrinoid syndrome following phaco-vitrectomy for PDR. (**a**) Baseline: No retinal detachment on B-scan. (**b**) Combined phaco-vitrectomy and IOL implantation was performed due to dense cataract obscuring the fundus. (**c**) The retina remained flat intraoperatively. (**d**) Day 3 postoperative: Significant vision loss. B-scan shows a classic funnel-shaped RD secondary to severe fibrinoid exudation

8.9 Summary

"Only a strategic protracted war is the sole path to final victory." The surgical management of advanced PDR is inherently complex, characterized by extended therapeutic timelines and significant variability in procedural difficulty. Achieving successful outcomes necessitates comprehensive perioperative care and a high level of technical proficiency to navigate frequent and multifaceted intraoperative and postoperative complications.

Novice surgeons should initially operate under the close supervision of senior mentors. It is essential to strictly adhere to surgical indications, prioritize clinical observation, and engage in continuous self-reflection and systematic case reviews. Independent management of severe PDR cases should only be undertaken after accumulating substantial surgical experience and demonstrating consistent clinical judgment.

Surgical Management of Epiretinal Membrane

9

Epiretinal membrane (ERM) is a common structural abnormality of the vitreomacular interface. It is characterized by the proliferation of collagen fibers on the inner retinal surface, resulting in varying degrees of fibrocellular tissue attachment to the macula. Clinically, ERM primarily manifests as decreased visual acuity and metamorphopsia. Optical coherence tomography (OCT) has become an essential tool for diagnosing ERM and provides critical evidence for determining surgical timing.

ERM is classified into two types: idiopathic and secondary. The former lacks a definitive clinical cause and remains a diagnosis of exclusion. (Etymologically, 'idiopathic' combines the Greek idios, meaning 'self' or 'private,' with the suffix -pathic, indicating a pathological condition). Secondary ERM, conversely, is directly attributable to specific ocular pathologies. This chapter explores the pathogenesis of ERM, with a focus on surgical management techniques and key clinical considerations.

9.1 Clinical Characteristics

9.1.1 Classification and Etiology of ERM

Idiopathic ERM: No definitive cause is identifiable, making it a diagnosis of exclusion. Before confirming this diagnosis, a comprehensive fundus examination and a thorough medical history review are mandatory.

Secondary ERM: This form is associated with various ocular pathologies, including retinal vein occlusion, diabetic retinopathy, uveitis, trauma, retinal detachment, hamartomas, and retinal angiomas. While identifying the primary disease is often straightforward, it is vital to meticulously examine the peripheral retina for breaks. If indicated, fluorescein angiography should be performed to assess vascular exudation.

Z. Zhang, U. Spandau, *Vitreoretinal Surgery*,
https://doi.org/10.1007/978-3-032-25271-5_9

"Iatrogenic" ERM: Though technically a subset of secondary ERM, it is highlighted here to underscore that ocular intervention is a frequent trigger. This includes ERM formation following retinal detachment repair, silicone oil tamponade, laser photocoagulation, or cryotherapy—typically driven by postoperative inflammatory activation.

9.1.2 Staging of Idiopathic Epiretinal Membrane

Idiopathic epiretinal membrane (iERM) peaks in incidence among individuals aged 60–70 years, with a slightly higher prevalence in women. According to the Gass classification, it is divided into three clinical stages:

- Stage 0 (cellophane maculopathy): Characterized by a thin, transparent membrane that produces a shimmering, cellophane-like reflex over the macula. At this stage, the membrane does not distort the underlying retina. Patients are typically asymptomatic, and the condition is often an incidental finding during routine examination (Fig. 9.1a). Because the risks of surgery significantly outweigh the potential benefits, surgical intervention is not recommended, and observation is the standard of care.

  Because the risks of surgery significantly outweigh the potential benefits, surgical intervention is not recommended, and observation is the standard of care.
- Stage 1 (Crinkled Cellophane Maculopathy): The membrane begins to contract, causing fine wrinkles or striae in the inner retinal layers. If contraction involves the fovea, patients may report mild decreased visual acuity or metamorphopsia. These symptoms are often subtle and may only be noticed during monocular testing—especially if the affected eye is non-dominant (Fig. 9.1b).

  For patients with stable, good visual acuity, surgeons should prioritize long-term monitoring over immediate surgery, tracking the progression of visual distortion.
- Stage 2: Stage 2 (macular pucker): The membrane thickens and becomes increasingly opaque, appearing translucent or grayish-white. Significant contraction results in full-thickness retinal folds, vascular tortuosity, and potential displacement of the fovea. Secondary clinical signs such as small hemorrhages, exudates, or cotton-wool spots may be present, and cystoid macular edema (CME) occurs in approximately 20%–40% of cases (Fig. 9.1c, d).

  Clinical symptoms do not always correlate perfectly with imaging findings in these patients; approximately 80% report decreased visual acuity or metamorphopsia. Prior to recommending surgery, surgeons must thoroughly evaluate the patient's primary complaints. Given the typically elderly demographic, concurrent conditions such as cataracts or dry eye syndrome should be considered. Surgical decisions must align with the patient's functional goals; intervention is rarely urgent if symptoms are mild or if the patient is hesitant.

Secondary and iatrogenic ERMs are not typically staged.

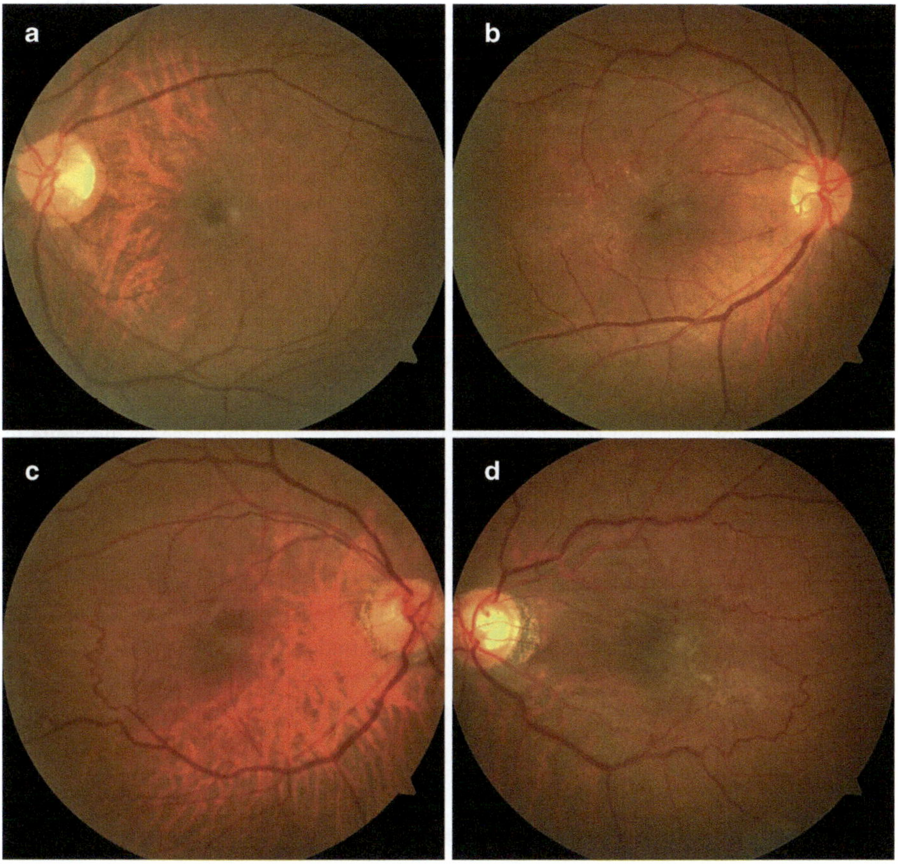

Fig. 9.1 Fundus photographs of ERM at different clinical stages (**a**) Cellophane-like reflection on the macula (Stage 0). (**b**) Mild contraction and wrinkling of the ERM (Stage 1). (**c**) Vascular tortuosity near the macula (Stage 2). (**d**) Thickened ERM with small hemorrhages (Stage 2)

9.2 Etiology of Epiretinal Membrane

While the precise initiating trigger for ERM remains elusive, the transdifferentiation of various precursor cells into myofibroblasts is considered a critical step in ERM formation. During this process, cells often lose their original markers, complicating definitive identification. However, immunohistochemical studies suggest that retinal glial cells and retinal pigment epithelial (RPE) cells are the primary contributors. The mechanism by which these cells migrate to the inner retinal surface is still debated, though three prominent theories have been proposed:

1. ILM dehiscence theory: Following a posterior vitreous detachment (PVD), minor defects or "breaks" in the internal limiting membrane (ILM) may allow retinal glial

cells to migrate onto the inner retinal surface. However, because visible ILM damage is rarely observed in idiopathic cases, this theory is not universally accepted.

2. Vitreous remnant theory: Following PVD, residual vitreous cortical cells (hyalocytes) remain on the retinal surface, where they proliferate and undergo metaplasia. A limitation of this theory is its inability to account for ERM cases occurring in the absence of a PVD.
3. Chronic traction theory: In eyes without PVD, chronic vitreomacular traction (VMT) may stimulate Müller cells, triggering glial proliferation and vascular leakage. Glial cells then migrate and proliferate along the posterior vitreous cortex, eventually forming the ERM.

Currently, no single theory comprehensively explains all clinical presentations of ERM formation.

Histologically, an ERM typically consists of two distinct layers:

- The outer layer: This layer is in direct contact with the ILM and is composed of an acellular extracellular matrix (ECM) secreted by the membrane's cellular components.
- The inner layer: This is the cellular component of the ERM, consisting of single or multiple strata of glial cells, RPE cells, fibroblasts, and immune cells. The specific cellular composition often reflects the underlying etiology and chronicity. For instance, ERM secondary to proliferative vitreoretinopathy (PVR) is typically RPE-dominant, whereas idiopathic ERM is primarily composed of glial cells.

9.2.1 Cellular Components of ERM

(1) Glial Cells

Microglia, astrocytes, and Müller cells are all implicated in the pathogenesis of ERM. The reactive proliferation of glial cells is a primary driver of both ERM and proliferative vitreoretinopathy (PVR). Upon migrating to the retinal surface, these cells proliferate to provide a scaffold for extracellular matrix (ECM) deposition. Glial cells can also transdifferentiate into myofibroblasts; furthermore, they secrete transforming growth factor-beta (TGF-β), which acts as a potent paracrine signal promoting the myofibroblastic transformation of other cellular constituents within the membrane.

(2) Hyalocytes

Hyalocytes are vitreous-resident mononuclear phagocytes primarily located within the posterior vitreous cortex and vitreous base. Within the ERM, these cells are characterized by long cytoplasmic processes and often cluster around fibroblasts. Research indicates that hyalocytes exhibit a robust contractile response to TGF-β2. Consequently, it is hypothesized that ERM may develop post-PVD due to the proliferation of residual premacular hyalocytes. If the posterior vitreous detachment occurs cleanly, completely separating the hyalocyte-containing layer from the macula, the likelihood of ERM formation may be reduced.

(3) Retinal Pigment Epithelial (RPE) Cells

RPE cells typically reach the inner retinal surface through retinal breaks, making them a dominant cellular component in PVR and ERM secondary to rhegmatogenous retinal detachment. While they are not a hallmark of idiopathic ERM, RPE cells on the retinal surface can differentiate into myofibroblasts under the influence of TGF-β2. While their migration pathway in idiopathic cases remains debated, one hypothesis suggests that other retinal cell types may undergo transdifferentiation into RPE-like cells.

(4) Macrophages

Macrophages are frequently identified in ERM secondary to vitreous hemorrhage. Although their exact role in membrane formation is not fully elucidated, they are known to secrete a variety of cytokines and growth factors that likely modulate the myofibroblastic transformation of surrounding cells.

(5) Fibroblasts and Myofibroblasts

The contractile properties of fibroblasts and myofibroblasts are responsible for the mechanical distortion of the underlying retinal architecture. This traction results in the formation of retinal folds, vascular tortuosity, and, in severe cases, the development of secondary macular holes.

9.3 Evaluation and Differential Diagnosis

While diagnosing ERM is often straightforward, surgeons must avoid "diagnostic monism." Because ERM predominantly affects the elderly, concurrent ocular pathologies are common. Misclassifying an ERM as idiopathic without a thorough evaluation can lead to overlooked details and potential medical disputes.

A comprehensive fundus examination and medical history are essential to distinguish between idiopathic, secondary, and iatrogenic types. Identifying the underlying etiology is critical for:

1. Patient communication: Providing an accurate diagnosis manages patient expectations and fosters a realistic understanding of their condition.
2. Comprehensive care: Facilitating the detection of associated abnormalities, such as peripheral vascular lesions or retinal breaks.
3. Optimizing outcomes: Identifying contraindications to surgery. For instance, in ERM secondary to uveitis, surgery should be deferred until inflammation is controlled.
4. Prognostic accuracy: Enabling objective predictions of visual recovery and complications, which is vital for informed consent.

The differential diagnosis of ERM includes: (1) Vitreomacular traction (VMT): High-resolution OCT easily distinguishes VMT from ERM by the presence of a continuous posterior vitreous cortex band. If VMT and ERM coexist, surgeons must exercise caution to avoid iatrogenic foveal traction; (2): Cystoid macular edema (CME): Centered on the fovea, CME appears as cystic intraretinal spaces on OCT, typically without vascular tortuosity. Fluorescein angiography (FA) may reveal characteristic "petaloid" leakage in late phases. If ERM and CME coexist (e.g., in retinal vein occlusion), surgeons should evaluate whether conservative treatments—such as anti-VEGF or corticosteroid implants—are indicated before proceeding with surgery.

9.4 Surgical Timing and Prognostic Factors

9.4.1 Surgical Timing

Historically, a best-corrected visual acuity (BCVA) of 20/100 (0.2) was the standard threshold for intervention, with metamorphopsia considered a secondary factor. However, the improved safety profile of minimally invasive vitrectomy (MIVS) and the increasing visual demands of modern lifestyles—particularly mobile device use—have made surgical indications more flexible. For novice surgeons, the following principles should be strictly observed before considering a more relaxed criteria:

1. ERM Severity and Baseline Visual Acuity
Denser membranes are typically associated with lower BCVA. While thick membranes are often easier to grasp and peel—facilitating the creation of an initial flap and a broader peeling range—they present unique challenges. If the ERM is highly concentrated or tightly adherent at the fovea (Fig. 9.2), the risk of mechanical retinal trauma significantly increases. In such cases, surgical intervention is not recommended for surgeons still in the early stages of their learning curve.

2. Patient Expectations
While ERM often causes moderate metamorphopsia, visual acuity frequently remains above 20/200 (0.1) in the absence of significant cataracts. Because pars plana vitrectomy is a specialized and costly intervention, patients typically harbor high expectations for functional recovery. If a patient's expectations are unrealistic or if they are intolerant of potential postoperative limitations, the surgeon must prioritize thorough communication. Avoiding overconfidence and ensuring informed consent are essential to prevent medical disputes—a common challenge when evaluating ERM patients in a clinical setting.

3. Primary Clinical Complaint
The patient's motivation for seeking care is a critical, yet often overlooked, factor. Patients may not notice metamorphopsia if the affected eye is non-dominant or if a

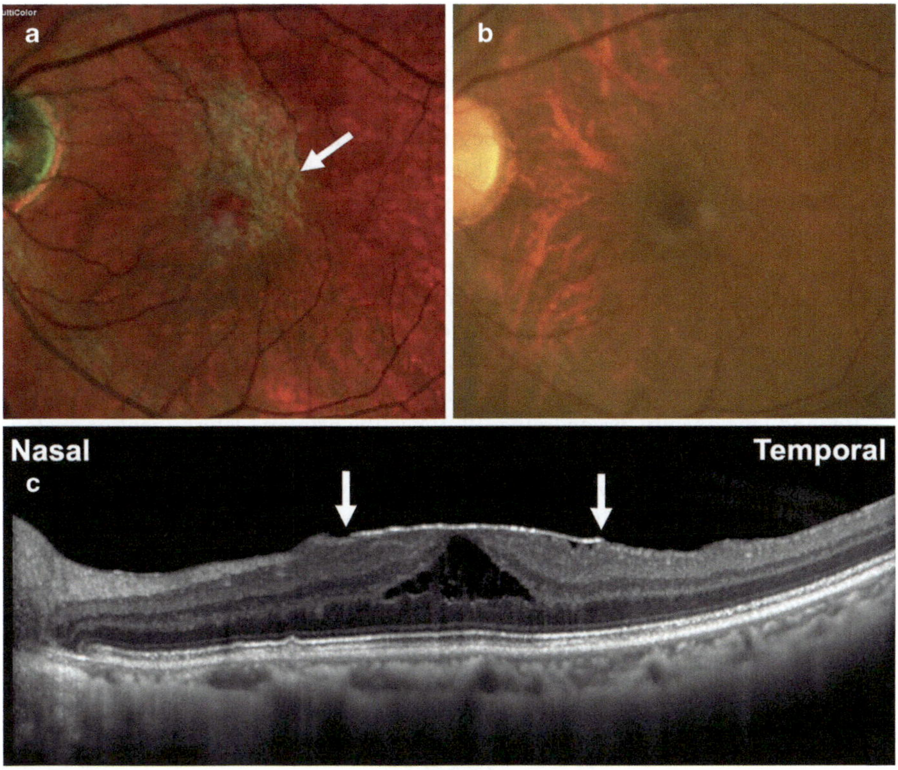

Fig. 9.2 Centrally localized ERM with high foveal adherence, increasing the difficulty of flap initiation. (**a**) Multicolor fundus imaging: Clearly delineates a localized ERM concentrated at the fovea with distinct, identifiable margins (white arrows). (**b**) Standard fundus photograph: The ERM boundaries are poorly visualized; the primary clinical sign is the loss of the foveal light reflex. (**c**) OCT: Confirms the localized nature of the ERM (demarcated by white arrows), showing focal traction and the loss of the physiological foveal depression

dense cataract masks macular symptoms. Such cases are frequently referred by cataract or general specialists after ERM is incidentally detected. In these scenarios, a conservative approach is often warranted. Initial management may include treating ocular surface issues (e.g., dry eye or foreign body sensation). If cataracts are significant, performing cataract surgery first may yield satisfactory visual improvement, potentially reducing the patient's desire for further retinal intervention.

Generally, ERM surgery has a high safety profile and is considered a foundational procedure in many specialized training programs. However, given the risk of irreversible macular damage during membrane peeling, it is traditionally performed by experienced vitreoretinal surgeons. Novice surgeons should adopt a graduated approach to training, prioritizing the principle of "Primum non nocere" (First, do no harm) before transitioning to independent practice.

9.4.2 Prognostic Factors

Most patients do not experience immediate visual improvement following surgery. Significant recovery typically occurs only after postoperative inflammation subsides and macular anatomy begins to stabilize. While approximately 60%–80% of patients eventually achieve improved visual acuity and reduced metamorphopsia, phakic patients frequently face progressive cataract formation (Fig. 9.3). This decline in vision can lead to patient anxiety during the recovery period. To mitigate this, surgeons must provide comprehensive preoperative counseling and ongoing reassurance during follow-up visits. Furthermore, clinicians should be aware that lens opacity can be underestimated without pupillary dilation; some patients may report transiently improved clarity once the pupil is dilated, highlighting the need for thorough monitoring of lens changes.

Beyond lens opacity, preoperative BCVA is the primary determinant of postoperative vision. High-resolution OCT allows surgeons to objectively quantify retinal involvement (Fig. 9.4). Key indicators of a limited visual prognosis include chronic duration, dense ERM, significant tractional elevation, and structural damage such as EZ disruption or inner plexiform layer thinning.

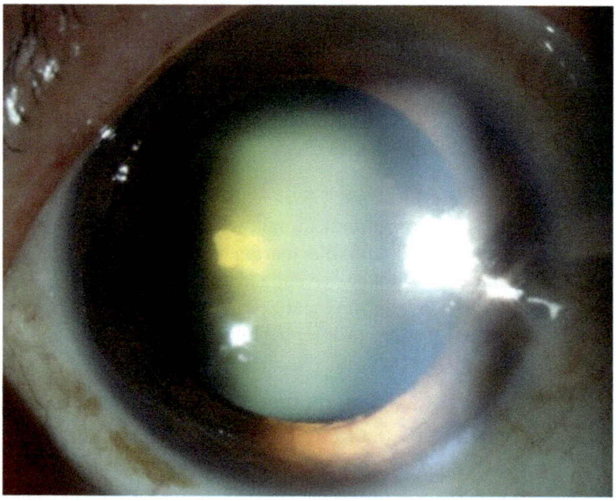

Fig. 9.3 Progression of nuclear cataract 6 months after ERM surgery. BCVA decreased from 0.6 (1-month post-op) to 0.1

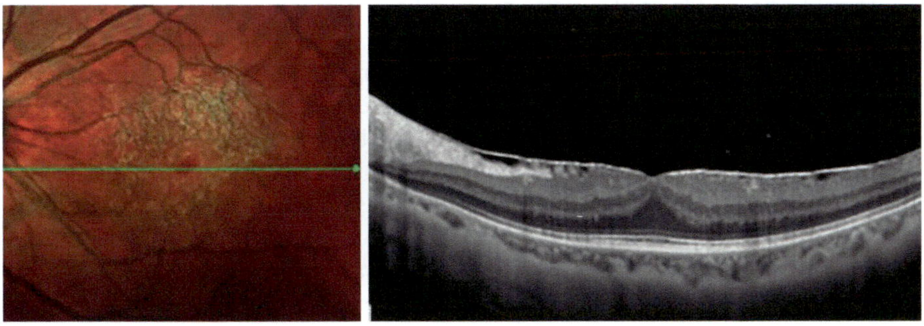

Fig. 9.4 Multicolor fundus photograph (left) and OCT (right) of a thin ERM with minimal retinal involvement and an intact ellipsoid zone. BCVA improved from 0.6 preoperatively to 0.9 following surgical intervention

9.5 Standard Surgical Steps

Approximately 60% of ERMs are associated with some degree of PVD at the time of diagnosis, which typically facilitates the surgical process. MIVS is currently the standard approach, with the 25-gauge platform offering an optimal balance between instrument rigidity, invasiveness, and surgical efficiency. Following the general principles of PPV, the procedure typically follows these steps:

1. Core vitrectomy: Resection of the central vitreous is performed, extending to the mid-periphery to create sufficient space for posterior pole maneuvers and PVD induction.
2. Confirm the presence of PVD: This step is essential for a thorough procedure. The use of triamcinolone acetonide (TA) is recommended to confirm the presence of PVD and to assist in subsequent membrane visualization.
3. Staining: Staining may be bypassed if ERM boundaries are clearly visible, allowing for direct peeling.
4. Initial flap formation: An initial flap is created at the edge of the ERM using ILM forceps. This step is considered a critical technical skill in the training of vitreoretinal surgeons.
5. Membrane peeling: The peeling is expanded with an emphasis on hand stability and controlled movements to ensure a smooth transition across the macula.
6. ILM peeling: The decision to remove the ILM remains a subject of clinical debate. The approach may be adjusted based on intraoperative findings, such as the presence of spontaneous ILM flaps.
7. Peripheral vitrectomy: Thorough shaving of the mid-peripheral vitreous is recommended to mitigate the risk of postoperative traction. Vitreous surrounding the trocar should be meticulously cleared to prevent vitreous incarceration at the incision sites.
8. Peripheral retinal examination: A 360° scleral indentation is performed to inspect the peripheral retina. Any identified retinal breaks or degenerative areas

should be addressed with surrounding vitreous removal and laser photocoagulation.
9. Intraocular tamponade: Balanced salt solution (BSS) is the standard tamponade; however, filtered air may be utilized based on surgeon preference. While some suggest air tamponade may help maintain dry incisions, this remains a theoretical benefit.
10. Incision closure: The requirement for sutures is determined by the integrity and seal of the scleral incisions. While beveled incisions are often self-sealing, suturing may be performed to ensure postoperative wound stability.

9.6 Use of Vital Dyes

In ERM surgery, staining is not strictly mandatory, as the membrane's morphology often provides sufficient contrast for dissection. However, vital dyes are frequently utilized to accentuate architectural details and ensure the safe identification of surgical planes.

Commonly used agents include triamcinolone acetonide (TA), indocyanine green (ICG), and brilliant blue G (BBG). Less frequent options include trypan blue, patent blue, and infracyanine green. It is important to note that the intraocular safety profile of these agents is dose-dependent, and surgeons must remain cognizant of potential retinal toxicity.

9.6.1 Triamcinolone Acetonide (TA)

TA suspension does not chemically stain the ERM. Instead, TA particles adhere to residual vitreous cortex or the viscous surface of the ERM, providing a "coating" effect that enhances textural details and contours.

Typically, 4 mg (0.1 mL) of TA is sufficient to visualize the posterior vitreous and membrane. A modified technique involves diluting 0.1 mL of the original suspension into 1.0 mL of balanced salt solution (BSS) prior to injection; this predilution facilitates more rapid intraocular clearance during irrigation. TA is considered highly safe for intraocular use, as it can be thoroughly aspirated during the procedure, leaving minimal residue.

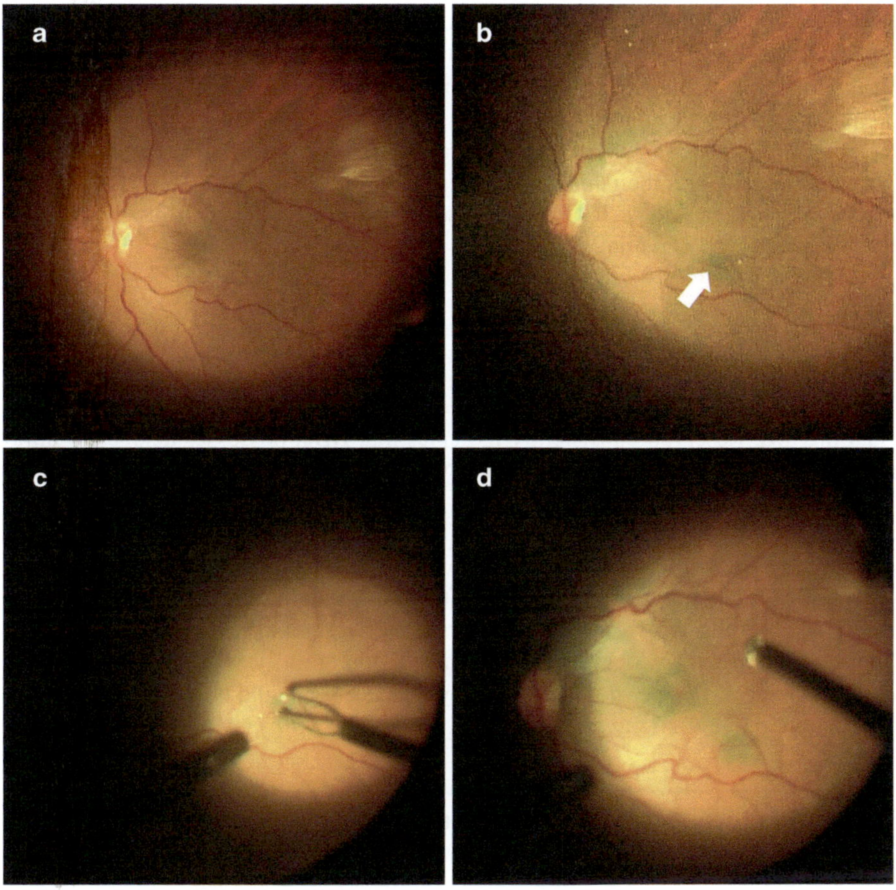

Fig. 9.5 Negative staining technique for ERM visualization. (**a**) Thin ERM with unclear contour even after TA injection, making flap initiation difficult. (**b**) After ICG injection, the ILM outside the ERM is stained, while the ERM itself is not—revealing the ERM edge (white arrows). (**c**) Successful flap initiation at the junction of the ILM and ERM using ILM forceps, with complete ERM peeling. (**d**) Reinjection of ICG after ERM peeling showing stained ILM around the fovea

9.6.2 Indocyanine Green (ICG)

ICG specifically binds to the ILM and has a negligible staining effect on the ERM itself. In ERM surgery, ICG is utilized for "negative staining" (Fig. 9.5): by staining the surrounding ILM, the non-stained ERM becomes clearly demarcated, outlining its borders for safer initiation of the peeling process.

In addition to TA, ICG is the most widely available vital dye in ophthalmic clinical practice. Its high affinity ILM has made it a preferred tool for many vitreoretinal surgeons. While a standard concentration of 5 mg/mL provides robust ILM staining, its potential retinal toxicity remains a subject of ongoing clinical debate. Four primary hypotheses have been proposed regarding ICG toxicity:

1. Osmotic imbalance: ICG may alter intraocular osmotic pressure, leading to cellular stress.
2. Phototoxicity: Intense light from the endoilluminator fiber optic may exacerbate the toxicity of the staining solution.
3. Direct retinal damage: High-concentration ICG may exert a direct toxic effect upon contact with the neurosensory retina.
4. Degradation products: ICG decomposes when exposed to light; its degradation byproducts are potentially toxic to the retina and RPE.

9.6.3 Brilliant Blue G (BBG)

BBG exhibits high affinity for the ILM and is typically utilized at a concentration of 0.25 mg/mL. Research consistently indicates that BBG possesses a superior intraocular safety profile compared to other dyes, leading to its U.S. FDA approval for intraocular use in December 2019.

In ERM surgery, vital dyes (other than TA) should be utilized judiciously and are generally reserved for cases where membrane planes are difficult to identify. When their use is necessary, surgeons must strictly manage both the concentration and the duration of exposure. To minimize the risk of phototoxicity, the endoilluminator should be directed away from the macula or temporarily withdrawn during the staining process. Furthermore, repeated dye injections should be avoided to prevent cumulative retinal toxicity.

9.7 Underlying Logic and Practical Skills of Membrane Peeling

While many professional textbooks detail ERM peeling, the majority emphasize the initial flap formation—indoubtedly the most critical phase of the procedure. However, for novice surgeons, pre-peeling preparation is equally vital. As previously noted, an epiretinal membrane is a structural abnormality with measurable elevation. To successfully leverage this physical characteristic, the surgeon must first clearly delineate the ERM margins. Establishing a distinct visual boundary significantly bolsters surgical confidence and enhances hand stability during these delicate intraoperative maneuvers.

9.7.1 Preparation

Before initiating the flap, the following conditions must be optimized:

1. Adequate anesthesia: Retrobulbar anesthesia should follow standard protocols, including sufficient orbital compression to ensure a complete block. This

minimizes patient anxiety and involuntary ocular movements, providing the stable environment necessary for delicate membrane peeling.

2. Optimal trocar placement: Strategic placement is critical for ergonomic stability. Hand movements during peeling are categorized into four components (Fig. 9.6):
   (a) Grasping: Force is generated by the thumb-index finger adduction.
   (b) Vertical Control: Controlled by wrist flexion and extension.
   (c) Horizontal control: Controlled by wrist abduction and adduction.
   (d) Rotational movement: Controlled by internal and external wrist rotation to expand the peeling range.

   The surgeon's hand should rest gently on the patient's forehead as a fulcrum, with joints above the wrist relaxed. Positioning the primary trocar at 10 o'clock (for right-handed surgeons) allows for a neutral, extended wrist. Deviation from this position forces compensatory wrist adjustments, which significantly reduces tip stability and increases the risk of "empty" or inaccurate grasping.
3. Optimizing visualization: Minimize anterior segment interference. In pseudophakic eyes with posterior capsule opacification (PCO), consider preoperative laser capsulotomy or an intraoperative clear zone creation with the vitrectomy cutter to clear the visual axis (Fig. 9.7a).

   Furthermore, remember that excessively high brightness does not necessarily enhance detail. Maintain illumination at a moderate level (e.g., 35%) and avoid placing the endoilluminator tip too close to the macula. This prevents 'overexposure,' which obscures membrane texture, induces surgeon eye fatigue, and increases the risk of phototoxicity (Fig. 9.7b).
4. Ergonomic and psychological relaxation: Sympathetic activation due to nervousness leads to muscle tension and tremors. Excessive effort to resolve macular details often leads to accommodative fatigue, shifting the focal plane anteriorly and blurring the view. For less experienced surgeons, this loss of clarity can cause undue stress and hinder the flow of the procedure.

   If tension arises, surgeons should: (1) Pause the procedure briefly to break the stress cycle; (2) Regulate breathing with deep, slow respirations; (3) Relax the posture by lowering the shoulders and momentarily looking away to ease eye strain; (4) Communicate briefly with the surgical team to help diffuse situational stress.

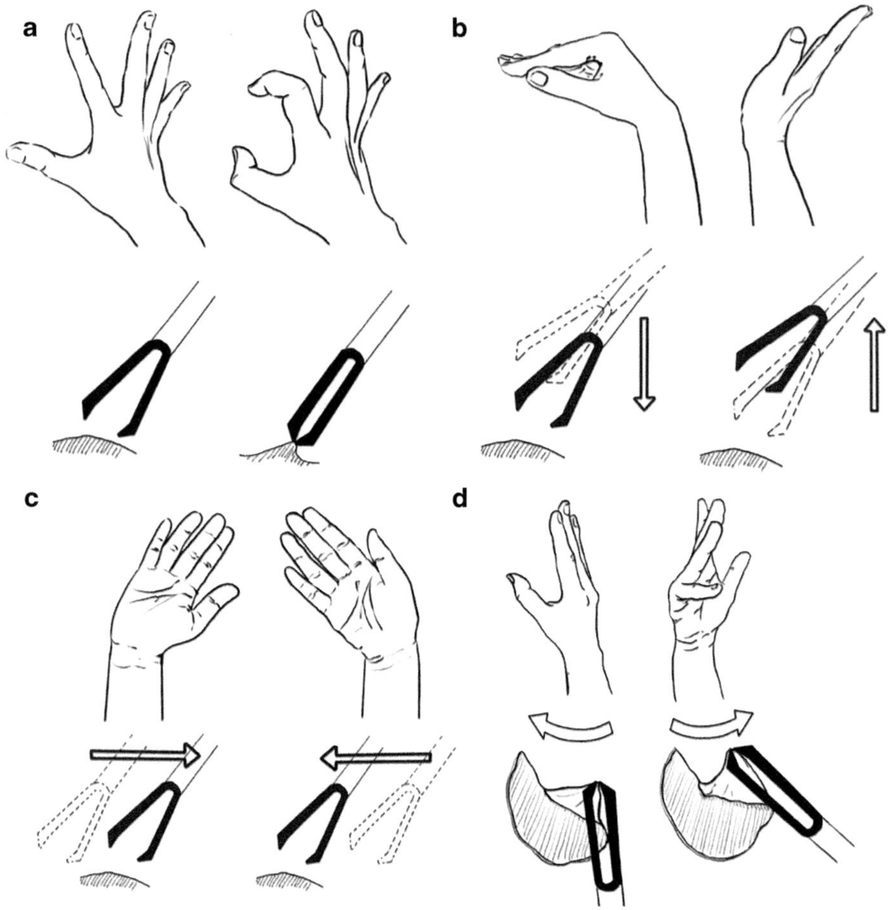

Fig. 9.6 Schematic of hand kinematics and intraocular forceps manipulation. (**a**) Grasping mechanism: Adduction of the first metacarpophalangeal (thumb-index) joint controls the opening and closing of the forceps tips. (**b**) Vertical positioning: Flexion and extension of the wrist regulate the vertical (anterior-posterior) depth of the forceps within the vitreous cavity. (**c**) Horizontal positioning: Abduction and adduction (radial and ulnar deviation) of the wrist control the horizontal (lateral) placement of the forceps. (**d**) Rotational control: Internal and external rotation (pronation and supination) of the wrist enables rotational maneuvering of the forceps, typically utilized for continuous curvilinear membrane peeling

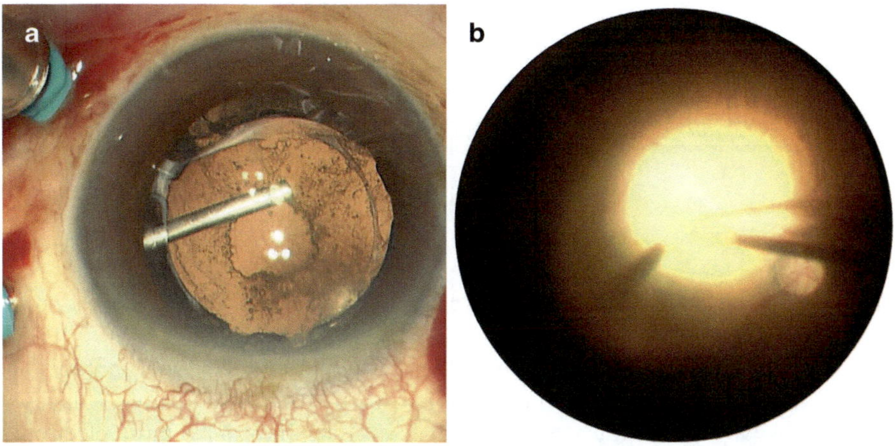

Fig. 9.7 Optimization of illumination and visualization for ERM peeling. (**a**) Clearing the visual axis: Intraoperative creation of a central opening in an opacified posterior capsule using a vitrectomy cutter to ensure an unobstructed view of the posterior pole. (**b**) Suboptimal illumination: The endoilluminator tip is positioned too close to the macula, resulting in "overexposure" (glare). This obscures fine membrane architecture while increasing the risk of surgeon eye fatigue and retinal phototoxicity

9.7.2 Flap Initiation Methods

The following techniques are essential for safe and effective flap initiation. Regardless of the chosen method, novice surgeons must prioritize safety: it is far better to "grasp thin air" (miss) than to "grasp incorrectly" (traumatize the retina).

1. Strict svoidance of high-risk zones: Flap initiation should always be performed away from retinal blood vessels. Furthermore, avoid the papillomacular bundle located between the fovea and the optic disc; injury to this area can lead to irreversible central vision loss.
2. Target the steepest margin: Selecting a "steep" or elevated ERM edge provides a more accessible target for forceps. This elevation increases the safety margin between the forceps tips and the underlying neurosensory retina (Fig. 9.8), reducing the risk of accidental retinal engagement.
3. Recognizing and halting inadvertent retinal grasping: Inadvertent retinal grasping is a risk even for experienced surgeons. Identifying this error depends on tactile feedback: the adhesion between an idiopathic ERM and the retina is typically much weaker than the attachment between the retina and the RPE. If the forceps encounter a "stiff or resistant" sensation, the surgeon must immediately release the grip to prevent a rctinal tear.
4. Avoiding sites of high adhesion: In areas where the ERM is firmly incarcerated into the retinal surface, forceful peeling can compromise retinal integrity. Indicators of excessive traction include the presence of retinal fragments on the peeled membrane or localized retinal whitening (pallor). If significant resistance is met, the surgeon should seek an alternative, less adherent initiation site.

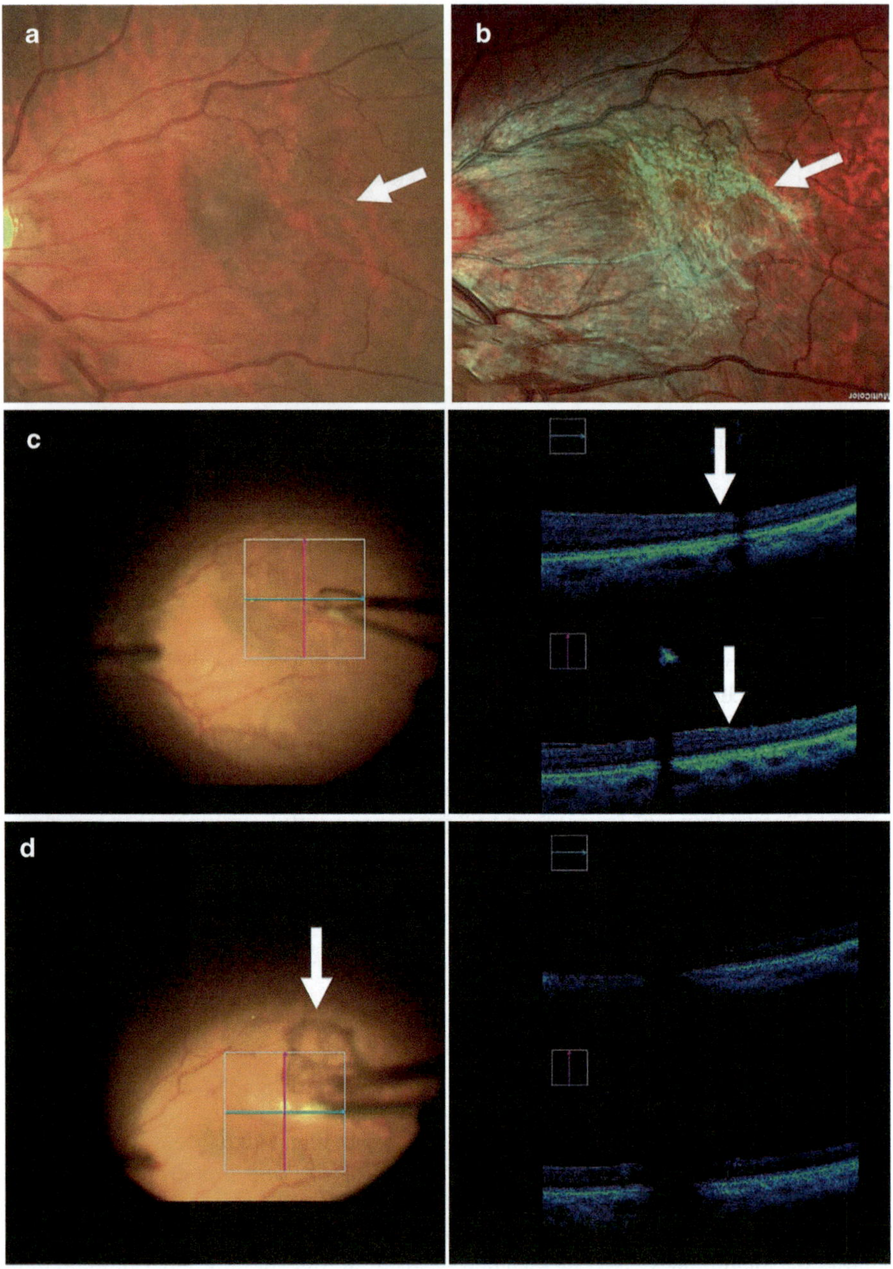

Fig. 9.8 Preoperative planning and selection of safe sites for ERM flap initiation. (**a**) Photograph suggesting a steep ERM edge approximately two-disc diameters temporal to the fovea (white arrows). (**b**) Multicolor fundus imaging confirming this observation. (**c**) iOCT verifying the predicted edge as an ideal flap initiation site, showing a steep ERM edge. (**d**) Successful ERM grasping, with iOCT confirming no residual ERM

9.7.3 Expanding the Flap

Once a flap is successfully initiated, the expansion phase is generally straightforward and carries a lower risk of iatrogenic retinal damage. For novice surgeons, the primary objective is to maintain continuous controlled movement, thereby minimizing the need for repeated re-grasping and additional flap initiations. During this process, precise wrist kinematics remain critical.

Expanding the flap relies predominantly on wrist extension and rotation, complemented by subtle radial or ulnar deviation (abduction/adduction) to modulate the trajectory. After engaging the ERM margin, the surgeon should translate the forceps in a plane tangential to the retinal surface. By avoiding vertical traction, the force is directed specifically toward the ERM–retinal interface, effectively lysing adhesions while minimizing mechanical stress on the underlying neurosensory retina.

9.7.4 Deciding Whether to Peel the ILM

ILM peeling is not always mandatory; often, portions of the ILM are sequestered and removed concurrently during ERM peeling. Whether routine ILM peeling should be performed remains a subject of ongoing clinical debate.

The potential benefits of ILM peeling include the complete removal of the scaffold for myofibroblast proliferation, which may reduce the rate of ERM recurrence. Conversely, the potential drawbacks include mechanical trauma to the superficial retinal nerve fiber layer (RNFL) and structural disruption of the Müller cell footplates.

Novice surgeons should not feel compelled to perform ILM peeling in every case. The guiding principle is pragmatic: if a vital dye has been utilized and the stained ILM is clearly visible, one may attempt to peel the identified areas. However, if no stain was used and the clinical outcome appears satisfactory, it is wise to follow the adage, "If it isn't broken, don't fix it." Avoid performing additional, potentially redundant maneuvers that require extra staining and surgical time unless clinically indicated.

9.8 Complications

9.8.1 Intraoperative Complications

(1) Hemorrhage

Unless major retinal vessels are compromised, intraoperative hemorrhage is typically punctate and self-limiting, requiring no specific intervention. Surgeons should avoid direct manipulation of the bleeding site with a flute needle or vitrectomy cutter, as mechanical irritation can exacerbate the hemorrhage and expand the area of involvement.

In rare instances of deep retinal or vascular trauma leading to significant vitreous hemorrhage, the surgeon should allow the clot to partially consolidate before attempting aspiration with a flute needle or vitrectomy cutter. Once the bleeding point is localized, hemostasis should be achieved via endophotocoagulation or cautery. Excessive energy or confluent laser applications must be avoided to minimize the risk of permanent visual field defects.

(2) Iatrogenic Retinal Breaks

The incidence of iatrogenic retinal breaks during ERM surgery is low, with most occurring during peripheral vitrectomy. These are manageable if identified early: the break should be surrounded by laser photocoagulation, followed by a filtered air or inert gas tamponade. Postoperative positioning should be dictated by the location of the break to ensure adequate internal tamponade.

(3) Lens Injury

Iatrogenic lens trauma during PPV is a known risk during the learning curve. While mild, peripheral lens touch may not impede the current procedure, severe injury requires primary intervention.

For significant lens damage, phacoemulsification is preferred over lensectomy to preserve the capsular bag, which is essential for stable intraocular lens (IOL) implantation. If secondary cataract surgery is deferred, the patient must be informed that lens opacity will progress rapidly. Regular B-scan ultrasonography is mandatory to monitor the posterior segment until the cataract is removed.

During subsequent cataract surgery in vitrectomized eyes, surgeons must account for reduced vitreous support. Maintaining anterior chamber stability and ensuring a meticulous capsulorrhexis and gentle hydrodissection are critical. Should the lens nucleus displace into the vitreous cavity, a repeat PPV is necessary for retrieval.

9.8.2 Postoperative Complications

(1) Cataract Progression

Cataract development is the most frequent postoperative complication of ERM surgery. Patients often report transient visual improvement followed by a gradual decline in acuity. This is primarily due to nuclear sclerosis, which significantly impacts vision and necessitates subsequent cataract surgery. Consequently, combined phacovitrectomy (simultaneous lens extraction and vitrectomy) is increasingly performed. However, for novice surgeons, the added complexity of a combined procedure increases intraoperative risk and is generally not recommended during the learning curve.

(2) Retinal Detachment

Although rare, postoperative retinal detachment (RD) can progress rapidly and cause severe visual loss; thus, meticulous prevention is paramount. The three primary etiologies include:

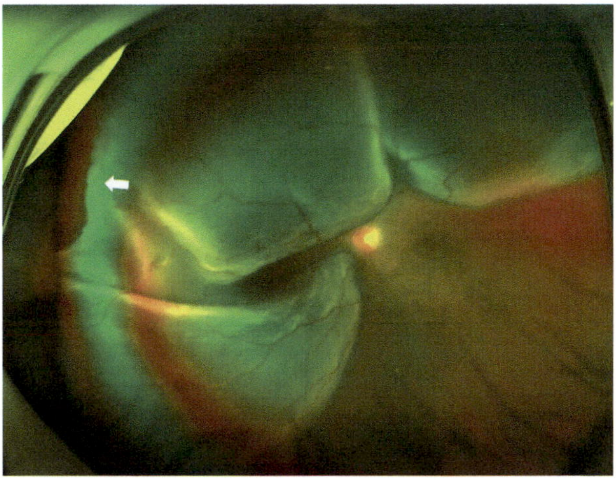

Fig. 9.9 Superior nasal retinal dialysis (white arrow) secondary to ERM surgery

1. Entry-site related breaks: Iatrogenic tears may occur if instrument tips inadvertently traumatize the peripheral retina during insertion through the trocars.
2. Undetected peripheral pathology: Inadequate 360° scleral indentation may lead to overlooked retinal breaks or pre-existing degenerative lesions.
3. Vitreous traction: Residual vitreous may become incarcerated in the scleral incisions or undergo contraction, leading to secondary retinal breaks (Fig. 9.9). Notably, the incidence of this complication has significantly decreased with the widespread adoption of small-gauge minimally invasive vitrectomy.

(3) ERM Recurrence

The long-term recurrence rate for epiretinal membrane is reported to be less than 20%. In most instances, recurrent ERM does not substantially impair visual acuity, and surgical re-intervention is typically not indicated. However, in cases of secondary ERM, the risk of recurrence may rise significantly if the underlying primary pathology—such as intraocular inflammation or vascular disease—remains poorly controlled.

9.9 Summary

ERM surgery is generally straightforward with a favorable prognosis, this high success rate often engenders elevated patient expectations—rendering surgical safety the paramount priority. Novice surgeons should adopt a deliberate approach to clinical practice, meticulously refining their maneuvers to develop techniques tailored to their individual skill sets. When encountering intraoperative challenges during membrane peeling, it is vital to adhere to the principle advocated by Steve Charles: "Be patient, be persistent, slow is better." As the saying goes, "The shortest way is often the most reliable one," reminding us that precision should never be sacrificed for speed.

Surgical Intervention of the Macular Hole 10

A macular hole (MH) is a lamellar or full-thickness defect of the neurosensory retina at the fovea. It predominantly affects individuals over the age of 50, with a higher prevalence in women and a bilateral incidence ranging from 20% to 30%. The primary clinical manifestations include diminished visual acuity, metamorphopsia, and central scotomata. Optical coherence tomography (OCT) has become the gold standard for diagnosing MH, providing precise imaging data essential for understanding its pathogenesis and evaluating surgical prognosis.

While surgical intervention for MH has existed for only three decades, high success rates have driven vitreoretinal surgeons to continuously refine techniques, significantly advancing the surgical paradigm. Notably, MH surgery is unique among vitreoretinal procedures as it is perhaps the only intervention capable of facilitating the anatomical restoration of a neurosensory tissue defect. Consequently, surgical management must prioritize the preservation of healthy retinal tissue. The ultimate goal is to achieve closure with minimal trauma, ensuring the restored macula can effectively perceive and transmit light—a fundamental principle for every vitreoretinal surgeon.

10.1 How Macular Hole Became a Curable Disease: Lessons for Surgeons

In 1869, the German-American ophthalmologist Hermann Knapp first reported a case of traumatic MH. Notably, he also founded the journal in which this case was published—*Archives of Ophthalmology* (now *JAMA Ophthalmology*)—that same year. In 1871, Henry Noyes, a New York-based physician, provided the first comprehensive clinical description of traumatic MH. The term "hole at the macula" was later coined in 1900 by the British surgeon F.M. Ogilvie. While MH was initially categorized as a degenerative condition, subsequent research identified vitreomacular traction as its primary etiologic factor. Donald Gass further advanced the field

Z. Zhang, U. Spandau, *Vitreoretinal Surgery*,
https://doi.org/10.1007/978-3-032-25271-5_10

with his seminal work on MH pathogenesis and the development of the widely adopted clinical staging system.

The transformation of MH into a surgically curable disease is credited to the pioneering work of American physicians Neil Kelly and Robert Wendel. On October 31, 1989, at the *American Academy of Ophthalmology* (AAO) meeting in New Orleans, they reported that MH could be successfully closed via pars plana vitrectomy (PPV). Despite initial skepticism from their peers, their subsequent research validated the high success rate of PPV, ushering in an era of rapid innovation and surgical refinement.

Medical progress often follows three stages of enlightenment: from innocence, through complexity, to enlightened simplicity. Every leap in science is born from the tension between conventional wisdom and the innovative spirit of the few. It is the twin engines of relentless exploration and rigorous validation that propel us through the doorway to new medical frontiers.

Before MH was recognized as curable, the internal limiting membrane (ILM) was long considered a vital structure that should remain undisturbed. Early observations during epiretinal membrane (ERM) surgery noted that inadvertent ILM peeling could occur, raising concerns about irreversible functional damage. However, clinical experiences with Terson syndrome demonstrated that removing the ILM to evacuate sub-ILM hemorrhages significantly improved visual outcomes without long-term complications. To solidify this evidence, electron microscopy confirmed that the membrane removed in these procedures was indeed the ILM.

Beginning in 1995, surgeons began deliberately peeling the ILM to improve MH closure rates. Subsequent multicenter studies confirmed its therapeutic value. Despite its recognized importance, the technique remained technically demanding due to poor ILM visualization and limited instrumentation.

In 2000, the introduction of indocyanine green (ICG) for ILM staining revolutionized the procedure, marking the beginning of the "staining era." While subsequent studies revealed potential retinal toxicity associated with ICG, it remains widely used due to its superior staining contrast. Conversely, research has confirmed the higher safety profile of brilliant blue G (BBG), which was approved by the U.S. FDA in late 2019 for intraocular use.

In 2010, Zosia Michalewska from Łódź, Poland, first published a randomized controlled study in *Ophthalmology* on the use of inverted ILM flap coverage for treating large-diameter MH, marking the beginning of the "ILM flap technology" era in MH treatment. Beyond innovations in ILM manipulation, attempts have also been made to fill MH with amniotic membrane, lens capsule, or retinal grafts to promote hole closure.

This evolution is a microcosm of the unique charm of retinal surgery. Its inherent delicacy and the need for intuitive solutions allow every surgeon to contribute to its progress. Often, the driving force for such innovation originates from clinicians who bridge the gap between bedside practice and scientific research.

10.2 Classification and Staging of MH

10.2.1 Classification

Macular holes are categorized into several distinct clinical types. Given that high-resolution OCT readily differentiates pseudomacular holes and lamellar MH, these subtypes are not detailed here.

1. Idiopathic macular hole (IMH): This is the most common form, typically age-related with no identifiable external etiology. IMH generally presents the lowest surgical complexity and the most favorable functional prognosis (Fig. 10.1).
2. Hypermyopic macular hole: A severe complication of pathological myopia, typically occurring in eyes with a refractive error exceeding −6.00 diopters (D) or an axial length greater than 26.5 mm. These holes are frequently associated with posterior staphyloma, choroidal atrophy, and macular retinoschisis. Surgical management is technically demanding, with lower primary closure rates and prolonged anatomical recovery compared to idiopathic cases (Fig. 10.2).
3. Traumatic macular hole: This results from blunt ocular trauma, where sudden anteroposterior compression leads to acute equatorial expansion. The resulting vitreoretinal traction and retinal tension cause a rupture at the fovea—the thinnest portion of the neurosensory retina. These cases are often complicated by retinal edema, vitreous hemorrhage, or commotio retinae. Traumatic holes are usually large, resulting in significant visual loss and dense central scotomata. Recently, macular injuries caused by laser pointers have emerged as an increasingly common subset of this category (Fig. 10.3).

10.2.2 Staging of Idiopathic Macular Hole (IMH)

The staging of IMH now primarily relies on OCT, which allows surgeons to determine optimal surgical timing and predict visual prognosis. In clinical research, documenting the specific stage and minimum hole diameter for each case is essential for data analysis. The classification system originally proposed by Gass remains the clinical standard; a concise overview is provided below:

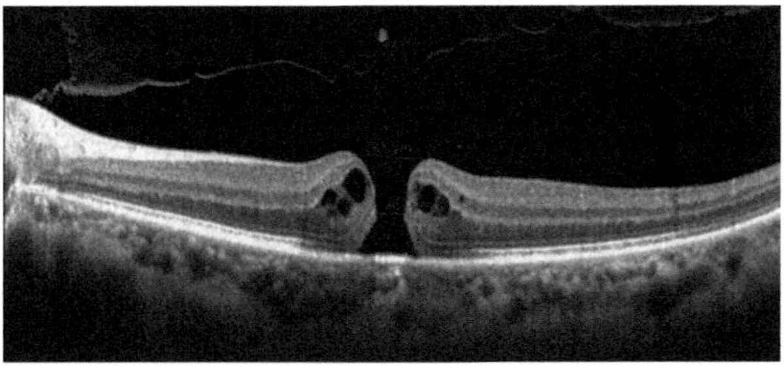

Fig. 10.1 OCT image of idiopathic macular hole

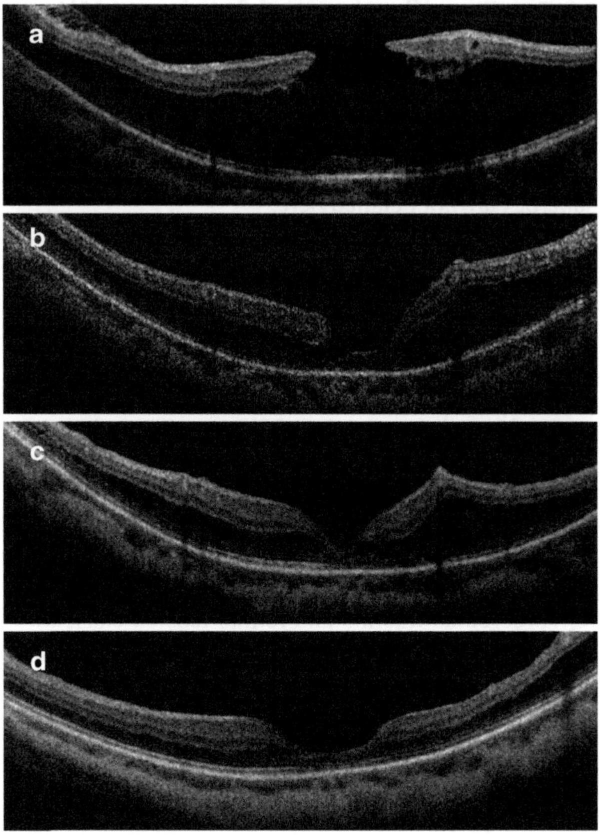

Fig. 10.2 Preoperative and postoperative OCT images of hypermyopic macular hole. (**a**) Preoperative OCT shows macular hole with extensive shallow retinal detachment in the posterior pole. (**b**) OCT at 2 weeks postoperatively shows partial closure of the macular hole and improvement of retinal detachment. (**c**) OCT at 1 month postoperatively shows nearly complete healing of the macular hole and almost resolution of retinal detachment. (**d**) Postoperative OCT shows complete closure of the hole and good retinal reattachment

1. Stage 1 (impending MH): This stage represents the earliest phase, characterized by a partial-thickness foveal detachment without a full-thickness break (Fig. 10.4). Surgical intervention is generally not indicated at this stage, but rigorous monitoring is essential, as approximately 50% of cases progress to full-thickness defects.
2. Stage 2: Characterized by a full-thickness retinal cleavage with a diameter <400 μm.These typically develop within weeks to months following Stage 1. Patients usually begin to experience symptomatic metamorphopsia and central scotomata, and surgical intervention is generally recommended.
3. Stage 3: A full-thickness hole with a diameter ≥400 μm in the absence of a complete posterior vitreous detachment (PVD). The hole is typically round, often accompanied by cystic edema at the margins and a visible operculum (hole cover). Despite the larger size, surgical closure rates remain high, and active intervention is advisable.
4. Stage 4: A full-thickness macular hole associated with complete PVD, clinically evidenced by a Weiss ring. Many patients are already at this stage upon initial consultation. While anatomical success rates remain high, prolonged duration or

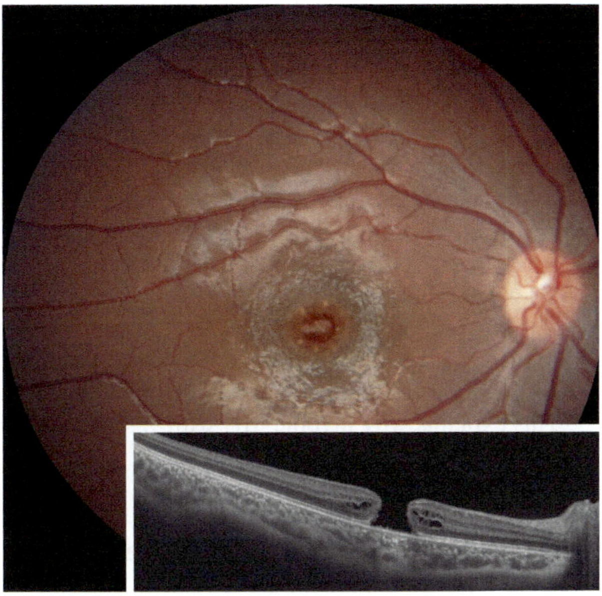

Fig. 10.3 Fundus photograph and OCT image of macular hole caused by direct laser pointer irradiation

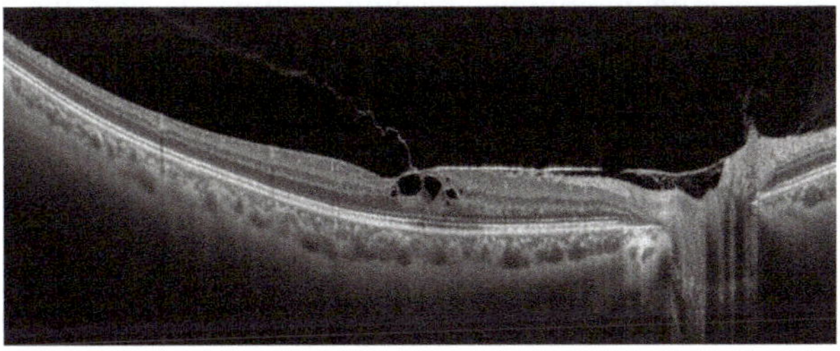

Fig. 10.4 OCT image of Stage 1 macular hole. The patient complained of metamorphopsia for 1 week

excessive hole diameter may limit the quality of visual recovery. Comprehensive preoperative counseling is essential to manage patient expectations regarding functional outcomes.

10.3 Etiology of Macular Hole

Modern understanding of macular hole (MH) pathogenesis remains rooted in Gass's 1988 theory, which posits that tangential traction from the posterior vitreous cortex drives hole formation. This hypothesis, later validated by OCT, suggests that alleviating this traction can prevent progression.

Beyond the Gass model, four primary factors are now recognized as contributors to the pathogenesis of idiopathic, traumatic, and myopic MH:

1. Vitreoretinal tangential traction: During incomplete PVD, the posterior vitreous cortex remains adherent to the thin foveal nerve fiber layer. Multidirectional

tangential forces exerted during ocular movement lead to foveal dehiscence. In early-stage MH, managing these forces is critical to prevent hole enlargement.
2. Vitreoretinal anteroposterior traction: Vitreous liquefaction and shrinkage can exert forward-pulling forces on the macula. This mechanism is particularly significant in myopic MH, where progressive posterior staphyloma exacerbates the destructive tractional role of the vitreous.
3. ILM contraction and tension: The significant improvement in closure rates following ILM peeling identifies ILM shrinkage as a key factor in MH development. In cases where the ILM is stiff and under tension, peeling often reveals a distinct separation from the underlying retina, typically correlating with a favorable surgical prognosis.
4. Vascular and epiretinal tension: Reduced elasticity of the retinal vessels or the ERM can restrict retinal extensibility, resulting in tangential stress on the fovea. This explains why myopic MH with vascular rigidity often exhibits suboptimal postoperative closure rates.

10.4 Routine Surgical Procedures

MH surgery is technically similar to ERM. The primary clinical distinctions lie in the specific membrane peeling techniques and the requirement for intraocular tamponade.

For novice surgeons, the most common challenges include iatrogenic lens injury and technical difficulty during ILM flap initiation or peeling.

1. PVD induction: Following core vitrectomy, the focus shifts to inducing PVD. Triamcinolone acetonide (TA) is utilized to visualize the posterior hyaloid. If the cortex is tightly adherent, a breakthrough point can be sought in the mid-periphery. By creating a small incision in the posterior cortex, irrigation fluid can enter the subhyaloid space, accelerating the separation and facilitating a complete PVD.
2. Staining: Prior to staining, the macular surface must be cleared of residual vitreous or ERM. While indocyanine green (ICG) remains common, its efficacy depends heavily on the interface condition (Fig. 10.5). If residual cortex or ERM covers the macula, ILM staining will be incomplete or absent. In such cases, TA should be used to identify and remove the overlying tissue before re-staining. Alternatively, if the visibility allows, the ERM and ILM can be peeled as a single complex.
3. Flap initiation: Using end-gripping forceps to create an initial ILM flap is the most demanding step for beginners. The technique and tactile feedback differ significantly from ERM peeling; specific maneuvers are detailed in subsequent sections.
4. Extending the ILM peeling range: Expanding the ILM rhexis requires higher precision than ERM peeling due to the fragile nature of the ILM and the risk of underlying retinal trauma.

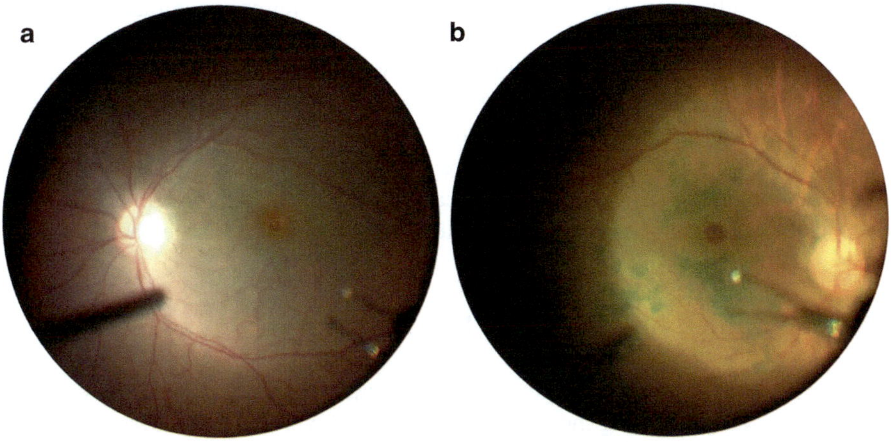

Fig. 10.5 ICG-stained ILM. (**a**) Uniform ILM staining: A consistent staining pattern typically suggests a clean vitreoretinal interface and lower peeling complexity. (**b**) Mottled ILM staining: Non-stained patches often indicate overlying residual vitreous cortex or epiretinal membrane (ERM), which increases surgical difficulty. Novice surgeons must maintain "3D anatomical layer awareness" throughout the procedure. It is essential to avoid premature flap initiation in poorly stained areas to prevent inadvertent trauma to the underlying neurosensory retina

5. Comprehensive peripheral vitrectomy and examination: Although partial vitrectomy is sometimes discussed, novice surgeons should perform a thorough peripheral vitrectomy under 360° scleral indentation. This mitigates risks associated with residual vitreous, such as: (1) Tangential traction on the fovea hindering hole closure; (2) Visual disturbances (floaters) from subsequent vitreous liquefaction; (3) Secondary retinal detachment resulting from peripheral vitreous contraction.
6. Air/fluid exchange: This can be achieved through passive aspiration via a flute needle or active aspiration with a vitrectomy cutter. For increased safety and control, a flute needle is recommended for beginners.
7. Intraocular tamponade: Long-acting gas is the standard choice. Following fluid-air exchange and wound closure, approximately 0.6 mL of pure C_3F_8 is typically injected. The patient must then adhere to a strict face-down position postoperatively.

10.5 Use of Dyes

10.5.1 Commonly Used Dyes

In clinical practice within China, the most frequently utilized dyes are ICG, trypan blue (TB), and brilliant blue G (BBG). Among these, BBG is recognized for its superior safety profile in both experimental and clinical research, typically applied at a concentration of 0.25%. Despite the advantages of newer agents, ICG remains the most widely used dye due to its exceptional staining contrast and broad availability.

While not strictly mandatory, vital dyes play a more critical role in MH surgery than in ERM procedures. Although the history of ILM staining spans only two decades, current evidence suggests that dye assistance significantly reduces surgical complexity, enhances anatomical closure rates, and contributes to superior functional outcomes. The specific biochemical properties and safety profiles of these dyes were detailed in the preceding chapter and will not be reiterated here.

10.5.2 Modified Approaches to ILM Staining

Unlike epiretinal membrane surgery, direct dye injection for macular holes carries a risk of the agent contacting the exposed nerve fiber layer and the underlying retinal pigment epithelium (RPE). Over the past two decades, awareness of dye toxicity has grown, leading to several methods aimed at enhancing intraocular safety:

1. Optimizing dye concentration: The standard concentration of ICG historically used in China is 0.25% (2.5 mg/mL). However, research has explored significantly lower concentrations, such as 0.125%, 0.05%, and 0.025%. Currently, 0.05% ICG is regarded as relatively safe, not only due to the reduced chemical load but also because its osmolarity (approximately 290 mOsm/L) is nearly isotonic to the vitreous.
2. Minimizing exposure time and surface area: Vital dyes should not remain in the vitreous cavity longer than necessary. When using high-concentration dyes (e.g., 0.5% ICG), the solution should be aspirated immediately after injection. For lower concentrations, a short retention period (typically under 30 seconds) is acceptable. To further reduce phototoxicity, the endoilluminator should be withdrawn or directed away during the staining phase.

   Additionally, Some surgeons dilute ICG with a 5% glucose solution (approximately 278 mOsm/L) to create an isotonic environment that protects the retina. The increased density of the glucose solution allows the dye to settle directly onto the posterior pole, minimizing dispersion. For example, mixing 0.25% ICG with 50% hypertonic glucose in a 9:1 ratio achieves the desired 5% glucose concentration, ensuring both isotonicity and localized delivery.
3. The "Yin-Yang" staining method: Pioneered by Rizzo, this technique involves placing a small droplet of heavy water (perfluorocarbon liquid) directly over the macular hole to act as a shield. Subsequently, 0.05% ICG (diluted with 5% glucose) is injected, and the eyeball is gently rotated. This ensures comprehensive ILM staining while preventing any direct contact between the ICG and the exposed RPE at the base of the hole.

Furthermore, the author (Zhang) have implemented an alternative 'Yin-Yang' staining technique (Fig. 10.6): following core vitrectomy and PVD induction, a small drop of TA suspension is injected directly into the MH to act as a temporary

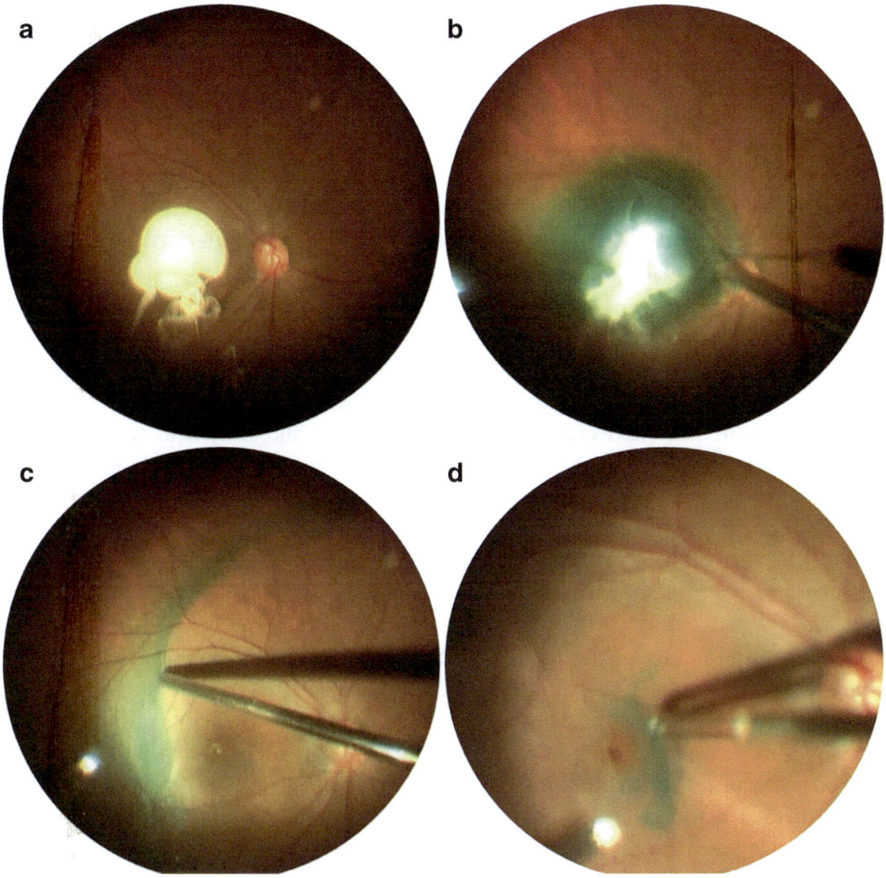

Fig. 10.6 "Yin-yang" staining method for ILM. (**a**) Injecting TA suspension to cover the macular hole and its surrounding area. (**b**) Injecting ICG dissolved in glucose to stain the area outside the TA coverage. (**c**) Aspirating ICG and TA, showing that the ILM covered by TA is unstained. (**d**) Initiating the flap from the stained area and extending the peeling range

plug. Subsequently, the ICG solution (0.25% ICG mixed with 50% glucose at a 9:1 ratio) is injected over the posterior pole for staining. Once the residual ICG is aspirated using a vitrectomy cutter or flute needle, the TA plug is removed from the MH. This refined approach provides exceptional ILM staining while providing a robust mechanical barrier against RPE toxicity.

It is crucial to recognize that the safety and efficacy of a staining agent depend on a multifaceted evaluation of its properties. Regardless of the surgical technique employed, the following factors must be comprehensively assessed. (1)Intrinsic toxicity: One must consider the chemical profile of both the vital dye and its solvent, as certain agents can cause direct cellular damage to the RPE or neurosensory retina; (2) Osmolarity: Often overlooked in clinical practice, the osmolarity of the solution is a critical determinant of safety. Non-physiologic osmolarity—particularly hypotonicity—can induce severe retinal stress and apoptosis; (3) Synergistic toxicity: It is essential to evaluate whether the interaction between the dye and its solvent produces or enhances toxic effects, especially when exposed to high-intensity endoillumination; (4) Efficiency of clearance: Rapid and complete aspiration minimizes the duration of toxic exposure and prevents long-term complications associated with residual dye.

10.6 Underlying Logic and Practical Skills of Internal Limiting Membrane Peeling

ILM is the basement membrane of the retinal Müller cell footplates, composed primarily of type IV collagen. Its thickness varies significantly across the retina: approximately 400 nm in the periphery, increasing to about 1,400 nm in the perimacular region. The ILM contributes nearly 50% of the structural rigidity of the retinal nerve fiber layer (RNFL). Unlike pathological epiretinal membranes, the ILM is a continuous, translucent, and smooth layer without pre-existing edges or folds. While the technique resembles the continuous curvilinear capsulorhexis in cataract surgery, the clinical priority is fundamentally different: the underlying neurosensory retina must be strictly preserved, whereas the lens cortex is intended for removal.

ILM peeling is one of the most demanding procedures in vitreoretinal surgery, characterized by a steep learning curve. As with epiretinal membrane surgery, the "flap initiation" phase is the most critical and technically challenging step for novice surgeons.

The mechanics of ILM flap initiation rely on applying tensile stress to the membrane surface using micro-forceps. By engaging the ILM at two minute contact points and applying traction, the surgeon induces focal strain. When this stress exceeds the membrane's tensile strength, a controlled tear occurs, allowing the flap to be initiated. Consequently, surgeons must focus on the precision and fluidity of the "pinching" and "lifting" maneuvers to achieve a successful flap without traumatizing the underlying retinal architecture.

10.6.1 Challenges for Novice Surgeons

Novice surgeons learning ILM peeling often face significant psychological pressure, which manifests in the following clinical challenges:

1. Exacerbated Hand Tremors: The physiological resting tremor of the human hand typically has an amplitude of 100 μm and a frequency of 6–12 Hz. Under surgical stress, both parameters increase significantly. Beyond psychological tension, factors such as fatigue, hunger, caffeine intake, and cold temperatures can further compromise hand stability.
2. Surgical field defocus: (Instrument Myopia and Defocus): When utilizing surgical microscopes, novices often unconsciously employ ocular accommodation,

shifting the focal plane anterior to the instrument's intended focal point (Fig. 10.7). This phenomenon, known as "instrument myopia," is inversely correlated with surgeon proficiency; less experienced physicians may induce 1–2 D of myopia. This subtle defocusing blurs the surgical field, severely compromising the extreme precision required for ILM peeling. Experienced surgeons mitigate this by maintaining relaxation and using the microscope foot pedal for micro-adjustments.

3. Depth Perception and Spatial Judgment: Because the ILM is a smooth, continuous layer lacking anatomical markers or folds, judging the vertical depth of intraocular instruments is exceptionally difficult. An overly superficial maneuver results in "empty" grasping, while excessive depth leads to retinal trauma and hemorrhage (Fig. 10.8). In severe cases, this can cause permanent visual field defects. The resulting "fear of injury" often leads to a cycle of anxiety and intraoperative stress.

These three negative factors often interact and reinforce one another, causing the procedure to stall during this critical phase. The solution lies in managing intraoperative stress through a deliberate approach: pause (rather than rushing), observe (confirming the clarity of ILM staining), and strategize (determining the optimal site for flap initiation and the precise manipulation of the end-gripping forceps).

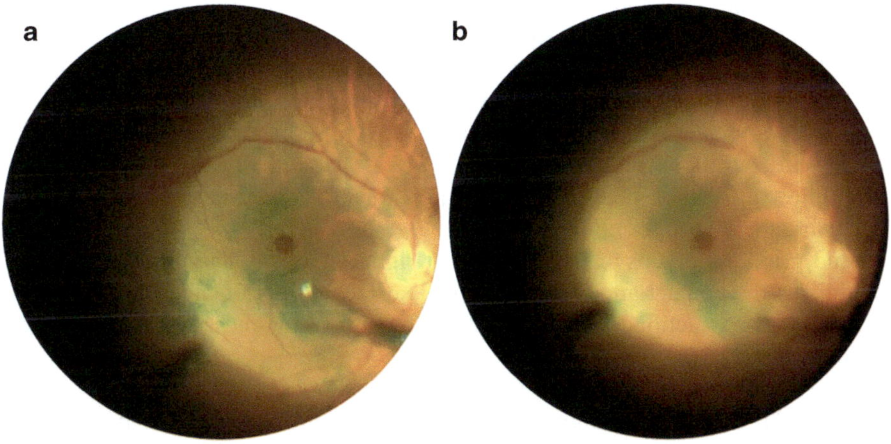

Fig. 10.7 Surgical field defocus caused by accommodative "instrument myopia." (**a**) Optimal visualization: Prior to the onset of instrument myopia, the image observed through the eyepieces remains in precise focus, matching the clarity of the digital capture from the integrated camera. (**b**) Induced defocus: When instrument myopia occurs, the surgeon's unconscious accommodation blurs the image within the eyepieces. To restore clarity, the surgeon must either refocus using the microscope foot pedal or compensate by adjusting the eyepiece diopter settings (typically by –1.0 to –2.0 D)

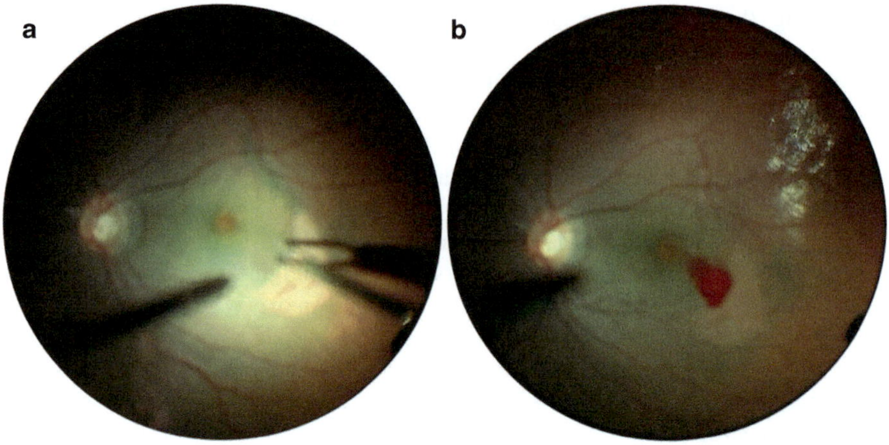

Fig. 10.8 Challenges in depth perception during ILM peeling. (**a**) Insufficient depth: The tips of the end-gripping forceps are positioned slightly above the ILM, resulting in an "empty" or failed grasp. (**b**) Excessive depth: The forceps are positioned too deep, traumatizing the underlying neurosensory retina. Although the ILM is successfully engaged, iatrogenic hemorrhage occurs as a result of mechanical injury

10.6.2 Flap Initiation Techniques

Flap initiation should avoid the nasal side of the macular hole to protect the papillomacular bundle, as injury to this area can lead to permanent central vision loss and scotomata. The preferred sites are the superotemporal or inferotemporal regions, approximately 1000–1500 μm from the hole margin (roughly one optic disc diameter). Proximity to the hole increases the risk of foveal trauma, while initiation too far into the periphery is hindered by the diminishing thickness of the ILM.

While various instruments are available, end-gripping forceps remain the most widely utilized tool for ILM peeling in the era of minimally invasive vitrectomy. The following section details the techniques for initiating and extending the ILM flap using these specialized forceps.

End-gripping forceps feature sharp, near-right-angle tips. This ergonomic design minimizes the contact area with the retinal surface during engagement, providing sufficient sharp traction to tear the ILM while minimizing mechanical stress on the underlying neurosensory retina.

1. Maintain a neutral, straight wrist and rest the ulnar side of the hand on the patient's forehead to ensure a stable fulcrum.
2. Adopt a "pen-grip" posture. As the forceps approach the macula, optimize microscope magnification and center the macular hole in the field of view to ensure focused illumination.
3. Calibrate the endoilluminator. Intensity should typically be maintained at 30%–35%. Avoid placing the light tip too close to the macula to prevent "overexposure" (glare), which obscures textural details and induces surgeon eye fatigue.

4. Slightly open the forceps and gently engage the ILM with the tip. While applying a controlled squeeze through the finger joints, lift the forceps by slightly extending the wrist. This "pinch-and-lift" motion creates a focal tear. The maneuver must be subtle and precise—evoking the image of a "dragonfly skimming the water" (Fig. 10.9).
5. After each pinch attempt, regardless of success, briefly pause and retract the forceps slightly to observe and assess the tissue response (Fig. 10.10).
6. If an attempt fails or results in a focal hemorrhage, select an alternative safe site to retry (Fig. 10.11).
7. Upon confirmation of a successful ILM tear, proceed to expand the peeling rhexis.

10.6.3 Extending the ILM Flap

1. If a clear separation exists between the ILM flap and the underlying retina, conventional peeling techniques may be employed: securely grasp the edge of the flap at its basal "platform" and steadily expand the peeling area (Fig. 10.12).
2. If only a focal tear is visible without an identifiable gap, continue applying the "pinch-and-lift" maneuver at the ILM margin. This subtle lifting action increases the sub-ILM space, facilitating a safer transition to continuous peeling (Fig. 10.13).
3. Should both maneuvers fail to yield an adequate flap, re-initiate the process at an alternative site. If necessary, re-apply vital dye to enhance contrast and ensure precise identification of the ILM.

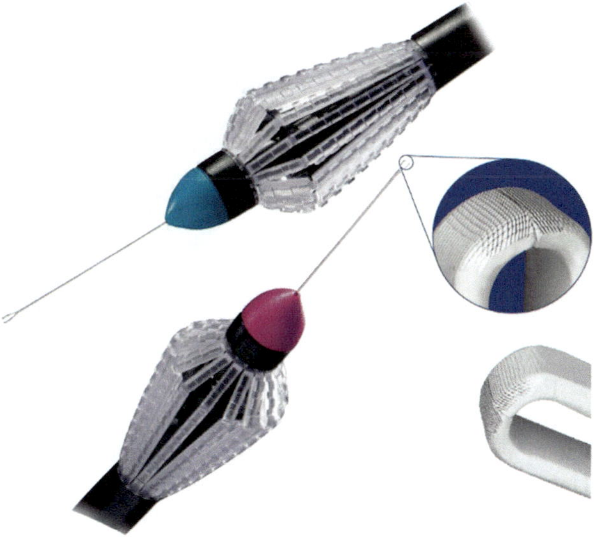

Fig. 10.9 Toothed end-gripping forceps. The right-angle tips at both ends are used for ILM flap initiation (photo courtesy of Alcon)

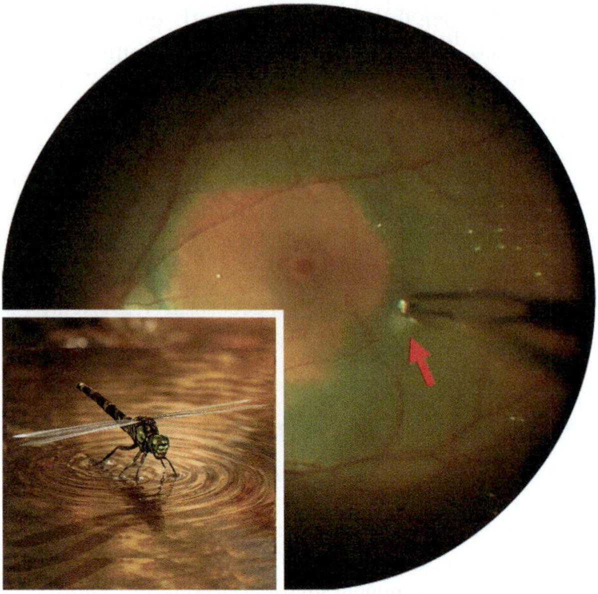

Fig. 10.10 Following "Yin-Yang" staining of the ILM with triamcinolone acetonide (TA) and indocyanine green (ICG), a subtle "pinch-and-lift" maneuver—delicate as a "dragonfly skimming the water"—is performed to initiate the flap at the margin of the stained area. The sharp tips of the end-gripping forceps engage the membrane with minimal surface contact, inducing a focal tear (red arrow) in the taut ILM

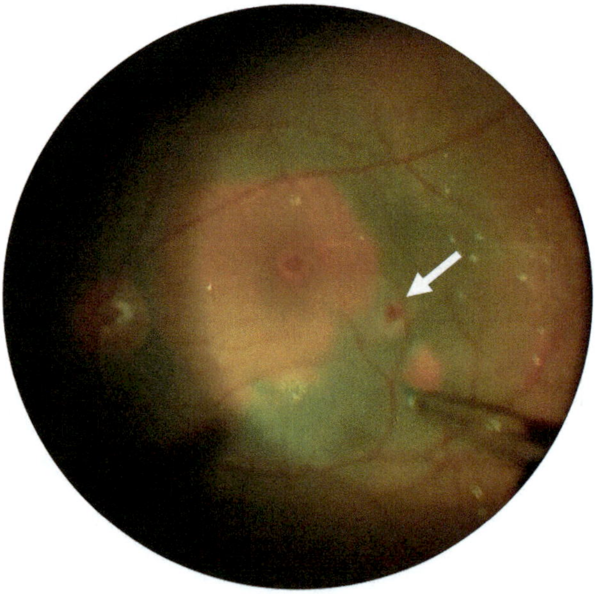

Fig. 10.11 A focal hemorrhage occurs at the initial attempt site (white arrow) due to mechanical trauma during ILM engagement. The site is promptly abandoned, and an alternative safe zone is selected for re-initiation of the flap

Extending the ILM peeling area typically requires a controlled maneuver analogous to "continuous curvilinear capsulorhexis" in cataract surgery. Utilizing internal or external wrist rotation helps maintain a steady, circular peeling motion. Unlike flap initiation, if the membrane tears or breaks during this stage, it generally does not significantly increase the surgical complexity, as the established flap edge can be readily re-engaged.

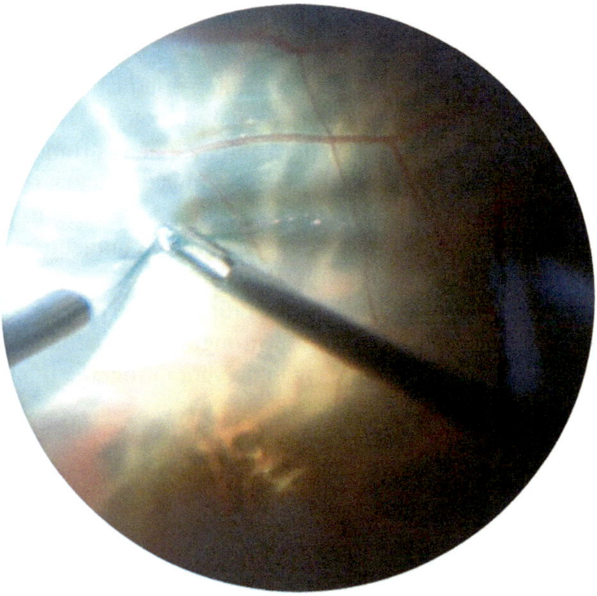

Fig. 10.12 This technique is ideal when the ILM is loosely adherent to the underlying neurosensory retina, providing a clear sub-ILM surgical plane. By gently grasping the flap's leading edge, the surgeon can steadily expand the peeling rhexis with minimal traction on the retinal architecture

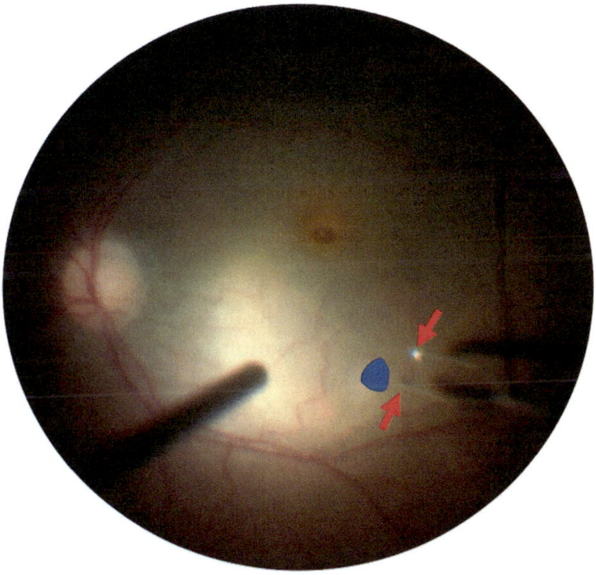

Fig. 10.13 Controlled "pinch-and-lift" maneuver to expand a focal ILM tear. A subtle "pinch-and-lift" motion is applied at the margin of the initial ILM tear (blue area, indicated by the red arrow) to elevate the membrane and develop a surgical plane. This technique is particularly effective when the ILM is highly adherent to the underlying neurosensory retina, lacking the spontaneous separation required for conventional grasping

In patients with high myopia (particularly those with an axial length ≥30 mm), both ILM flap initiation and extension are exceptionally challenging. These difficulties stem from: (1) Poor ILM staining contrast; (2) The presence of adherent macular retinoschisis or residual cortical vitreous; (3) Extreme axial length, which may exceed the reach of standard intraocular instruments; (4) Posterior staphyloma, which creates a steep, irregular contour that lacks a stable operating plane for the temporal ILM. To manage these challenges, surgeons may consider switching from a wide-angle viewing system to a corneal contact lens for higher magnification and better depth perception. If standard forceps are too short, one may utilize specialized long-reach forceps or temporarily remove the trocar to extend the instrument's effective intraocular length. Throughout the procedure, maneuvers must be executed with extreme delicacy to prevent iatrogenic injury to the thinned, fragile neurosensory retina.

10.6.4 ILM Flap Techniques

Advanced ILM flap techniques, such as coverage and insertion maneuvers, have revolutionized the management of complex macular holes. Mastery of standard ILM peeling remains a prerequisite for exploring these specialized approaches. For large or chronic macular holes, these flap-based strategies significantly improve primary surgical success by providing a biological scaffold for anatomical repair (Fig. 10.14).

10.7 Complications

While complications for MH and ERM surgery are generally similar, MH procedures involve more intensive use of vital dyes, necessitating close monitoring for dye-related retinal toxicity and visual field loss. Precision during ILM peeling is critical, as iatrogenic damage from forceps can lead to irreversible functional deficits. For cases involving non-closure or recurrence, the decision to re-operate should be based on a realistic evaluation of potential benefits. Furthermore, specialized macular hole tamponade or 'massage' maneuvers must be approached with caution due to their potential for further retinal trauma.

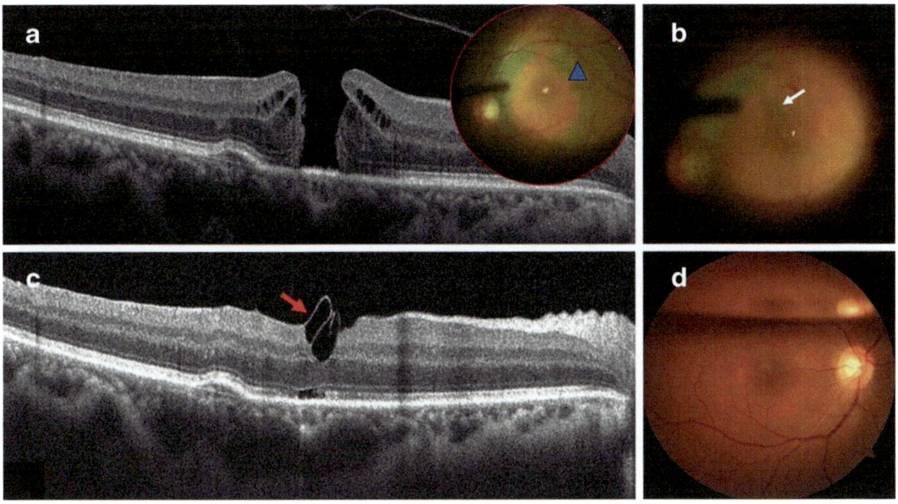

Fig. 10.14 Combined application of ILM "Yin-Yang" staining and flap coverage technique. (**a**) Preoperative minimum macular hole diameter: 425 μm; corrected visual acuity: 0.15. Intraoperative ILM "Yin-Yang" staining shows unstained ILM at and around the fovea (red circle). Flap initiation starts from the stained inferotemporal area. (**b**) Intraoperative view shows the peeled ILM flap covering the macular hole, with a small amount of ICG-stained ILM flap visible at the edge (white arrow). (**c**) OCT at 10 days postoperatively shows closed macular hole with the ILM flap still overlying it; corrected visual acuity: 0.5. (**d**) Fundus photograph shows residual gas and no obvious abnormalities in the posterior pole retina

10.8 Summary

As suggested in the ancient allegory, "Great oaks from little acorns grow," the ultimate success or failure of macular hole surgery often hinges upon the subtlest of details. From the precision of the initial incision and the gentle calibration of intraocular illumination to the fluid dynamics of a single-pass ILM peel, each minor maneuver acts as a seed for the final outcome.

For the retina surgeon, there are no 'small' steps; a microscopic tremor or a moment of misplaced traction can alter a patient's visual prognosis entirely. Therefore, meticulous attention to every procedural nuance is not merely a technical requirement but a fundamental philosophy essential to achieving a consistently successful anatomical and functional result.

11 Prevention and Management of Proliferative Vitreoretinopathy

Proliferative vitreoretinopathy (PVR) is a complex intraocular condition characterized by pathological cellular proliferation, resulting from an aberrant wound-healing response following vitreoretinal injury. As a frequent complication of rhegmatogenous retinal detachment (RRD), ocular trauma, or previous vitreoretinal intervention, PVR markedly increases surgical complexity and remains the primary etiology of anatomical failure in retinal detachment repair.

The incidence of PVR secondary to RRD is estimated at 5%–10%. Currently, there are no clinically proven pharmacologic therapies for its prevention or treatment. Once PVR manifests, the majority of patients require salvage vitreoretinal surgery. This chapter explores the underlying pathogenesis of PVR, with a primary focus on the essential surgical principles and maneuvers required for successful management.

11.1 Etiology

11.1.1 Cell Composition of Proliferative Vitreoretinopathy

PVR membranes are heterogeneous, consisting of various cell types that contribute to membrane formation and contraction, including:

- Retinal glial cells: Primarily Müller cells, microglia, and astrocytes.
- Epithelial cells: Retinal pigment epithelial (RPE) cells and ciliary epithelial cells.
- Vitreous cells: Primarily hyalocytes.
- Inflammatory/immune Cells: Macrophages, lymphocytes, and neutrophils.

Z. Zhang, U. Spandau, *Vitreoretinal Surgery*,
https://doi.org/10.1007/978-3-032-25271-5_11

During the progression of PVR, these precursor cells undergo epithelial-mesenchymal transition (EMT) or transdifferentiation into contractile myofibroblasts, which drive the mechanical shortening of the membrane and subsequent retinal traction.

11.1.1.1 RPE Cells

The transformation of RPE cells through EMT drives the development of PVR. While normally quiescent, RPE cells are activated by the disruption of the blood-retinal barrier during RRD. Cytokine exposure causes these cells to shed their epithelial characteristics—such as tissue polarity and tight junctions—and transdifferentiate into mesenchymal cells. These newly formed cells are highly migratory, resistant to apoptosis, and serve as the primary source of extracellular matrix (ECM) production within PVR membranes.

11.1.1.2 Glial Cells

PVR is essentially an exaggerated wound-healing response to retinal injury, with Müller cells serving as central mediators. Müller cell activation begins within 24 hours of retinal detachment. By day 3, these cells migrate into the subretinal space, collaborating with RPE cells and immune cells (microglia/macrophages) to form subretinal proliferative strands.

Pathological changes include the downregulation of inwardly rectifying potassium channels, triggering a loss of cell polarity and subsequent proliferation. The resulting glial-neuronal unit dysfunction and Müller cell depolarization lead to neuronal degeneration and characteristic retinal thinning. Furthermore, activated Müller cells secrete pro-inflammatory cytokines that sustain a feedback loop of cellular migration and extracellular matrix deposition, ultimately forming contractile PVR membranes.

11.1.1.3 Macrophages

Disruption of the blood-retinal barrier allows systemic macrophages to enter the vitreous and subretinal spaces, where they secrete pro-inflammatory cytokines and regulate photoreceptor cell death. Experimental induction of PVR via intravitreal macrophage injection confirms their role: the membranes formed are macrophage-rich, with the cells exhibiting fibroblastic transdifferentiation. Consequently, macrophages are increasingly recognized as critical initiators of the PVR cascade.

11.1.2 Regulation of Cell Proliferation and Migration

Blood-retinal barrier disruption allows hematic components to enter the vitreous and subretinal spaces, fueling PVR via several mechanisms:

- Thrombin induces glial proliferation and RPE-to-mesenchymal transdifferentiation (EMT).
- Fibronectin acts as a chemoattractant for glial cells and mediates ECM.
- Plasmin upregulates the production of platelet-derived growth factor (PDGF).

Beyond blood-derived regulators, activated RPE and glial cells secrete a diverse array of cytokines that drive PVR progression. These include platelet-derived growth factor (PDGF), vascular endothelial growth factor (VEGF), epidermal growth factor (EGF), transforming growth factor (TGF), basic fibroblast growth factor (bFGF), colony-stimulating factor (CSF), insulin-like growth factor (IGF), and monocyte chemoattractant protein-1 (MCP-1).

11.1.3 Extracellular Matrix Remodeling

Composed of proteins like collagen and fibronectin, the extracellular matrix (ECM) serves as a dynamic scaffold that regulates cell behavior through continuous feedback loops. Cells both respond to and remodel the ECM via protein secretion. In PVR, this process becomes dysregulated, leading to a progressive increase in ECM deposition. The fibrous contraction and maladaptive remodeling of the ECM are the terminal pathological events that drive retinal traction in PVR.

11.1.4 Susceptibility Genes

While PVR lacks a mendelian inheritance pattern, genetic associations have been established through case-control studies. Identified risk-associated genes are predominantly involved in cytokine regulation, cell cycle control, and programmed cell death, highlighting the role of individual genetic backgrounds in PVR development.

11.2 Clinical Classification and Staging of PVR

11.2.1 Clinical Manifestations

11.2.1.1 Characteristic Retinal Changes

The hallmark manifestations of PVR include retinal shortening, reduced elasticity, full-thickness fold formation, and the development of fibroproliferative membranes. These pathological changes progressively restrict retinal mobility, eventually culminating in retinal detachment with a wide-funnel or closed-funnel configuration.

Severe preoperative PVR not only complicates the primary surgical repair but also significantly elevates the risk of postoperative recurrence. Preoperative PVR is an established anatomical state that cannot be reversed prior to surgical intervention. Consequently, the surgeon's focus must be on maximizing intraoperative reattachment and implementing strategies to mitigate postoperative proliferative responses.

Direct consequences of postoperative PVR include the following:

1. Reopening of primary retinal breaks (Fig. 11.1)
2. Formation of new retinal breaks
3. Preretinal proliferative membranes (Fig. 11.2)
4. Subretinal proliferative membranes or strands (Fig. 11.3)
5. Retinal stiffness and shortening

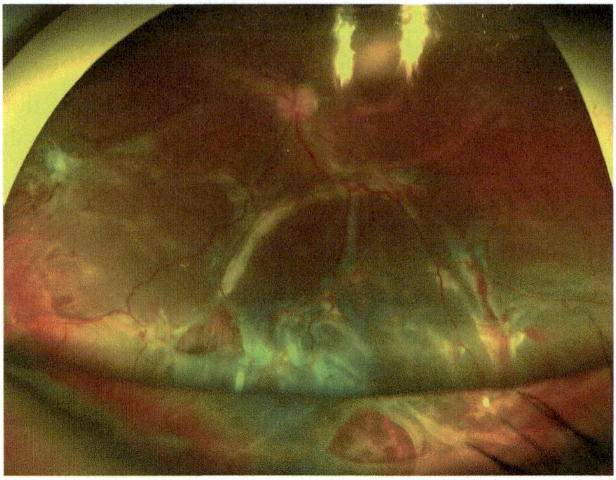

Fig. 11.1 Recurrent PVR under silicone oil tamponade resulting in the reopening of inferior primary breaks. The peribasal retina is characterized by marked stiffness and longitudinal shortening, representing one of the most challenging manifestations of postoperative PVR. Several high-risk factors contributed to this outcome: (1) young age (20 years), (2) the presence of two large, inferiorly located breaks, and (3) significant vascular permeability accompanied by localized microhemorrhages

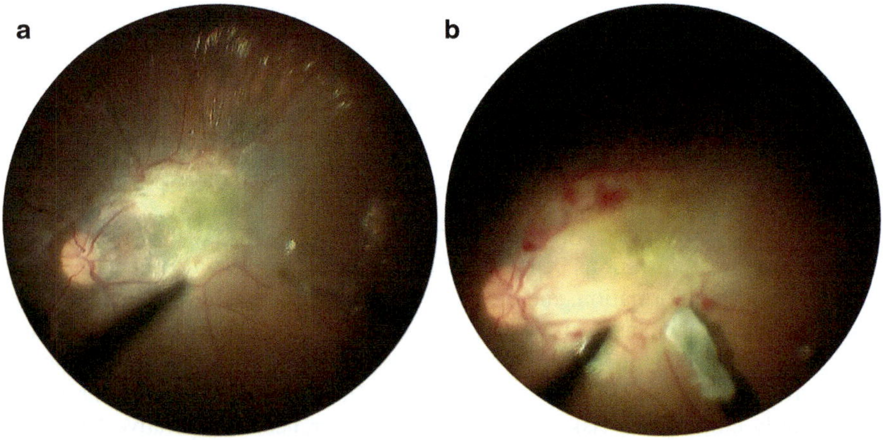

Fig. 11.2 Epiretinal proliferative membrane following vitrectomy and silicone oil tamponade. (**a**) Intraoperative visualization: A dense epiretinal proliferative membrane is shown, exerting significant traction and causing marked vascular distortion. (**b**) Following complete removal of the proliferative membrane, the underlying macular is fully exposed and the tractional distortion is relieved

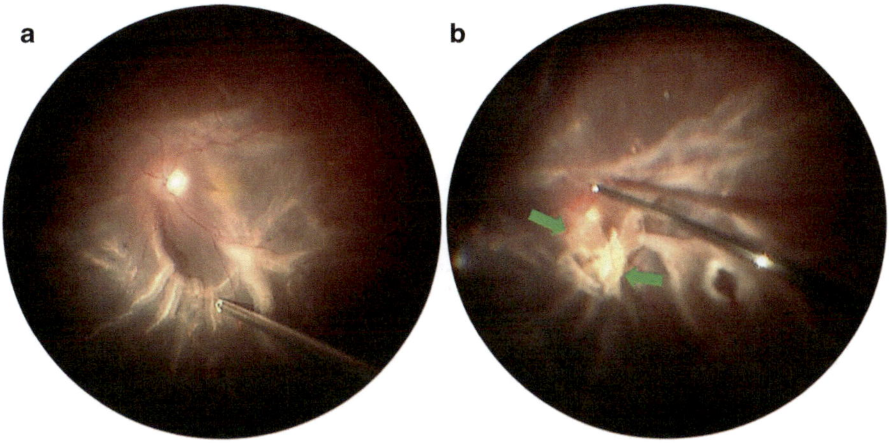

Fig. 11.3 Subretinal "napkin ring" proliferative strands in PVR. (**a**) Tractional deformity: Circumferential subretinal proliferative strands resulting in significant "napkin ring" constriction and apparent retinal shortening. (**b**) Surgical management: A localized retinotomy is performed to facilitate the extraction and removal of the dense subretinal strands (green arrow), allowing for retinal mobilization

11.2.1.2 Anterior Segment Manifestations

PVR can affect the anterior segment to varying degrees:

- PVR without prior vitrectomy typically causes mild anterior segment involvement.
- PVR after vitrectomy (especially with silicone oil tamponade) often leads to more severe anterior segment involvement.

Nevertheless, both situations may present the following symptoms. Novice surgeons must understand how these accompanying clinical signs can complicate surgical maneuvers:

1. Posterior iris synechia: This may impair both preoperative examination and intraoperative visualization. Synechiae can typically be lysed intraoperatively while maintaining lens integrity (Fig. 11.4). If needed, intracameral epinephrine can be administered to enhance pupillary dilation. When using a wide-field viewing system, a clear pupillary aperture of approximately 3 mm is usually sufficient for adequate fundus visualization.
2. Lens opacification: If cataracts significantly obstruct the view of the posterior pole, lens extraction is required. However, if visualization remains adequate, concurrent lensectomy is generally discouraged. A ruptured posterior capsule necessitates a peripheral iridectomy, which increases the risk of postoperative silicone oil migration into the anterior chamber, potentially triggering secondary complications and complicating management.

   Fluctuations in IOP can induce corneal epithelial edema, significantly compromising fundus visibility. Debridement of the edematous epithelium using toothed forceps can effectively restore intraoperative clarity (Fig. 11.5).

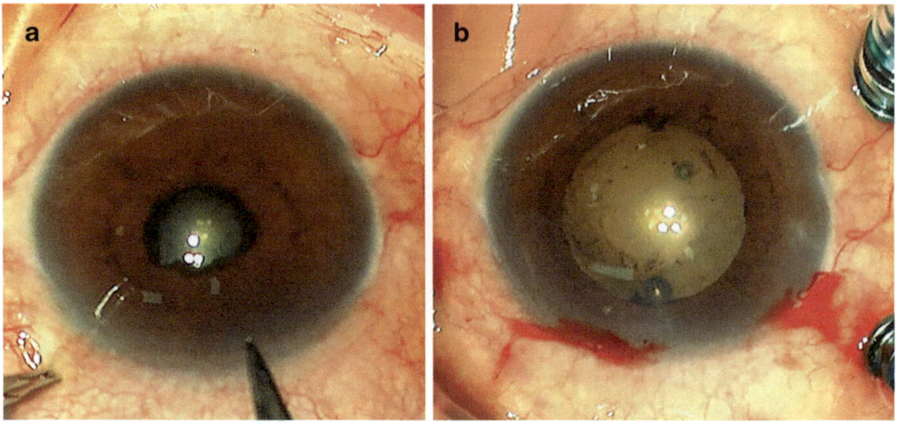

Fig. 11.4 Management of posterior iris synechia in PVR. (**a**) Extensive 360° posterior iris synechiae resulting in a significantly constricted, non-reactive pupil. (**b**) Intracameral injection of viscoelastic is utilized to lyse the synechiae and expand the pupil, thereby restoring adequate visualization and providing an optimal surgical field for vitreoretinal intervention

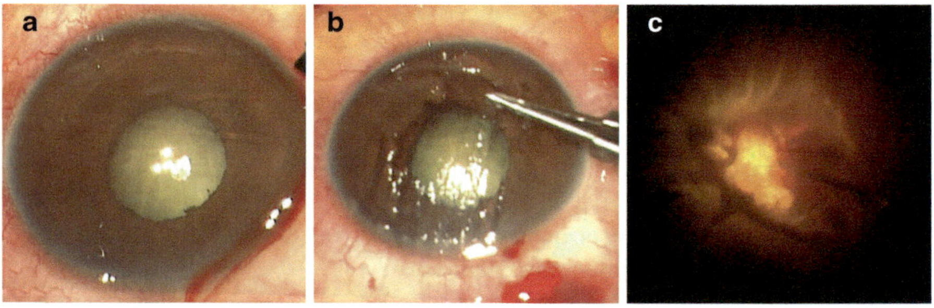

Fig. 11.5 Epithelial debridement to restore intraoperative visualization. (**a**) Acute corneal edema: Significant corneal epithelial edema developed rapidly following an intraoperative increase in intraocular pressure (IOP) via irrigation (baseline preoperative IOP: 6 mmHg) (**b**) Epithelial debridement: Utilizing toothed forceps to meticulousy scrape the edematous epithelium within the pupillary axis. (**c**) Restored clarity: A clear fundus view is achieved, facilitating safe intravitreal maneuvers (endoilluminator brightness set at 35%)

3. Ciliary injection: This must be carefully differentiated from infectious conjunctivitis to ensure appropriate perioperative management.
4. Anterior chamber Flare: Frequently observed postoperatively, this indicates significant intraocular inflammation and requires aggressive anti-inflammatory therapy.
5. Reduced iris elasticity: This often results in inadequate mydriasis. If combined with cataract surgery, the restricted operating space increases the risk of posterior capsule rupture during capsulorhexis and phacoemulsification.
6. IIris neovascularization (rubeosis iridis): Although rare, this condition carries a high risk of intraoperative hyphema and intractable postoperative ocular hypertension.

Table 11.1 Grades and clinical manifestations of PVR

	Grade	Clinical signs	
A	Minimal	Vitreous haze and pigment clumps	
B	Moderate	Surface retinal wrinkling, rolled edges of the retina, retinal stiffness, and vessel tortuosity	
C	Marked	Full-thickness fixed retinal folds in	
		(i) C-1	(i) one quadrant
		(ii) C-2	(ii) two quadrants
		(iii) C-3	(iii) three quadrants
D	Massive	Fixed retinal folds in four quadrants that result in	
		(i) D-1	(i) a wide funnel shape
		(ii) D-2	(ii) a narrow funnel shape
		(iii) D-3	(iii) closed funnel without view of the optic disc

11.2.2 Grading

In clinical practice, the classification system proposed by The Retina Society (USA) in 1983 remains a foundational tool (Table 11.1). This system categorizes PVR into four grades—ranging from mild to severe—based on the progressive stages of fibrocellular proliferation following rhegmatogenous or traumatic retinal detachment. By providing a standardized quantitative framework for assessing the severity of vitreoretinal proliferation, this system has significantly advanced the understanding, research, and surgical management of PVR within the global ophthalmic community.

The primary strengths of this system are its simplicity and ease of clinical application, which facilitate clear communication among vitreoretinal surgeons. While subsequent modifications have been proposed, they have seen limited adoption in routine clinical practice. However, this foundational grading system has notable limitations: it lacks a detailed description of subretinal proliferative tissue and fails to account for the anteroposterior localization of PVR, which is a critical factor in determining surgical strategy.

11.3 Risk Factors of Occurrence and Development of PVR

PVR can manifest within days following the onset of rhegmatogenous retinal detachment (RRD), whereas postoperative PVR typically develops within weeks following surgical intervention. The primary risk factors for its development and progression include:

1. Prolonged duration of rRD: Persistent patency of retinal breaks provides a continuous pathway for the migration and dissemination of RPE cells into the vitreous cavity. Progressive vitreous liquefaction further facilitates the accumulation of pro-inflammatory cytokines, leading to advanced wide-funnel or closed-funnel configurations (Fig. 11.6).

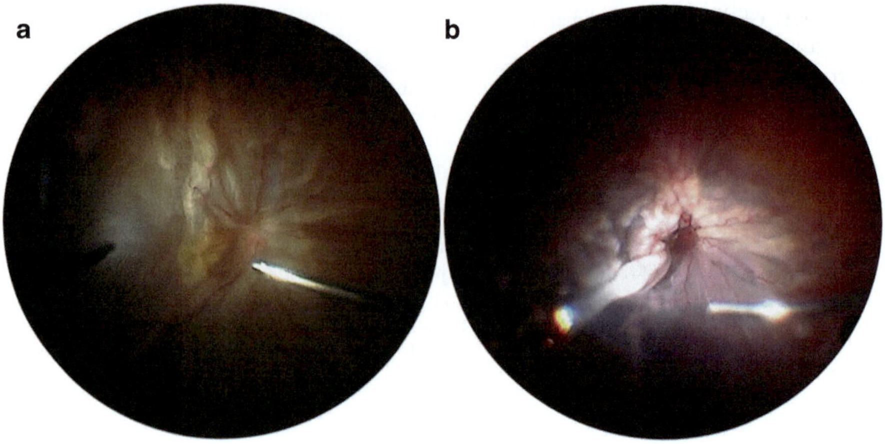

Fig. 11.6 Morphological variations of funnel-shaped retinal detachment. In both wide and closed configurations, surgical management prioritizes the meticulous resection of posterior pole proliferative tissue to facilitate retinal mobilization. (**a**) Wide-funnel retinal detachment: Observed in a patient with a 6-month history of progressive vision loss; the configuration allows for relatively better intraoperative visualization of the posterior pole. (**b**) Closed-funnel retinal detachment: Observed in a patient following 2 years of chronic vision loss; the tight, constricted configuration significantly increases surgical complexity and poses a higher risk of iatrogenic injury during dissection

In younger patients with an intact vitreous and small breaks, epiretinal PVR may be delayed; however, subretinal PVR can still manifest as multiple fibrous strands, a finding relatively common in pediatric and adolescent RRD cases.

From a surgical perspective, established preoperative PVR is unmodifiable. Therefore, when a "fresh" retinal detachment is diagnosed, prompt surgical intervention is paramount to forestall PVR progression. Surgeons should maintain flexibility in their schedules to accommodate these urgent cases.

Notably, many ophthalmic centers in China have prioritized these cases by establishing "Retinal Detachment Fast Tracks," significantly improving the chances of visual recovery through timely intervention.

2. Large retinal breaks: Giant retinal tears (GRTs) are the classic example. Large breaks facilitate massive RPE cell liberation. Because liberated RPE cells tend to settle inferiorly due to gravity, excessive intraoperative manipulation of the inferior RPE should be avoided, and the margins of the break must be protected to prevent iatrogenic enlargement.
3. Intraoperative and postoperative hemorrhage: Both epiretinal and subretinal hemorrhages are potent triggers for PVR. Blood components facilitate the influx of cytokines and act as a biological scaffold for membrane proliferation.

   Meticulous hemostasis is essential. Hemorrhage must be controlled intraoperatively to mitigate PVR risk, which underscores the benefit of preoperative anti-VEGF therapy in complex proliferative diabetic retinopathy (PDR) cases.

Procedures such as retinotomy or retinectomy require precise hemostasis. Inadvertent damage to the underlying RPE or choroid can lead to extensive hemorrhage. Timely and accurate endodiathermy is critical; missing the window for effective hemostasis can significantly jeopardize the surgical outcome.

4. Systemic or immunological predispositions: This includes RRD secondary to Stickler syndrome, FEVR, or uveitis. While anatomical reattachment is achievable, the underlying inflammatory milieu increases the risk of recurrent PVR.

   For these high-risk patients, iatrogenic trauma (e.g., unnecessary retinotomies) should be minimized. Comprehensive vitrectomy and thorough laser photocoagulation of all suspicious areas are advised. Silicone oil tamponade is generally preferred to sequester inflammatory mediators and inhibit cellular dissemination.

5. Absence of PVD or excessive residual vitreous: Frequently encountered in young patients, this presents as extensive vitreoretinal adhesion (Fig. 11.7), increasing the risk of iatrogenic breaks during hyaloid induction.

   Although some literature may not explicitly categorize residual peripheral vitreous as a standalone risk factor, the clinical necessity of a complete PVD and thorough peripheral shaving is well-recognized in PVR prevention.

6. Multiple previous vitreoretinal interventions: Repeated surgeries (excluding simple injections) often lead to a chronic breakdown of the blood-ocular barrier. Management should involve a careful analysis of previous failures and may necessitate adjunctive therapies, such as scleral buckling (encircling) or the off-label use of pharmacological agents like methotrexate or triamcinolone.

7. Excessive cryotherapy or excessive laser photocoagulation: Both modalities, if used immoderately, can exacerbate intraocular inflammation and barrier disruption, fueling the proliferative response.

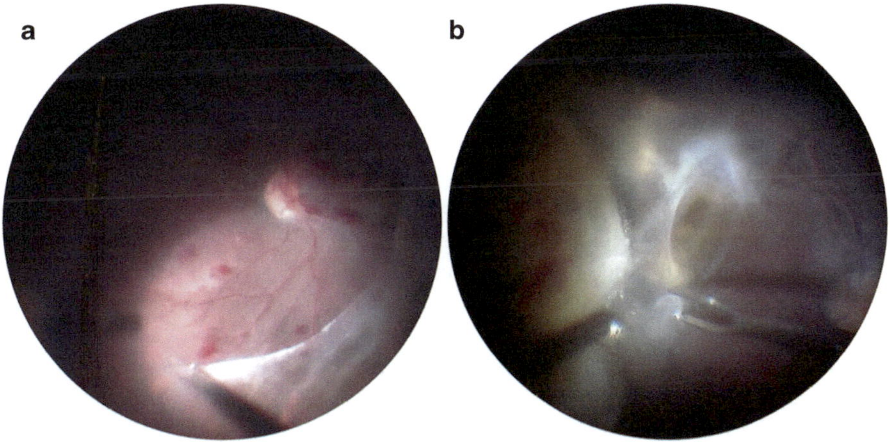

Fig. 11.7 PVR caused by residual vitreous. (**a**) Residual sheet-like peripheral vitreous with mild hemorrhage during peeling. (**b**) Extensive residual vitreous in the posterior pole, mixed with emulsified silicone oil droplets. Retinal breaks occurred during peeling

For novice surgeons, the most common pitfalls in retinal photocoagulation include applying excessive laser energy and creating overly dense, confluent treatment patterns. This tendency toward overtreatment is often driven by the concern that any missed pathology may lead to surgical failure. However, through systematic training and meticulous peripheral retinal examination, surgeons can refine their precision and strategically minimize total energy delivery without compromising safety.

11.4 Surgical Strategies for Improving Long-Term Outcomes in Severe PVR

The primary objective of PVR intervention is to alleviate all tractional forces while strictly avoiding mechanical retinal injury. For novice surgeons, mastering additional specialized skills is essential; these include the peeling of preretinal and subretinal proliferative tissue and the placement of a scleral buckle or encircling band. These procedures are crucial for restoring retinal mobility and will be discussed below.

11.4.1 Identification and Release of Preretinal Proliferation

Preretinal proliferation is classified into two types based on visibility:

- Early stage: Immature proliferative membranes (rich in vitreous content) are typically transparent, soft, and shapeless (Fig. 11.8).
- Mid-to-late stage: Mature proliferative membranes (rich in fibroblast content) are visible, firm, and well-defined (Fig. 11.9).

Complete intraoperative resection of proliferative tissue is essential, except in cases where the membranes are so firmly incarcerated into the underlying retina that removal would pose an unacceptable risk of iatrogenic trauma.

Early-stage proliferative membranes are often translucent and difficult to visualize. The following clinical indicators and techniques can facilitate their identification

1. Anatomic landmarks: Proliferative membranes are typically localized at the apices or the most constricted segments of retinal folds.
2. Perfluorocarbon Liquid (PFCL) challenge: Incomplete retinal flattening following PFCL injection indicates persistent traction in the corresponding area (Fig. 11.10).
3. Vital dyes: While agents such as indocyanine green (ICG), triamcinolone acetonide (TA), or brilliant blue G (BBG) can be utilized, staining efficacy is often limited for immature or hypocellular membranes.

Early-stage epiretinal proliferative membranes can generally be managed using standard intraocular forceps, as they often lack significant adherence to the underlying retina.

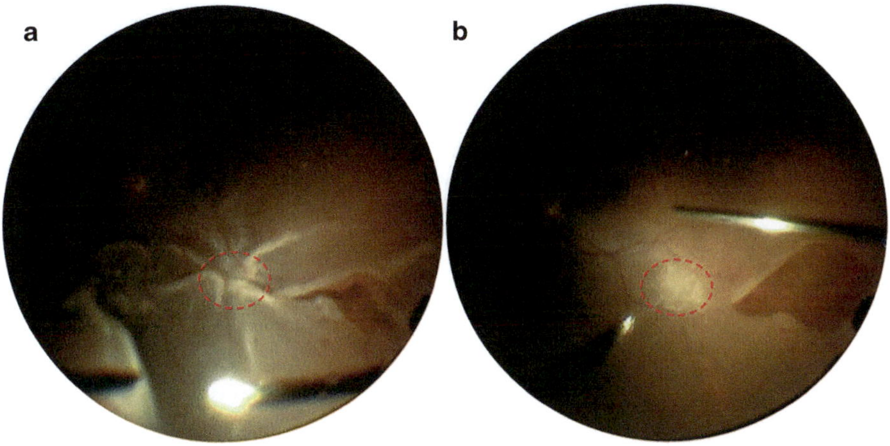

Fig. 11.8 Immature preretinal proliferative membrane. (**a**) "Napkin ring" folds (within the red dashed line), but the proliferative membrane is not visible. (**b**) After peeling the unformed proliferative membrane at the center of the folds, heavy liquid completely flattens the folds (red circle)

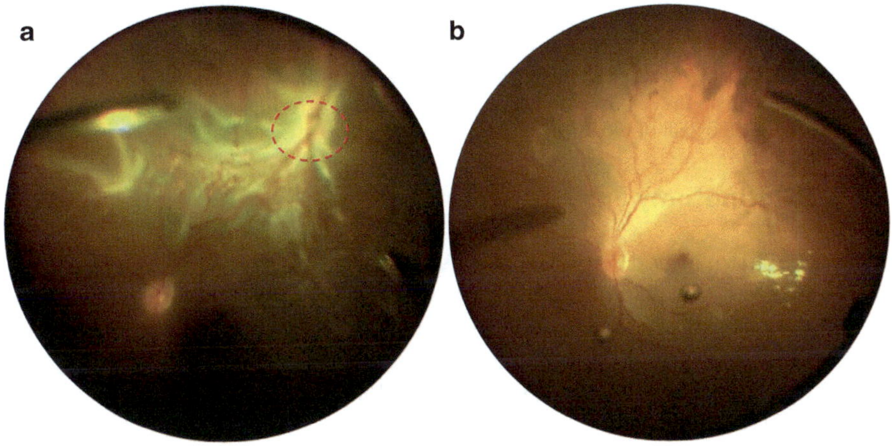

Fig. 11.9 Mature preretinal proliferative membrane. (**a**) "Canyon-like" folds (red circle), with a brown formed proliferative membrane visible in the fold center. (**b**) After membrane peeling, heavy liquid injection completely flattens the folds

In mid-to-late stage PVR, proliferative membranes are typically opaque and well-defined, making identification straightforward. While these membranes do not generally present significant technical challenges for dissection, the surgeon must exercise precise control over the tractional force during peeling. Because these membranes are often densely adherent, excessive force can easily lead to iatrogenic retinal breaks or mechanical trauma to the fragile neurosensory retina.

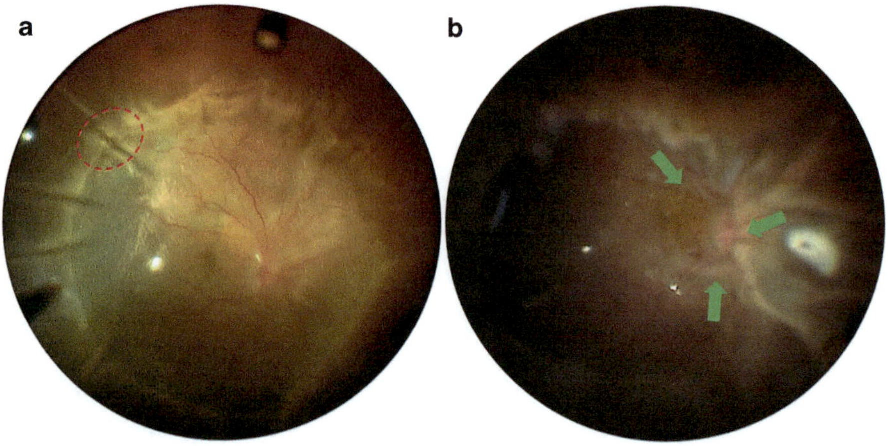

Fig. 11.10 Utilizing perfluorocarbon liquid (PFCL) to detect residual proliferative tissue. (**a**) Identification of peripheral traction: Following PFCL injection, the posterior pole is successfully flattened; however, persistent fixed folds remain visible in the periphery (demarcated by the red dashed line), indicating the presence of residual epiretinal membranes. (**b**) Detection of subretinal "napkin ring" strands: After the removal of the epiretinal membranes, further PFCL injection fails to achieve complete retinal apposition. Fixed folds persisting around the optic disc and the nasal retina suggest the presence of circumferential subretinal "napkin ring" strands (green arrow). A localized retinotomy is indicated to facilitate the removal of these strands and ensure successful retinal reattachment. In such cases, the surgeon must strategically design the retinotomy site based on the anatomical extent of the subretinal involvement

11.4.2 Retinotomy and Retinectomy

11.4.2.1 Differences Between the Two Procedures

These two frequently conflated concepts were pioneered by Machemer in the late 1970s, with their safety and efficacy since well-established. Both are invasive maneuvers intended to restore retinal mobility in cases of severe shortening. The primary technical challenge lies in the meticulous prevention and management of intraoperative hemorrhage.

The clinical distinction is rooted in their etymology:

- "-otomy" denotes a surgical incision into an organ or tissue (e.g., tracheotomy), where the structure remains intact.
- "-ectomy" refers to the surgical excision or removal of a tissue or organ (e.g., appendectomy).

In vitreoretinal surgery:

- Retinotomy: The creation of a focal retinal opening to provide access for subretinal maneuvers, such as the drainage of subretinal fluid or the extraction of subretinal proliferative strands.

- Retinectomy: The surgical excision of irreparably contracted retinal tissue (typically in the periphery) to eliminate traction and facilitate the anatomical reattachment of the remaining retina.

11.4.2.2 Retinotomy

Retinotomy is the creation of a focal retinal opening using intraocular instruments, most commonly the vitrectomy cutter. This maneuver is typically indicated in the following clinical scenarios:

1. Drainage of subretinal fluid (SRF): In rhegmatogenous retinal detachment (RRD) repair, if the primary break is located in the far periphery, a posterior or mid-peripheral drainage retinotomy may be created to facilitate the evacuation of SRF during fluid-air exchange.
2. Management of subretinal pathology: To provide access for the extraction of subretinal proliferative strands or membranes.
3. Evacuation of subretinal hemorrhage: To facilitate the removal of extensive or organized subretinal clots.
4. Release of focal traction: To mobilize the retina in areas where proliferative membranes are firmly incarcerated or too adherent to the underlying neurosensory tissue for safe dissection (Fig. 11.11).

11.4.2.3 Retinectomy

Retinectomy refers to the en bloc excision of a specific retinal area—typically in the far periphery—utilizing intraocular instruments such as the vitrectomy cutter. This procedure is generally indicated in the following clinical scenarios:

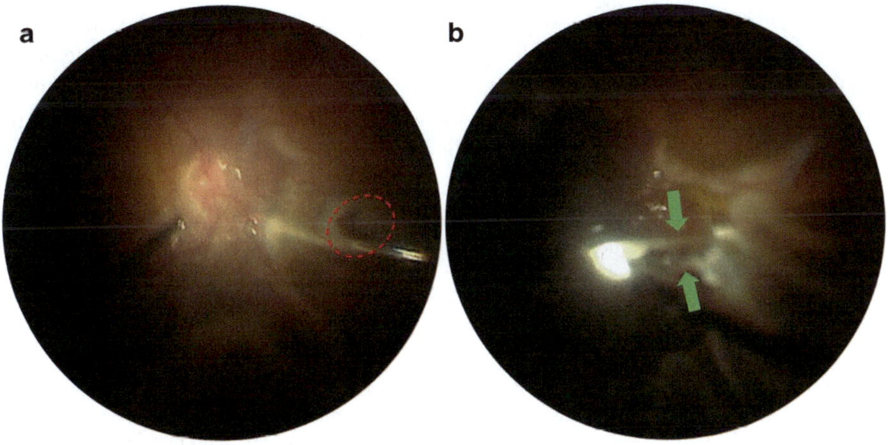

Fig. 11.11 Retinotomy. (**a**) Nasosuperior retinotomy (red circle) performed to insert forceps and remove "napkin ring" proliferative strands adjacent to the optic disc. (**b**) Large quantities of proliferative strands extracted through the retinotomy site

1. Severe retinal foreshortening: Cases where the peripheral retina is so stiff and contracted that it fails to achieve anatomical apposition even under the weight of perfluorocarbon liquid (PFCL).
2. Extensive subretinal proliferation: When subretinal membranes or strands are widely distributed and cannot be adequately managed via localized retinotomy. In these instances, a peripheral retinectomy is performed to mobilize the retina, providing the necessary exposure to identify and extract subretinal proliferative tissue using intraocular forceps (Fig. 11.12).

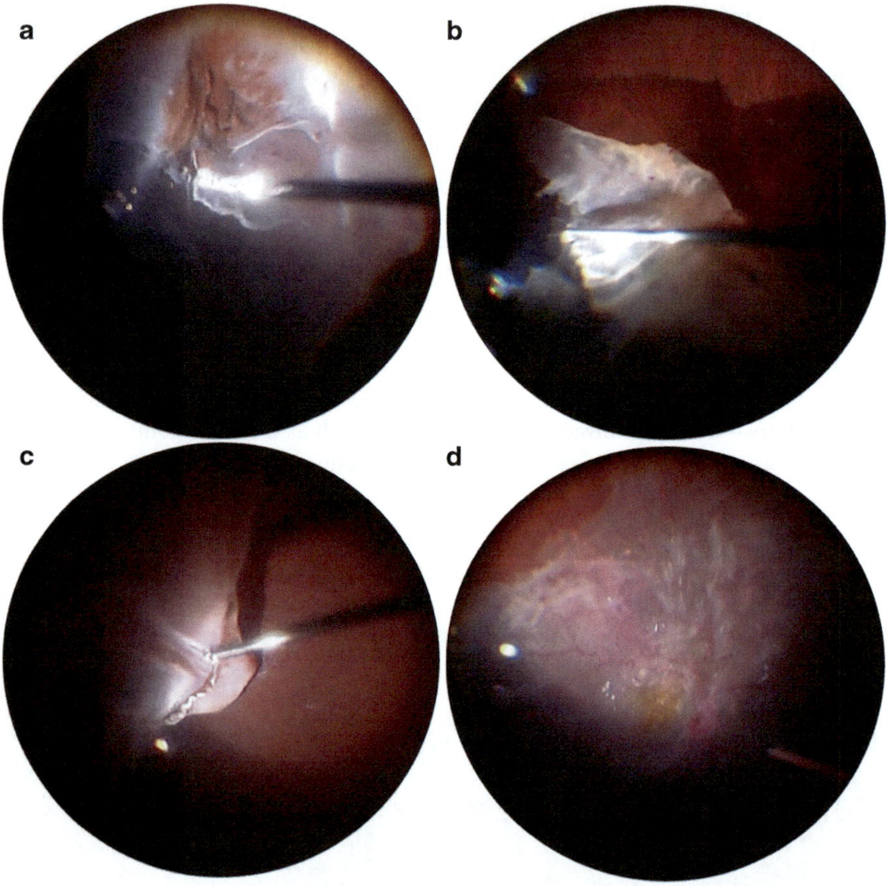

Fig. 11.12 Retinectomy. (**a**) Extensive preretinal proliferative membranes, retinal shortening, and tight adhesion between the membrane and retina (unremovable via peeling). (**b**) Vitrectomy cutter used to remove the stiff, shortened retina. (**c**) Retinal flap lifted to peel “napkin ring” proliferative strands adjacent to the optic disc. (**d**) Heavy liquid injection ultimately flattens the retina

11.4.3 Radial Retinotomy

Pioneered by Professor Xiaofeng Lin (China) in 2016, this technique addresses the clinical dilemma of whether to excise or preserve severely contracted retinal tissue. It provides an optimized "utilization" strategy, particularly for cases involving advanced inferior PVR where retinal shortening is most pronounced.

This approach adopts a "using the problem to solve the problem" philosophy: by leveraging the residual elasticity of the diseased retina, the creation of multiple relaxing radial incisions effectively reduces overall retinal tension and enhances pliability. This restoration of significant retinal mobility enables complete anatomical reattachment during fluid-air exchange or perfluorocarbon liquid (PFCL) injection. Furthermore, the preserved retinal tissue between these incisions provides an ideal substrate for endophotocoagulation, maximizing the potential for anatomical success. Clinically, this technique avoids the extensive RPE exposure associated with large-scale retinectomy—a known driver of recurrent PVR—and reduces the risk of postoperative ocular hypotony (Fig. 11.13).

11.4.4 Scleral Encircling and Buckling

The primary objective of scleral buckling in PVR management is to alleviate vitreous base traction. This approach is particularly effective for cases involving inferior retinal breaks. However, from a pathophysiological standpoint, the success of buckling is predicated on the complete neutralization of retinal traction; as a standalone procedure, it often fails to achieve stable anatomical reattachment in the presence of advanced proliferative forces.

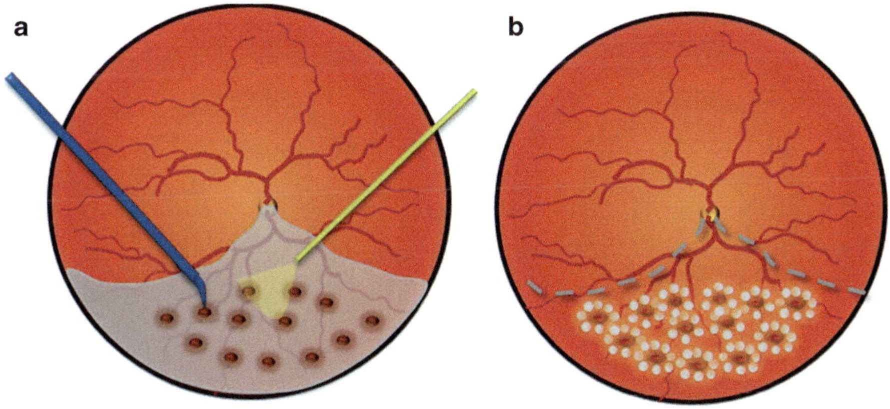

Fig. 11.13 Schematic diagram of radial retinotomy. (**a**) Multiple radial incisions made in the stiff, shortened inferior retina. (**b**) Retinal reattachment achieved via heavy liquid injection or air-fluid exchange. Laser photocoagulation applied around the incisions to fix the inferior retina. The area of exposed RPE is significantly reduced, maximizing retinal integrity

11.5 Summary

"Persistence and precision are the twin pillars of surgical mastery." For novice surgeons, the perioperative management of proliferative vitreoretinopathy (PVR) represents far more than a technical hurdle; it is a defining rite of passage that tests the very core of one's surgical foundation. The central mission of PVR surgery is the comprehensive neutralization of retinal traction—a task that demands not only steady hands but also a sophisticated level of clinical judgment. Intraoperative decision-making is a multi-dimensional process that primarily involves the following critical aspects: (1) Anatomic mapping. Accurately identifying the precise location, morphology, and extent of both epiretinal and subretinal proliferation; (2) Tissue preservation. Maximizing the protection of viable ocular structures while minimizing iatrogenic trauma during highly invasive maneuvers; (3) Strategic intervention. Selecting the optimal surgical maneuvers—ranging from meticulous membrane peeling to relaxing retinotomies—required to effectively release tractional forces; (4) Tamponade dynamics. Determining the appropriate timing and selection of intraocular tamponades (gas vs. silicone oil) to provide sustained anatomical support.

PVR is an enduring adversary that remains an inescapable reality throughout a vitreoretinal surgeon's career. Rather than viewing it with trepidation, beginners should approach PVR with a sense of composure and resilience. By confronting its complexities with rigorous scientific methodology and refined technical proficiency, surgeons can systematically overcome these challenges. The mastery of PVR management is not merely about achieving reattachment; it is about the relentless pursuit of excellence in the face of our most formidable surgical opponent.

Vitreoretinal Surgery in Children and Adolescents

12

Vitreoretinal surgery in the pediatric and adolescent population represents a formidable frontier, constituting a critical subspecialty within the field. Its complexity stems not only from the intricate and technically demanding nature of intraoperative maneuvers but also from the diagnostic ambiguity and the prognostic uncertainty of functional recovery. Effective management mandates a multidisciplinary approach, requiring seamless collaboration across various medical specialties. In clinical practice, the surgical and perioperative challenges escalate in inverse proportion to the patient's age.

The rapid advancement of medical technology in China has inspired an increasing number of vitreoretinal surgeons to specialize in this demanding field, driving its continuous development and refinement. When treating younger populations, surgeons must proactively adapt both their clinical mindset and technical approach. In this surgical context, the term 'younger patients' extends beyond chronological age—including children and adolescents—to encompass any patient whose vitreous body remains in a 'youthful' state, characterized by minimal liquefaction and significant structural clarity.

12.1 General Characteristics and Unique Challenges

In the pediatric and adolescent population, vitreoretinal conditions necessitating surgical intervention are primarily categorized into three groups: (1) vasoproliferative disorders (Fig. 12.1), including retinopathy of prematurity (ROP), familial exudative vitreoretinopathy (FEVR), and Coats disease; (2) parasitic infections, such as ocular toxocariasis (Fig. 12.2); and (3) traumatic injuries, specifically traumatic retinal detachment.

Although the diagnosis of these conditions is often straightforward, their symptoms are insidious and frequently bilateral. Once the optimal treatment window is missed, surgery becomes not only more difficult but also associated with a poorer prognosis. Due to age and cognition, patients often cannot or will not express their

Z. Zhang, U. Spandau, *Vitreoretinal Surgery*,
https://doi.org/10.1007/978-3-032-25271-5_12

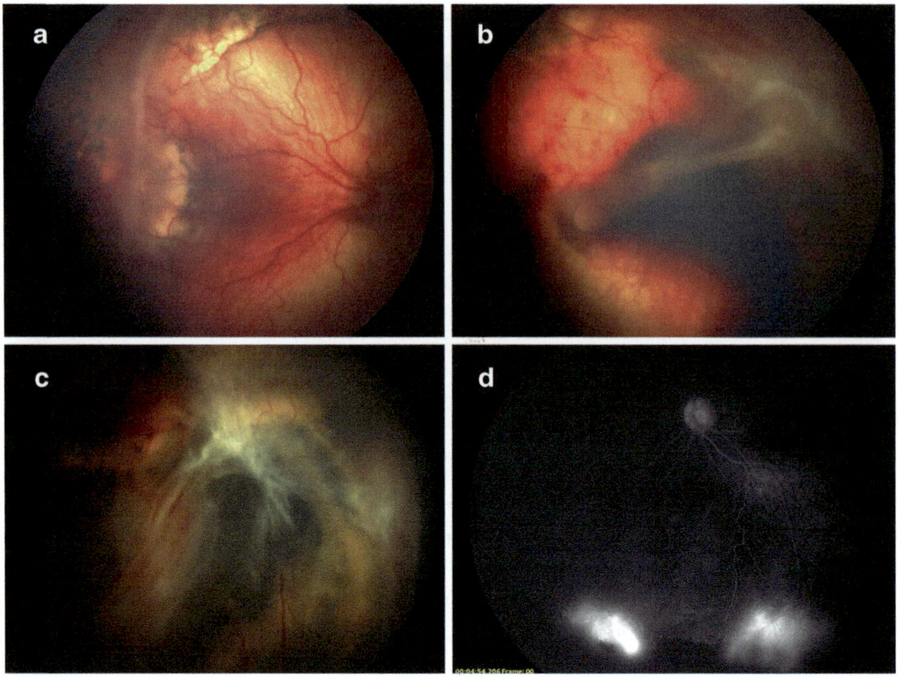

Fig. 12.1 Typical pediatric retinal detachment (**a**) Fundus photograph of stage 4A retinopathy of prematurity (ROP) with plus disease (characterized by tortuous posterior pole vessels) in the right eye. (**b**) Fundus photograph of stage 4B ROP with plus disease in the left eye. (**c**) Extensive retinal detachment secondary to familial exudative vitreoretinopathy (FEVR) in the right eye. (**d**) Fluorescein angiography of the fellow eye (left eye) of the patient in C shows peripheral avascular retina and dye leakage

concerns directly, but this invisible pressure is often expressed in the seemingly tough and hopeful eyes of parents. From the beginner's point of view, there is often nothing that can be done due to the limitations of surgical experience and the objective conditions, which is a frequent dilemma for both doctors and patients.

While parasitic vitreoretinal diseases may show signs in the anterior segment, symptoms are often subtle. Closely linked to hygiene and lifestyle—such as lack of deworming in pets and poor hand hygiene—they are more common in remote rural areas. Patients often present late with significant vision loss, and recovery of useful vision is generally limited. However, surgery can sometimes restore relatively normal intraocular structure.

Trauma-induced vitreoretinal lesions vary widely in form and severity. When multiple ocular structures are involved, multidisciplinary teamwork and multiple surgeries may be needed to partially restore vision. For beginners, advanced surgical management is challenging without adequate team support and trauma experience. However, the following less complex trauma-related conditions are more manageable: ① dialysis of the ora serrata; ② lens dislocation into the vitreous cavity;

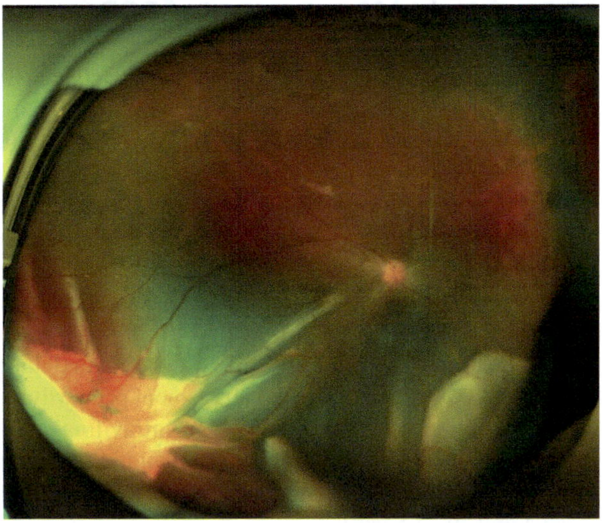

Fig. 12.2 Tractional retinal detachment in the right eye secondary to ocular toxocariasis, with a white inflammatory mass noted inferiorly. At presentation, the best-corrected visual acuity was 0.06. Laboratory testing revealed a markedly elevated aqueous humor toxocara IgG titer of 39.76 U/L (normal <3 U/L) and a serum toxocara IgG titer of 32.34 U/L (normal <9 U/L). The patient had a pet dog at home that had not received regular deworming treatment

③ rhegmatogenous retinal detachment without significant proliferative changes; and ④ laser-induced traumatic macular hole. These conditions follow more predictable surgical approaches, and standard vitreoretinal procedures often lead to favorable outcomes.

Vitrectomy in children and adolescents presents several key characteristics:

1. Diagnosis often relies on imaging, genetics, molecular biology, or pathology, especially to rule out retinoblastoma, unless clear causes or signs are present.
2. Preoperative and postoperative vision can vary significantly and may not correlate closely with anatomical abnormalities, with assessment sometimes being difficult.
3. The eye is not simply a smaller version of an adult eye—its structure and proportions are still developing, requiring different surgical approaches.
4. Vitreous liquefaction or posterior detachment is often absent, making adequate vitreous removal challenging.
5. Special tools like viscoelastic, intraocular scissors, or chandelier—not commonly used in adult surgery—may be needed to achieve our surgical goals; and choices for intraocular tamponade are more limited—for example, silicone oil is usually avoided in ROP cases without iatrogenic breaks, while viscoelastic may be used to separate membranes (though its use remains off-label). Additionally, if retinal breaks exist at the inferior, tamponade with gas or silicone oil tends to be less effective due to poor posturing compliance and may even worsen proliferation.

12.2 Surgical Management of ROP

ROP was first clinically described in 1942. Between 1941 and 1953, an estimated 12,000 newborns worldwide were affected, many of whom suffered devastating vision loss. Despite the rising incidence, the underlying etiology remained elusive for nearly a decade. In 1951, the Australian pediatrician Kate Campbell (1899–1986) made a landmark observation. Comparing two Melbourne hospitals, she noted that the well-funded facility—which provided ample supplemental oxygen to premature infants—had a higher incidence of ROP than the resource-limited hospital. Campbell concluded that excessive oxygen concentration was a primary driver of the disease, a causal link subsequently validated by rigorous clinical trials. As the complex pathogenesis of ROP is extensively documented in existing literature, it is not detailed here. Modern clinical management primarily involves three therapeutic pillars: (1) Pharmacological tntervention: Intravitreal anti-VEGF injections. (2) Laser therapy: Indirect retinal laser photocoagulation performed under indirect ophthalmoscopy. (3) Surgical intervention: Advanced vitreoretinal surgery reserved for stage 4 and stage 5 cases.

12.2.1 Overview of the Third Edition of ROP Classification

(i) The Reason for the Upgraded Version

In 1984, the International Classification of Retinopathy of Prematurity (ICROP) Committee was established, which led to the first multicenter clinical study on ROP. The results demonstrated that cryotherapy could effectively treat the condition, confirming that ROP is both preventable and manageable, with timely screening being a key measure for prevention and treatment. In 2021, the third edition of the ICROP guidelines was published in Ophthalmology. The update was driven by four main factors: ① certain aspects of the previous version were considered subjective; ② continuous advances in ophthalmic imaging technology; ③ the promise and challenges introduced by anti-VEGF therapy; and ④ the earlier version did not fully encompass the diverse disease presentations observed across different regions.

(ii) ROP Partition

The retina is divided into three concentric zones extending from the optic disc to the ora serrata. The posteriormost extent of retinal vasculature or ROP lesions defines the zone of involvement, and the extent of disease is recorded in clock hours (Fig. 12.3).

1. Zone I: This is the most posterior zone, defined as a circular area centered on the optic disc with a radius equivalent to twice the distance from the disc center to the center of the fovea.
2. Zone II: This is a concentric ring extending from the outer edge of Zone I to a circular boundary whose radius is the distance from the optic disc center to the nasal ora serrata. The peripheral portion of Zone II adjacent to Zone I—a band

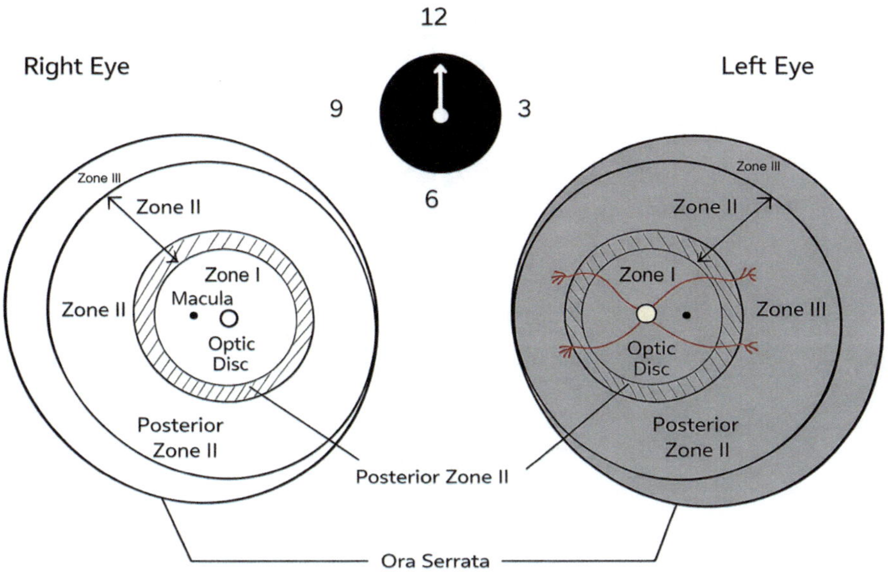

Fig. 12.3 The ICROP classification

approximately 2 disc diameters wide—is designated as posterior Zone II. ROP in posterior Zone II is noted to potentially be more severe and requires closer attention than disease in the more peripheral parts of Zone II.

3. Zone III: This is the remaining crescent-shaped, anterior retinal area outside Zones I and II.

(iii) ROP Staging

1. Stage 1 (Demarcation line): A clear line separates the vascularized from the avascular retina.
2. Stage 2 (Ridge): The demarcation line elevates, widens, and thickens to form a ridge.
3. Stage 3 (Ridge with extraretinal fibrovascular proliferation): The ridge is accompanied by growth of fibrovascular tissue beyond the retinal surface (Fig. 12.4).
4. Stage 4 (Partial retinal detachment): 4A is macula-on, and 4B is macula-off.
5. Stage 5 (Total retinal detachment): 5A is open funnel detachment, 5B is closed funnel detachment with non-visible optic disc, and 5C is stage 5B with simultaneous abnormalities of the anterior segment of the eye.

(iv) Long-Term Sequelae

Infants with a history of prematurity may develop long-term complications even without manifestations of ROP. This requires us to inquire about the medical history

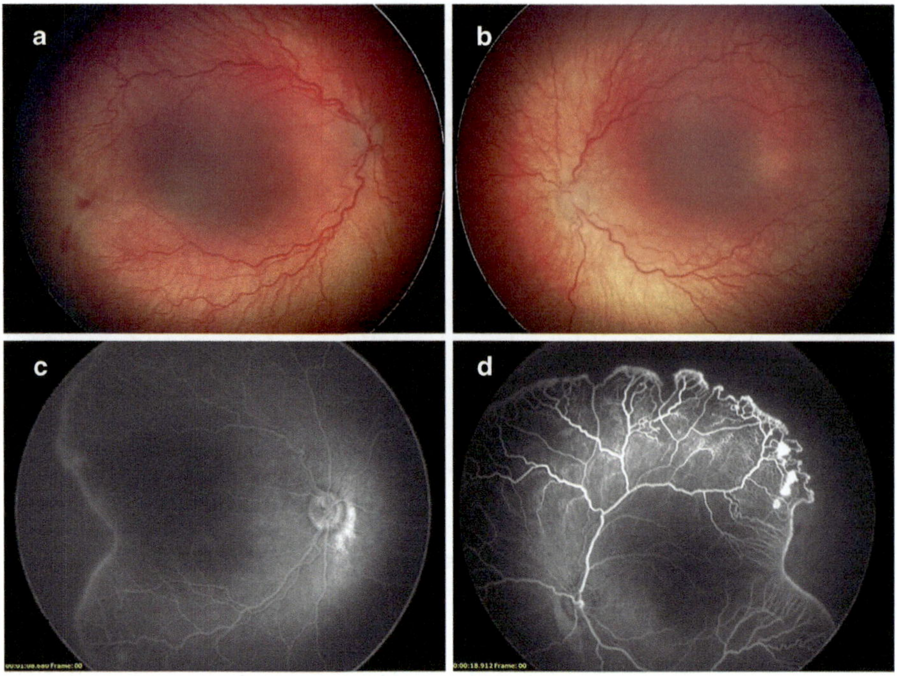

Fig. 12.4 Fundus photographs of Stage 3 ROP (**a**) wedge-shaped avascular area is visible in the peripheral retina of the right eye, with a ridge showing mild extraretinal fibrovascular proliferation, accompanied by plus disease. (**b**) The left eye of the same infant also exhibits Stage 3 ROP with Plus disease. (**c**, **d**) Fundus fluorescein angiography (FFA) images of both eyes in the same patient

when performing fundus examinations on adolescents, as these sequelae may only manifest in adulthood. The main sequelae include the following aspects:

1. Delayed tractional, rhegmatogenous, or less commonly, exudative retinal detachment.
2. Retinoschisis caused by chronic traction from regressed Stage 3 lesions, which may involve the macula and impair visual field and visual acuity without causing retinal detachment.
3. Residual avascular retinal areas, which are prone to retinal thinning, holes, and lattice degeneration, and may be associated with subsequent retinal detachment.
4. Macular abnormalities, including reduction in the size of the foveal avascular zone and blunting or disappearance of the foveal depression.
5. Retinal vascular changes.
6. Patients with a history of ROP may develop secondary angle-closure glaucoma in the later stage.

12.2.2 Anti-VEGF Intraocular Injection

(i) Comparison with Retinal Laser Photocoagulation

Intravitreal injection of anti-VEGF provides a relatively simple and feasible option for the timely treatment of ROP. Current research focuses on comparing the advantages and disadvantages between anti-VEGF and retinal laser photocoagulation, with no consensus reached in many aspects. However, in terms of operation by physicians and medical institutions, anti-VEGF has higher universality. Nevertheless, we should pay more attention to its limitations. The following table compares the advantages and disadvantages of anti-VEGF and laser in several major aspects (Table 12.1).

Table 12.1 Comparison of the advantages and disadvantages of anti-VEGF and laser therapy for ROP

	Anti-VEGF	Laser	Preferred option
Treatment success rate	Higher success rate for zone I lesions	The success rate of zone II lesions is on par with anti-VEGF	Anti-VEGF
Surgical difficulty	Lower requirements for equipment and operator proficiency; lower requirements for anesthesia and monitoring	Higher requirements for equipment and operator proficiency; longer learning curve; higher requirements for anesthesia and monitoring	Anti-VEGF
Intraoperative complications	Lower, decreasing to a lower level with increased operational experience	Higher, but decreasing to a lower level with increased operational experience	Anti-VEGF
Recurrence and follow-up	Increased recurrence and prolonged follow-up	Low recurrence and short follow-up	Laser
Favorable outcome	High	Reduced due to difficult laser photocoagulation	Anti-VEGF
Vision	Intact visual field	Reduced visual field and myopia	Anti-VEGF
Refractive changes	Lower chance of developing high myopia	Higher chance of developing high myopia	Anti-VEGF
Retinal detachment	Short term: low risk Long term: unknown	Short term: low risk Long term: unknown	Theoretically, and taking into account the residual avascular area of the retina, the laser has a stronger preventive effect on retinal detachment
Systemic side effects	There is no clear report; it is only a theoretical speculation	No systemic effect	Both are equivalent

(ii) Injection Technique

1. Dosage: The axial length of a newborn's eye is approximately 16–17 mm, while that of a normal adult eye is about 23–24 mm. In addition, the lens accounts for a larger proportion of the newborn's eye. A rough estimate shows that the vitreous cavity volume of a newborn is about 1/5 to 1/3 that of an adult. Theoretically, if the adult dosage is used (e.g., 0.5 mg of ranibizumab for treating AMD), the intravitreal concentration of anti-VEGF in newborns may be 3–5 times higher than that in adults.

   Although there is no clear medical evidence that adult dosage leads to higher postoperative complications, considering that higher anti-VEGF may hinder the normal development of retinal blood vessels and may affect the vascular development in other organs, the actual applied dosage should be slightly lower than that for adults.

   Many studies have also explored the differences between different doses in terms of therapeutic effectiveness and re-injection rates, and the more consistent conclusion is that retinal neovascularization can be significantly inhibited at lower doses, but the number of re-injections also increases accordingly. In practice, more attention should be paid to the precise control of the dose than in adult surgery. The recommended dose is 0.02 mL of ranibizumab.
2. Preinjection preparation: If under topical anesthesia, 1–2 trained nurses should be available to assist in fixing the child's trunk and head (which is crucial for surgical safety). The skin around the surgical eye should be disinfected in the same way as in adults. Before the injection, we recommend that 5% povidone-iodine to be instilled into the conjunctival sac (left for at least 1 min). After placing a pediatric eyelid speculum, rinse the povidone-iodine thoroughly with saline solution.
3. Eyeball fixation: The surgeon holds serrated forceps in one hand to grasp the conjunctiva at the limbus. The hand should have a stable support to avoid tremor.
4. Injection site: Use a caliper to select the injection site 1–1.5 mm posterior to the limbus.
5. Injection: This is the most difficult step. Beginners are advised to complete the drug injection with the assistance of a nurse. After the operator fixes the position of the syringe, ask the nurse to gently inject the drug. Due to the large proportion of the lens in the infant's eye, following the method in adult surgery is likely to damage the lens (this phenomenon is not uncommon). Unlike adults, if the child has been lying flat and fixed, the injection direction should be nearly perpendicular to the ground, and attention should also be paid to the depth of needle that into the vitreous cavity (Fig. 12.5). The usage of a microscopes is recommended.
6. Eye patching and postoperative local medication are basically the same as those for adults.

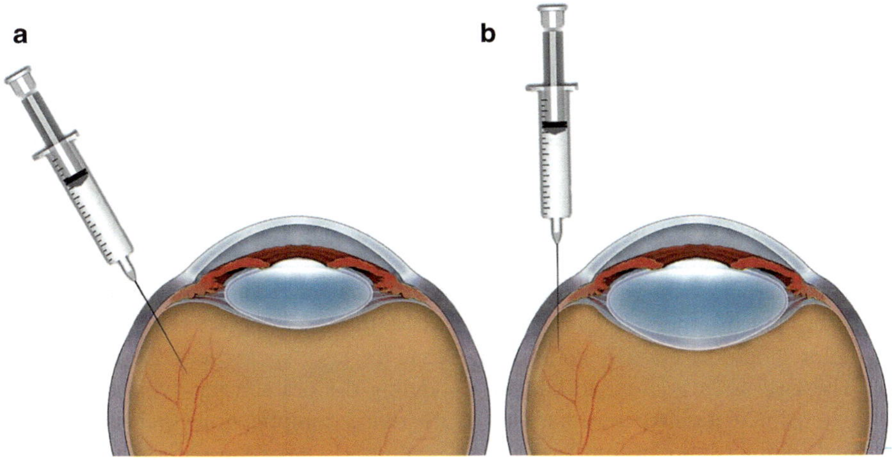

Fig. 12.5 Difference in the angles when the syringe needles entering into the vitreous cavity between adults and children (**a**) The safe range for intravitreal injection in adults is relatively large, and the injection direction can be toward the center of the vitreous cavity. (**b**) The safe range for intravitreal injection in children is relatively small. To avoid iatrogenic damage to the lens, the injection direction must be slightly perpendicular to the ground

12.2.3 Retinal Laser Photocoagulation

It must be performed under an indirect ophthalmoscope, with a relatively long learning curve. Beginners can first master the use of indirect ophthalmoscopes in daily outpatient work and adult external surgeries and then gradually transition to laser treatment of ROP. The key points in the operation are (1) treating the entire avascular zone to avoid skipped areas; (2) ensuring no lesions within the avascular zone are missed—the laser spots should extend anteriorly to the ora serrata; and (3) avoiding direct laser application to the ridge at the interface between the vascular and avascular retina.

When operating, the operator should pay attention to the following issues:

1. Maximal pupil dilatation. The pupil dilates after 20 min if you drop the eye extensively (every minute) with all available dilating eye drops.
2. Prolong the time when the refractive medium is sufficiently transparent as much as possible, in addition to adequate pupil dilatation before surgery, the strength and magnitude of the extra-scleral parietal pressure should be paid attention to during surgery to avoid the sharp changes of intraocular pressure, resulting in corneal edema and pupil narrowing.
3. The amplitude of eyeball rotation should be as small as possible. Due to the small corneal diameter and large curvature of newborns, if the angle between the light of the indirect ophthalmoscopes and the visual axis is too large, the aberration in the peripheral part will increase significantly. Therefore, the light of the indirect ophthalmoscopes should be as close to the vertical direction as possible,

and then cooperate with the scleral indentator to complete laser photocoagulation.

4. Proceed from easy to difficult, generally extending from the base of the ridge to the periphery, and gradually reducing the laser energy.
5. In the process of extending to the periphery, clearly identify the ora serrata before performing laser. The position and shape of the ora serrata in newborns are quite different from those in adults. It is located about 1 mm behind the limbus, a white area with leathery or shiny texture, adjacent to the dark brown area of the ciliary body.
6. The laser spots should not be too dense or too strong, with an interval of 1–1.5 laser spot distances (beginners often make the laser spots too dense), and the color should be grayish white (lighter than the laser spot reaction in adults).
7. The laser area is close to but not exceeding the ora serrata, avoiding anterior extension to damage the ciliary body, otherwise, complications such as hypotony and cataracts may occur.
8. The laser device has three settings: power, duration and interval. The critical setting is duration. A too high duration results in vitreous bleeding and progress of ROP. Always begin with a duration of 100 ms and maximize power before increasing the duration to 200 ms. Remark: In new laser devices, 100 ms duration is sufficient; in old laser devices 200 ms duration is required. 300 ms is too high.

12.2.4 Vitreoretinal Surgery

For ROP stage 4A, surgical treatment is not generally required. The therapy of choice is an anti-VEGF injection. We recommend to examine the eye in general anesthesia. If the eye has been pretreated with laser, then try to find skip lesions and treat these skip lesions with laser.

For ROP stage 4B, a vitrectomy is generally required, which is quite different from that of adults, and the focus should be on understanding its pathological anatomical features, access selection, surgical intent, and the corresponding surgical instruments.

(i) Pathologic Anatomical Features

The main manifestation is retinal detachment by traction and comparing it with severe PDR can help us better understand the pathological-anatomical features of ROP (Table. 12.2).

(ii) Choice of Surgical Approach

The choice of approach is determined by the severity of retinal detachment and the age of the child, as well as the operator's preference. The method of choice is a lens-sparing vitrectomy because the removal of the lens results in severe amblyopia. In advanced cases peripheral membranes develop and pull the retina toward the lens.

Table 12.2 Pathoanatomical features of ROP (≥4 stages) and severe PDR

	ROP	PDR
Vitreous state	Basically no liquefaction, delamination-like changes, and all-round adhesion to the retina below, there is great difficulty in posterior detachment	There may be partial or complete liquefaction, and adhesions to the underlying retina are well separated at the posterior pole and mid-periphery
Precipitating factor	Presence of avascular areas in the peripheral and mid-peripheral retina	Poor retinal perfusion, ischemic changes affecting the entire retina
Typical change	The ridge exists at the interface between the vascular and avascular areas of the retina	Fibrovascular membranes are present at the posterior pole and mid-periphery
Retinal detachment	From light to heavy, it can be expressed as peripheral shallow detachment, and full detachment can be wide-funnel or closed-funnel	After the detachment, the limited detachment of the pole is mainly, and it can also be expressed as a wide bucket or a closed bucket
Treatment time window	Extremely short	Longer
Operating space	Narrow	Spacious
Intraoperative complications that are difficult to manage	Iatrogenic break	Bleeding

Table 12.3 The distance between the posterior scleral incision and the corneal limbus

Month/age	0	1~6 month	6~12 month	1~3 age	3~6 age	6~18 age
Distance from limbus(mm)	0.5~1.0	1.5	2.0	2.5	3.0	3.5

The anterior pulled retina prevents access to the vitreous. In this case a lens removal is required.

The distance of the scleral incision from the corneal limbus is determined by the age of the child, usually starting at 0.5 mm, but the preoperative axis of the child and the degree of retinal detachment should be understood and adjusted (Table. 12.3).

Pars plana approach for ROP stage 4: The greatest advantage is that the clear lens is expected to be preserved, which is important for the visual development of the child.

One of the main problems encountered by beginners is the deformation of the eye during trocar insertion, mainly due to two major factors: (1) soft sclera and (2) the toughness of the conjunctiva and Tenon's capsule (associated with age). If both factors are present, the puncture becomes significantly more difficult, and the puncture step is like a "downward spiral" for the surgeon. We recommend therefore a perpendicular and not diagonal insertion of trocar cannulas. An additional help when inserting the trocar cannulas is to fixate the sclera with a forceps. An alternative is the opening of conjunctiva before you insert the trocar cannulas.

The pars plana approach is generally chosen for infusion. The biggest problem with pars plana infusion is that the trocar may swing toward the lens, injure the lens or prolapse backward, which can cause hypotony and choroidal detachment if not detected in time. To prevent this from happening, we recommend to tape the infusion cable onto the drape so that the infusion cannula is directed into the middle of the eye.

(iii) Basic Surgical Steps

1. Insertion of trocar cannulas
2. Insertion of infusion
3. Removal of the central vitreous
4. Removal of the peripheral vitreous
5. Decide whether to laser treat the retina
6. Partial fluid against air exchange
7. Inject anti-VEGF
8. Withdraw trocars
9. Check the scleral incision for tightness

In stage 5 ROP vitrectomy becomes very difficult. A pars plana (plicata) access is not possible. The only possible access is through the anterior chamber. The instruments are inserted through the limbus, the lens is removed, and then the closed retina is cautiously opened. The difficulty of this surgery is extremely high, and the postoperative results are very low so that surgery of stage 5 ROP is questionable.

Anterior approach: Insert the puncture knife at the corneal limbus, through the iris root, and let the puncture knife insert into the lens, with the angle of the two trocar being large enough, near 3 and 9 o'clock, respectively, to ensure sufficient space for both hands to operate; place the perfusion tube through the clear corneal incision; and remove the vitreous humor after the lens is removed; a clear corneal incision is generally chosen. The intraocular pressure is maintained by placing a perfusion tube, and care should be taken to avoid damage to the corneal endothelium.

For Stage 5 ROP, in addition to the above basic steps, a two-handed approach is often required, which may require a ceiling light, intraocular scissors, intraocular forceps, and "blunt" separation with viscoelastic if the vitreous is tightly adherent to the retina.

12.3 Rhegmatogenous Retinal Detachment Secondary to FEVR

12.3.1 Overview

Familial exudative vitreoretinopathy (FEVR) was first proposed and named by Criswick and Schepens in 1969. The lesion is similar to ROP without a history of prematurity or oxygen uptake and is inherited in autosomal dominant, autosomal recessive, and X-linked recessive forms. It is characterized by bilateral, slowly progressive vitreoretinal anomalies, dense distribution of peripheral retinal vessels, retinal neovascularization or intraretinal or subretinal exudation, optic disc or macular displacement, and in some cases, retinal detachment of retinal origin by traction or retinal break.

12.3.2 Clinical Staging of FEVR

In 2014, Kashani et al. proposed a new clinical staging method for FEVR based on the results of fundus wide-field fluorescence imaging, which differs from ROP in that the clinical symptoms of FEVR vary widely among individuals.

(i) Stage 1: no peripheral vascularity or abnormal intraretinal vascularization (1A: no exudation or fluorescein leakage; 1B: presence of exudation or fluorescein leakage)
(ii) Stage 2: peripheral retinal avascular area with extraretinal vascularization (2A: no exudation or fluorescein leakage; 2B: presence of exudation or fluorescein leakage)
(iii) Stage 3: retinal detachment without macular involvement (3A: no exudation or fluorescein leakage; 3B: presence of exudation or fluorescein leakage)
(iv) Stage 4: retinal detachment involving the macula, but not yet total detachment (4A: no exudation or fluorescein leakage; 4B: presence of exudation or fluorescein leakage)
(v) Stage 5: total retinal detachment (5A: open bucket shape; 5B: closed bucket shape)

In addition to retinal detachment requiring surgical treatment, related studies have shown that the presence of fluorescein leakage is a precursor to the occurrence of retinal leakage. For stage IB and 2B lesions, laser treatment should be performed promptly to close the leakage area and the avascular area to stop the progression of the lesion.

12.3.3 FEVR and RRD

Rhegmatogenous retinal detachment (RRD) in adolescents is not uncommon, but we often overlook the genetic factors behind it, the most typical example being FEVR.

FEVR is an underestimated disease in our country. In fact, among the majority of young patients with rhegmatogenous retinal detachment (RRD) who undergo scleral buckling in our practice, the underlying cause is eventually revealed to be FEVR after thorough fundus examination and screening of their family members.

Because retinal detachment due to FEVR often spreads gradually from the peripheral to the posterior pole, patients generally have no obvious subjective symptoms until the macula is involved, which is why many patients with FEVR may have been ill for a long time when they come to the clinic, and some may even have multiple subretinal bands or membranes visible. In recent years, there are also patients who were discovered during dilated pupil for fundus examination when seeking myopic laser surgery.

12.3.4 Principles of Surgical Management

(i) Laser photocoagulation, cryopexy, and anti-VEGF: Laser photocoagulation and anti-VEGF are the treatment of choice for FEVR. Perform a 360° laser photocoagulation from the ora serrata to the posterior pole. In young patients a treatment in general anesthesia is recommended. In the case of inferiorly located vasoproliferative tumors, a cryopexy can be added. The disadvantage of cryopexy is that an exudative detachment may develop which takes several months to resorb. It is therefore advisable to avoid cryopexy and if necessary to use it cautiously. Repeated anti-VEGF injections are recommended.

(ii) In the case of an exudative detachment, we recommend an external drainage of subretinal fluid and then treatment with laser photocoagulation or cryopexy. The healing time after treatment is long and may take 1–2 years.

(iii) Vitrectomy

For Stage 5 FEVR with obvious preretinal or subretinal proliferation or exudation, vitrectomy is generally required.

If the patient is young, no retinal tear is found, and the lesion is mainly exudate and traction; it can be treated basically according to the ROP internal surgery method, and postoperative attention should be paid to the treatment of residual avascular area, supplemented with laser or anti-VEGF intraocular injection if necessary.

If the patient is older and has retinal tears and proliferation, it should be treated according to RRD combined with severe PVR. The main difficulties of the operation are as follows:

1. Posterior vitreous detachment is difficult, and vitreous remains at the posterior pole.
2. Peripheral vitreous adhesions. It is very difficult to excise a sufficient amount. During the process of excision and stripping of the proliferative membrane, iatrogenic breaks are likely to occur.
3. If heavy water is used improperly, heavy water residues under the retina are likely to occur. If it is decided to perform vitrectomy, in order to better ensure the long-term success rate, episcleral cerclage can be performed at the same time to relieve the possible concentric traction caused by the residual vitreous in the peripheral area.

(iv) Scleral buckling

In our clinical work, most of the adolescent FEVR patients are often seen with mild or chronic retinal detachment. If RRD is not accompanied by obvious preretinal proliferation, regardless of whether the macula is involved or not, or whether there are subretinal proliferation strips, scleral buckling is generally recommended, which is what beginners need to focus on, and the main reasons include the following.

(a) Better closure of the breaks: retinal breaks are mostly atrophic and in the more peripheral area, which is less difficult to operate and easy to, especially when the primary break is located below, scleral buckling has a strong advantage.

(b) The degree of retinal shortening is lower: it is generally not necessary to perform subretinal fluid drainage, and the effect of scleral buckling is better, which can more precisely apply cryotherapy on the breaks and does not cause excessive eye wall and retinal damage.

(c) "Multiple benefits in one stroke": encircling and buckling can not only effectively close the retinal break, but also when there are multiple peripheral small breaks in the neighboring areas, scleral buckling can easily "close" all these breaks, so that the maximum effect can be obtained with the minimum amount of surgery. At the same time, it is less difficult to supplement retinal laser photocoagulation later because of the presence of scleral ridge."

(d) "Addressing both the primary breaks and the underlying avascular pathology": since the pathology of FEVR is based on the presence of avascular areas at the peripheral, scleral buckling not only closes the primary breaks but also treats these avascular areas with extra-scleral indentation, which largely relieves vitreous traction on the peripheral retina, and also prevents the progression of FEVR (if intraoperative cryotherapy or postoperative photocoagulation is applied).

It is worth noting that because the peripheral retina is relatively thin, the intensity and scope of intraoperative cryotherapy should be strictly controlled, otherwise it may cause retinal atrophy, which may lead to secondary retinal redetachment, and the risk of postoperative PVR may increase, making the second stage of treatment significantly more difficult.

We can apply laser photocoagulation around the degenerative retina in the undetached area before surgery, and then moderately perform cryotherapy intraoperatively around the primary break. 1~2 weeks after surgery, we can then perform laser photocoagulation on the retina in all peripheral degenerative areas in office.

12.4 Retinal Detachment Secondary to Stickler Syndrome

Stickler syndrome is a predominantly autosomal dominant disease of the connective tissues of the body characterized by a defect in collagen production due to a genetic mutation. It manifests as abnormalities in organs or systems such as the eyes, hearing, mouth and face, bones and joints, and heart.

12.4.1 Typology of Stickler Syndrome

Stickler syndrome generally includes four subtypes (Table 12.4), and the one closely related to ophthalmology is type 1, accounting for about 80%–90%.

12.4.2 Clinical Features of Stickler Syndrome

Patients with Stickler syndrome may have a series of abnormalities in appearance during childhood and adolescence, such as flattened face, anterior nostril tilt, wide or flat nasal bridge, jaw deformity (small or receding), joint hyperextension, kyphosis, etc. These external features can help us make preliminary diagnosis, but the gold standard for diagnosis requires genetic testing.

The abnormalities of Stickler syndrome in the eye are mainly manifested as follows: (1) congenital myopia with continuous increase; (2) premature liquefaction of the vitreous, which may be accompanied by curtain-like or string-like degeneration; (3) paravascular retinal degeneration and pigmentation; (4) focal lens cortical clouding; and (5) different types of retinal detachment.

Stickler Syndrome and Retinal Detachment

The lifetime probability of retinal detachment in patients with Stickler syndrome is about 50%–65%, but in the past, retinal detachment in this group of patients was often attributed to high myopia. With the advancement of our understanding of the disease and the development of genetic testing technology in recent years, more and more adolescents are diagnosed with the disease.

There are three common types of retinal detachment caused by Stickler syndrome: (1) giant retinal tear (GRT), (2) rhegmatogenous retinal detachment, and (3) retinal detachment without a clearly visible fissure. The recommended surgery is encircling band, vitrectomy and tamponade with gas or silicone oil. A prophylactic cryotherapy or laser photocoagulation of the fellow eye is recommended.

Table 12.4 Four subtypes of Stickler syndrome

Genes	Typing	Mode of inheritance	Clinical manifestations	Proportion
COL2A1	1	Autosomal dominant	Vitreous membrane like degeneration, congenital macroglossia, arthropathy, hearing impairment, cleft palate, etc	80%–90%
COL11A1	2	Autosomal dominant	Fibrous or beaded vitreous degeneration	10%–20%
COL11A2	3	Autosomal dominant	No general eye involvement	Rarely
COL9A1/ COL9A2	4	Autosomal recessive	Vitreous membrane like degeneration, congenital macroglossia, no systemic involvement seen	Rarely

(i) GRT

1. For fresh GRT without obvious PVR, because the vitreous liquefaction at the posterior pole is obvious and the mobility of the detached retina is high enough, vitrectomy is usually not so difficult, but the following details should be noted: (1) adequate removal of the peripheral vitreous to relieve the traction; (2) because mobility of the retina is high, iatrogenic damage caused by the intravitreal instruments should be avoided; and (3) if fluid/air exchange is required, the eye position should be adjusted appropriately to avoid rolling and slippage of the retinal flap.

   If you choose to fill with silicone oil, you can directly choose the oil/liquid exchange method to prevent slippage of the retinal flap; some patients can also choose to short- or medium-term tamponade of heavy liquid, and the patient can maintain the supine position after surgery, and then remove the heavy liquid 7~10 days after the initial surgery.
2. With obvious PVR mainly because of the longer duration, the surgery is more difficult and easy to have iatrogenic damages. Encirling can be considered as a supplementary option to prevent slippage of the peripheral retina.

(ii) Rhegmatogenous Retinal Detachment

Unlike common rhegmatogenous retinal detachment, the primary break is often multiple, and the crumpled and degenerated vitreous membrane-like tissue will adhere tightly to the retina, so attention should be paid to the strength and scope when peeling off the proliferative membrane during surgery, otherwise it will cause new fissures or enlargement of fissures.

Some patients with long-standing occult disease may have different degrees of subretinal proliferative tissues, which are often in the peripheral part, so the retina can be flattened with heavy water to determine the area where the subretinal retractive cords are located, and then the retinotomy site can be reasonably designed, and finally the proliferative cords or membranes can be pulled out with intraocular forceps. The key to this step is the design of the retinal incision site, which is generally close to the superior and mid-periphery.

In younger patients, simultaneous scleral episcleral ligation is generally recommended.

(iii) Retinal Detachment Without Visualization of the Break

The main cause of detachment is diffuse vitreous crinkling degeneration with extensive adhesions to the underlying retina, and the primary fissure is not visible although the retina is extensively detached preoperatively.

The surgical focus is to remove the vitreous proliferative membrane in the posterior pole and mid-periphery, inject TA and ICG if necessary to better label the residual vitreous, and strive for adequate removal of the crinkled vitreous. A retinotomy is often required, with the superior and mid-peripheral areas preferred. In younger patients, concomitant scleral episcleral ligation is generally recommended to relieve the centripetal pull that may be associated with the circumferential vitreous.

12.5 Summary

"The surgeon who operates without understanding the nature of the disease is like a traveler who journeys without a map." In the demanding field of pediatric retina, adhering to basic surgical protocols is merely the baseline; true mastery requires a profound comprehension of the underlying pathophysiologic mechanisms unique to the developing eye. This deep understanding enables the surgeon to transition from a generalized approach to a highly targeted surgical strategy, tailored to the specific vascular and tractional dynamics of each case. Furthermore, in the delicate environment of a child's eye, the prevention of iatrogenic trauma is paramount—precision must be absolute to avoid complications of medical origin. When managed with this level of expertise, modern vitreoretinal technology provides a powerful means to effectively salvage and preserve vision that was once deemed lost.

Complex pathologies such as Retinopathy of Prematurity (ROP), Familial Exudative Vitreoretinopathy (FEVR), and Stickler Syndrome represent some of the most formidable challenges in ophthalmology. These conditions are not only rare but technically exhausting to treat, characterized by aggressive vitreoretinal traction and fragile anatomical structures. Mastery of these pathologies necessitates a tripartite foundation: a comprehensive intellectual grasp of the disease's evolution, the refinement of advanced surgical skills, and the utilization of specialized, high-performance equipment. Only through this integration can the surgeon navigate these difficult cases with the confidence and precision required for success.

Editing and Presentation of Surgical Videos

13

"Seeing is believing." With the growing vitality of international ophthalmological academic exchange and the rapid expansion of digital platforms, surgical videos have become increasingly indispensable for academic dissemination. Along with traditional printed materials, these videos now constitute a core component of scholarly literature, offering a depth of information—particularly in the visualization of intricate operative details—that remains unparalleled by traditional print media. (1) Enhanced visualization of micro-surgical maneuvers; (2) Rapid dissemination across global academic networks; and (3) Intuitive learning experiences that bridge the gap between theory and practice.

A vast array of desktop and mobile software is now available for video production, most of which are highly accessible and capable of meeting basic surgical documentation needs. However, many practitioners still lack a comprehensive grasp of the essential concepts and technical nuances required to create professional surgical media. (1) Selection of appropriate hardware and recording systems to ensure high-definition clarity; (2) Implementation of standardized editing workflows to optimize operative time and educational value; and (3) Adherence to ethical guidelines, particularly regarding patient anonymity and data security. By starting with the fundamental elements of high-quality media, this chapter utilizes practical examples to guide the reader through the entire process of editing and presenting vitreoretinal surgical videos.

13.1 Unique Characteristics of Vitreoretinal Surgical Videos

Unlike other ophthalmological subspecialties, vitreoretinal surgery possesses distinct advantages for video production, characterized by the following features:ophthalmological subspecialties, vitreoretinal surgery has distinct advantages for video production, including the following:

Z. Zhang, U. Spandau, *Vitreoretinal Surgery*,
https://doi.org/10.1007/978-3-032-25271-5_13

1. Complex and diverse surgical maneuvers that provide a wealth of material for clinical demonstration
2. A wide spectrum of surgical difficulty, making these videos suitable for diverse audiences and academic events at all levels
3. A vast variety of pathologies with well-defined themes, allowing for diverse presentation styles and a high degree of novelty
4. A clear and continuous narrative structure that guides the viewer through the procedure, providing inherent educational value
5. An extensive operational scope with distinct anatomical layering, where the progression and switching of intraoperative views significantly enhance the video's engagement and visual appeal

13.2 Core Elements of Surgical Videos

A standard surgical video must include the following four core elements:

(1) Clarity
As the most fundamental element of a surgical video, clarity is the prerequisite for showcasing all other features. It mainly depends on three factors:

1. Hardware support (e.g., microscope resolution and camera pixel count)
2. Parameter settings (e.g., microscope magnification and focus adjustment)
3. Refractive media (e.g., opacification of the cornea or lens significantly reduces video clarity)

(2) Educational Value
As the core and soul of any surgical video, educational value dictates that the images are not merely simple recordings but essential carriers of surgical theories and techniques. To maximize this value, editors should focus on the following: (1) Identifying and extracting specific clinical problems encountered during the procedure; (2) Proposing clear, evidence-based solutions to these challenges; and (3) Utilizing concise video segments to help viewers intuitively understand and master complex surgical knowledge.

(3) Coherence
Surgical videos follow a linear timeline, sequentially presenting clinical challenges and highlighting critical intraoperative details. To effectively convey embedded knowledge within a limited timeframe, the production should adhere to the following principles: (1) Ensuring all surgical segments are highly relevant to the primary theme; (2) Maintaining a continuous and logical narrative flow to guide the viewer's cognitive process; and (3) Focusing on the seamless integration of visual evidence and theoretical explanations to enhance educational impact.

(4) Storytelling

A surgical video without a clear narrative structure risks presenting disjointed content, thereby failing to convey a compelling message. Each surgical case represents a unique clinical narrative, and many exceptional cases are overlooked due to a lack of effective presentation. Video editing provides the opportunity to transform these outstanding cases into compelling stories, thereby amplifying their educational impact. Consequently, before commencing the editing process, editors should undertake the following steps: (1) Conduct a thorough analysis of the case's key characteristics and clinical significance; (2) Strategically consider the intended display scenario and target audience; and (3) Ultimately, present a cohesive and impactful final product that seamlessly integrates medical expertise with artistic presentation techniques.

13.3 Basic Parameters of Surgical Videos

(1) Frame

The basic unit of a video. Continuous playback of static images creates the illusion of motion in the human eye (due to visual persistence); each static image is one frame.

(2) Frame Rate

A key parameter for video submissions, as different platforms may have varying frame rate requirements. It refers to the number of frames played per second, measured in frames per second (fps). A higher frame rate makes the video smoother, but it is not always better—24 fps is generally sufficient for good smoothness.

(3) Aspect Ratio

The ratio of a video's horizontal length to its vertical length, which determines the video's shape. The 4:3 aspect ratio is rarely used for surgical videos today; the most common is 16:9. This ratio feels natural for daily viewing, fully displays image information, and matches the aspect ratio of most modern electronic displays, making it widely accepted. However, for ophthalmic surgeries, the 16:9 ratio leaves large black areas on both sides of the video—these areas can be used to add video details and increase information content.

(4) Resolution

Refers to the pixel dimensions of a video image, usually expressed as width × height, such as 1920 × 1080 pixels. When a video is enlarged several times, small squares (pixels, the basic units of the image) become visible. In video terminology, "4K" generally refers to a horizontal resolution of approximately 4,000 pixels, although consumer 4K/UHD commonly uses 3840 × 2160 pixels. Higher resolution improves clarity but requires better device performance and longer time for transmission and downloading. Thus, excessive pursuit of high-resolution during video storage may cause device lag.

Unless specified otherwise, the common resolution for vitreoretinal surgery videos is 1920 × 1080 (1920 pixels horizontally and 1080 pixels vertically). This resolution fully displays surgical details and is well-supported by most electronic devices, ensuring smooth playback.

(5) Bitrate

The amount of data transmitted per unit time, usually measured in kilobits per second (kbps). A higher bitrate generally preserves more image information and produces a file closer to the original recording. Bitrate is proportional to video quality and file size; exceeding a certain bitrate has little effect on improving image quality.

For 1080P videos, the recommended bitrate is 5000–8000 kbps. To ensure optimal quality, the selected bitrate should match the camera's recording bitrate as closely as possible.

(6) Codec

A codec is a method or standard used to encode and decode video data, primarily to compress file size for easier storage and transmission.

The most common codec for surgical videos is H.264/AVC, a video compression standard established in 2003 with high compression efficiency, strong error resilience, good network adaptability, and high video quality. The newer H.265/HEVC standard (officially adopted in 2013 to expand H.264/AVC) offers even higher compression efficiency, reducing storage space for high-resolution videos and improving playback speed. It is expected to become mainstream as device performance improves.

(7) Format

Format selection is a common yet easily solvable issue in surgical video editing. The current general requirements are MP4 or MOV formats:

- MP4: A widely used multimedia container format that can store video, audio, subtitles, and other data. It is commonly encoded with codecs such as H.264 or H.265. Note that MP4 is not equivalent to MPEG-4—MPEG-4 can be used in formats like MP4, MOV, and AVI. MP4 is supported by most electronic devices and takes up less storage space; it is the default choice unless specified otherwise.
- MOV: Developed by Apple Inc., it has a slightly lower compression ratio than MP4 and higher video clarity. Like MP4, it has good cross-platform compatibility but is less widely supported. It works well for playback and editing on Apple devices.

A common problem for beginners is that the editing software does not support original video formats (e.g., AVI and MPG). Format conversion software is required, but this often reduces clarity or causes segment loss. The best solution is to set the original video format to the universal MP4 or MOV from the start to maximize editing efficiency and video clarity.

(8) Depth of Field (DOF) of the Microscope
Also called focal depth, it refers to the range within which the image remains clear when adjusting the distance between the objective lens and the sample surface (during microscopic observation or recording). Since the human eye's adjustment ability varies, DOF can differ between individuals.

13.4 How to Adjust Your Camera and Microscope

(1) Adjustment of Focus and Refraction
Microscopes are designed with a DOF; in vitreoretinal surgery, a larger DOF is highly advantageous as it minimizes the need for frequent manual focus adjustments. Ideally, the microscope's built-in camera has a fixed focus that is parfocal with the eyepieces. If the surgeon maintains an emmetropic state throughout the procedure, the images seen through the oculars and captured by the camera will share the same clarity, requiring only standard adjustments via the foot pedal.

However, many surgeons—particularly younger ones during delicate macular or anterior segment maneuvers—frequently experience instrument-induced myopia (or instrument accommodation). In this state, emmetropic individuals develop temporary myopia, while myopic individuals experience a transient increase in their refractive error. To compensate for this subjective blur, the surgeon often inadvertently adjusts the microscope's focus via the foot pedal to offset the refractive deviation. This action shifts the focal plane relative to the fixed-focus camera, resulting in a recorded image that is significantly blurred despite the surgeon seeing a sharp field (Fig. 13.1). Although this phenomenon does not hinder the surgical execution itself,

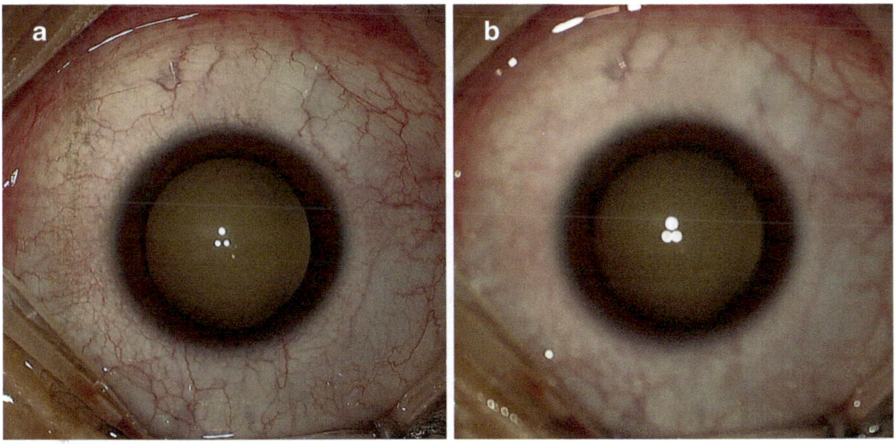

Fig. 13.1 Blurred display image due to microscope focus adjustment after the surgeon develops instrument-induced myopia. (**a**) Before instrument-induced myopia: The display image and the image seen by the surgeon through the microscope eyepiece have nearly the same clarity; (**b**) After instrument-induced myopia: Adjusting the microscope focus causes mild defocusing of the display image, but the image seen by the surgeon through the eyepiece remains clear—the surgeon is unaware of the blurred camera image

it severely compromises video quality, a technical flaw that is often only discovered—much to the surgeon's regret—during post-editing.

To solve this problem: First, adjust the display image to maximum clarity. Then, adjust the diopter on the microscope eyepiece to offset instrument-induced myopia (usually −1.00 to −3.00 diopters).

If the microscope is equipped with an external camera, simply adjust the camera's focus manually (no need to adjust the eyepiece diopter) to obtain a clear image.

To record a clear surgical video throughout the process, the surgeon and assistant should dynamically adjust the setup based on the display image at all times to avoid missing important operational details.

(2) Brightness Adjustment

Brightness is critical to video clarity: insufficient brightness causes excessive noise, while excessive brightness leads to overexposure and loss of details. Brightness adjustment mainly involves two scenarios:

1. For anterior segment surgery: Adjust the microscope brightness to clearly visualize iris texture.
2. For posterior segment surgery: Adjust the brightness of the light guide fiber. The fiber's end should not be too close to the retina. With a non-aging bulb, the brightness is generally set to 35%–40% of the maximum.

(3) Magnification Adjustment

Too low magnification limits the surgical field to a small area of the video. Cropping during postediting will enlarge the image, reduce overall resolution, and cause noise. Too high magnification may make the surgical field exceed the video frame, resulting in lost details. For posterior segment surgery, adjust the microscope magnification so that the upper and lower edges of the surgical field are slightly close to the upper and lower edges of the video frame

13.5 Choosing the Right Editing Software for Efficiency and Quality

For surgical video editing, regardless of the software type (Table 13.1), the following points should be noted:

1. Do not reduce video quality.
2. Allow cropping to center the surgical field.
3. Have moderate hardware requirements.
4. Use appropriate artistic elements (e.g., transitions and titles)—avoid being too dull or overly fancy to maintain academic rigor.

Table 13.1 Advantages and disadvantages of common video editing software

Software type	Advantages	Disadvantages	Operating system	Recommendation
Adobe Premiere Pro	Versatile, wide application range, strong image editing functions, meets almost all surgical video editing needs	High system requirements, prone to computer lag; requires frequent saving; relatively high operation difficulty; paid	Windows, MacOS	Medium
CapCut	Easy to use, free, fully functional, meets almost all surgical video editing needs	Artistic effects tend to be entertainment--oriented	Windows, MacOS	High
Final Cut Pro	Professional-level editing, simple operation, stable performance, smooth running; auto-saves edited files; supports multiple effects via plugins	Paid; only supports a few formats (e.g., MP4 and MOV); other formats require conversion first	MacOS	High
iMovie	Easy to use, stable performance, autosaves edited files; meets basic surgical video editing needs (suitable for general editing or rough cutting, with further processing via other software)	Monotonous artistic effects; only supports a few formats (e.g., MP4 and MOV); other formats require conversion first	MacOS	Medium
MOV AVI	Clean and user-friendly interface; built-in multiple video processing effects; supports multiple formats	Paid; high system requirements; prone to lag; entertainment--oriented artistic effects	Windows, MacOS	High
Corel VideoStudio	Simple operation, streamlined editing process, user-friendly interface, high system stability	Paid; monotonous effects; entertainment--oriented	Windows, MacOS	Medium
Windows Movie Maker	Preinstalled on Windows; very easy to use; smooth performance; supports multiple formats	No longer updated; limited functions; difficult to download	Windows	Low

Various software options are available (briefly introduced below). For beginners, it is often difficult to create high-quality surgical videos with a single software in a short time. Combining multiple software (leveraging each strengths) can achieve twice the result with half the effort.

13.6 Fundamental Steps and Matters Needing Attention

Taking CapCut Desktop Version as an example, this section explains the basic process and precautions for surgical video editing. Beginners can choose multiple editing software based on their habits to meet different needs and scenarios.

(1) Video Shooting and Storage

Surgical videos are usually recorded by the microscope's built-in camera and stored in real time on a computer hard drive or cloud system. To ensure compatibility with playback and editing software, it is recommended to set the original video format to the mainstream MP4 or MOV to avoid clarity loss or segment loss during post-conversion.

For videos to be edited, use a large-capacity hard drive (usually ≥1 TB) for timely storage and backup. Rename and archive the files promptly for easy retrieval.

(2) Starting Editing

After preparing the videos, open the software and click "Start Creating" (Fig. 13.2) to enter the workspace (Fig. 13.3).

(3) Importing Materials

Click "Import" in Area A, select the original video and other media to be integrated into the video from the hard drive, and drag the video from Area A to Area D (Fig. 13.4).

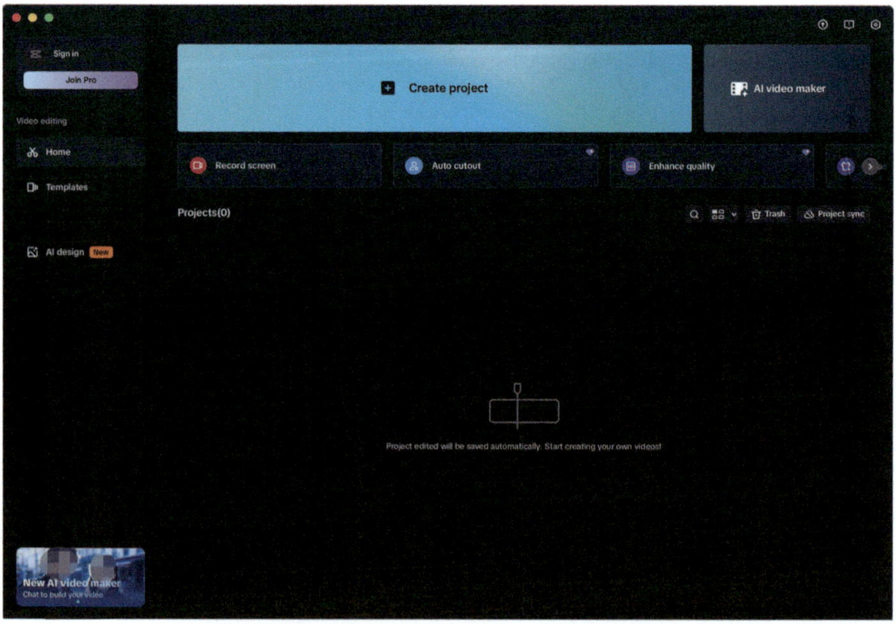

Fig. 13.2 Opening interface of CapCut Pro: Click "Start Creating" to enter the workspace

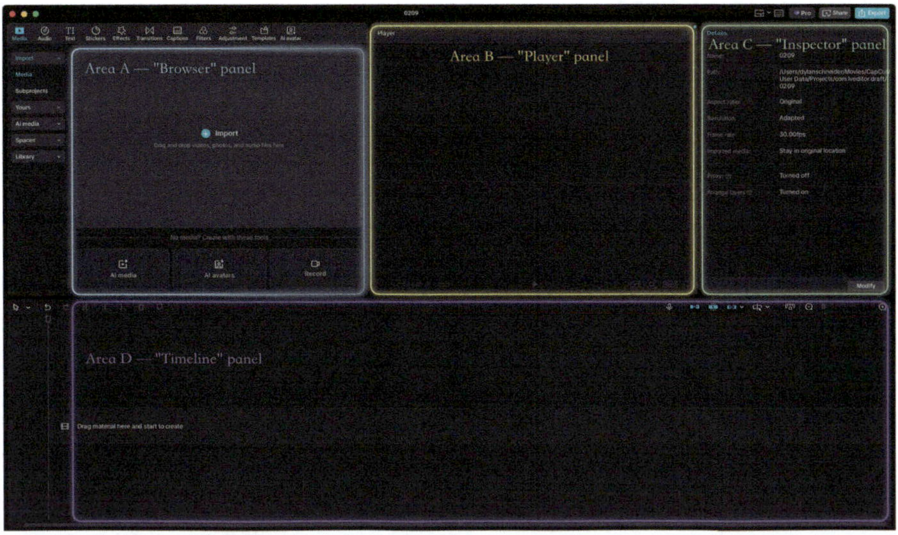

Fig. 13.3 Four workspaces of the software. Area A ("Browser" panel): Manages materials, imports videos, audio, images, etc. Area B ("Player" panel): Views video editing details in real time. Area C ("Inspector" panel): Views metadata, adjusts parameters, edits subtitles, etc. Area D ("Timeline" panel): Edits and processes all media

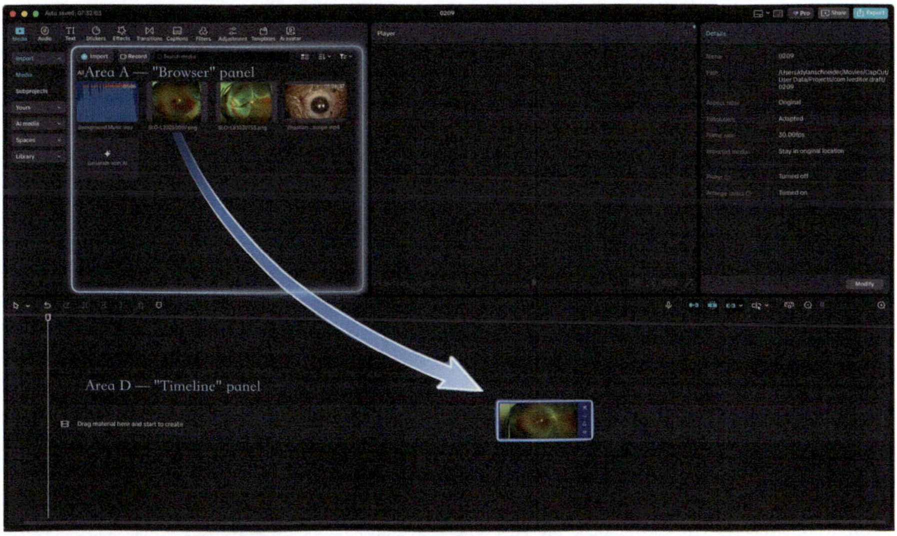

Fig. 13.4 Drag media files from Area A to Area D to start editing

(4) Rough Video Editing

In Area D, use the video split tool to divide the original video into segments, and then delete unnecessary parts. This is the most time-consuming and patience-requiring step in surgical video editing (Fig. 13.5).

(5) Image Adjustment

1. Image cropping: Due to magnification adjustments and surgical field shifts, continuous cropping is often needed to keep the surgical field centered (Fig. 13.6),

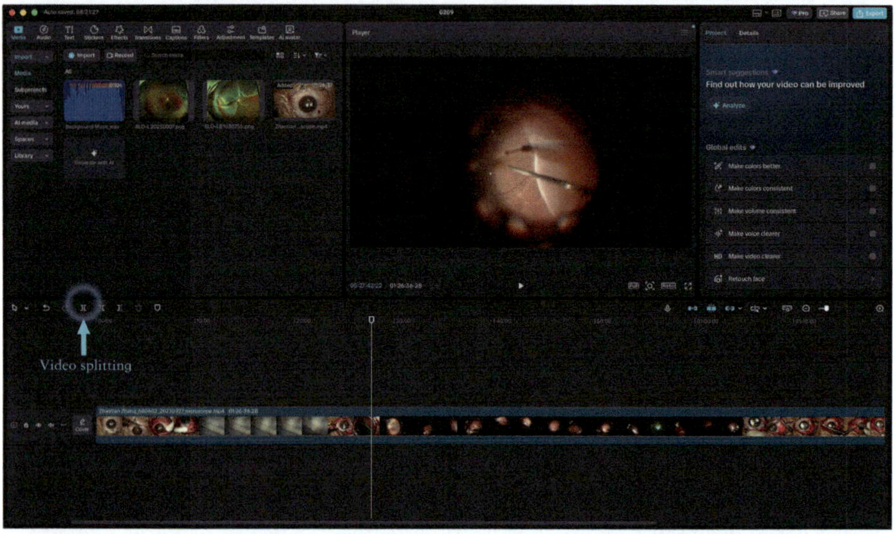

Fig. 13.5 Area D has multiple function buttons for splitting, cutting, and deleting video segments

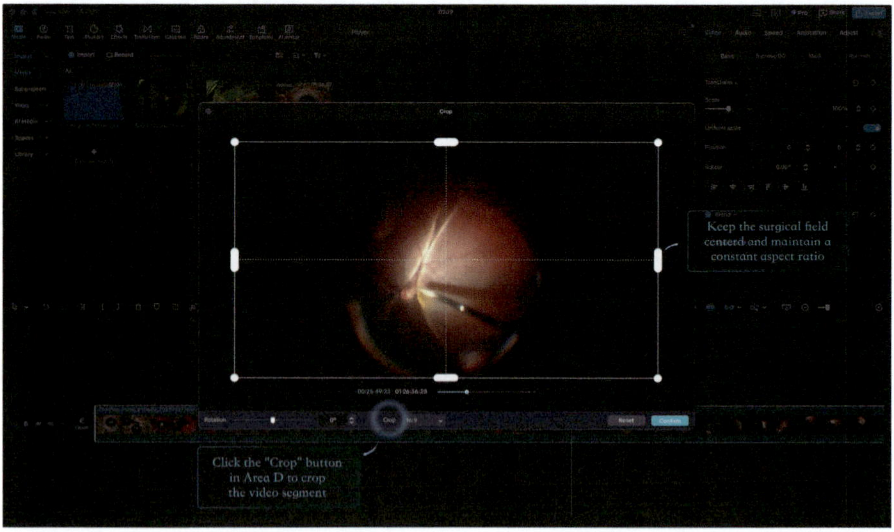

Fig. 13.6 Click the "Crop" button in Area D to crop the video segment; keep the surgical field centered and maintain a constant aspect ratio

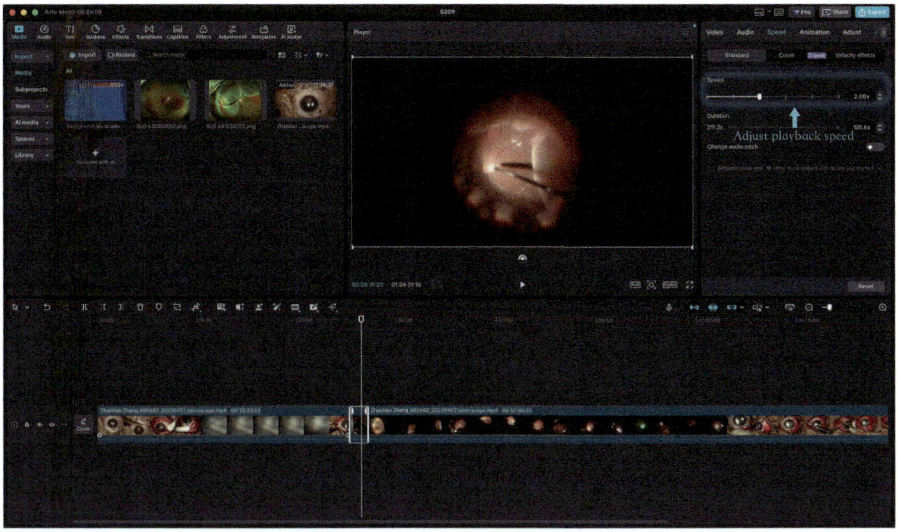

Fig. 13.7 Double-click the video segment in Area D to adjust the playback speed in Area C

which improves video quality. Note: If the original video has too low magnification, post-cropping will reduce clarity and may cause noise.

2. Playback speed: Adjusting playback speed is another key part of image adjustment. Based on long-term experience, doubling the original speed (2×) is optimal; dynamic adjustments can be made for key steps (Fig. 13.7).

(6) Adding Transitions

Transitions connect different surgical steps, improve video fluency, and attract viewers' attention (Fig. 13.8).

(7) Adding Subtitles

Subtitles play an important role in surgical video presentation. They should be accurate and concise, with no excessive effects (Fig. 13.9).

(8) Adding Audio or Narration

Audio and narration are not mandatory for surgical videos—editors can decide whether to add them based on specific needs. Audio enhances the video's atmosphere and viewers' immersion, but its style and volume should be appropriate to avoid overshadowing the main content. If needed, add narration: it should be concise and progress with the video's plot (Fig. 13.10).

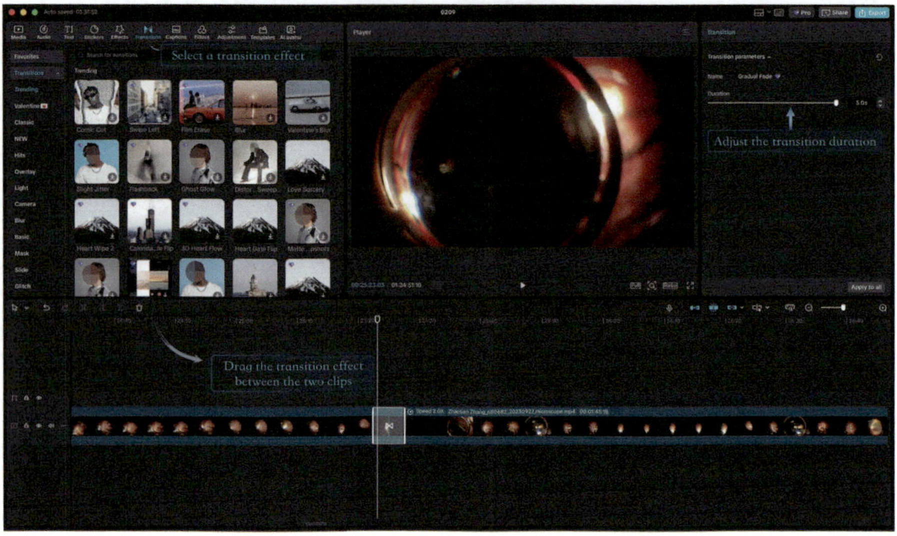

Fig. 13.8 Select a transition effect in Area A, drag it between two video segments in Area D, and adjust the transition duration in Area C

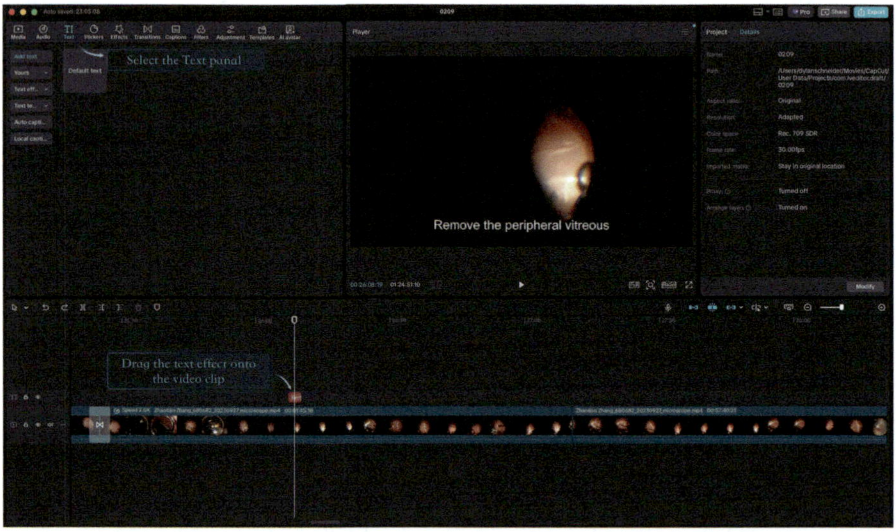

Fig. 13.9 Select a subtitle template in Area A, drag it above the video segment in Area D, enter the subtitle content and adjust its size/position in Area C; view the adjusted effect in Area B

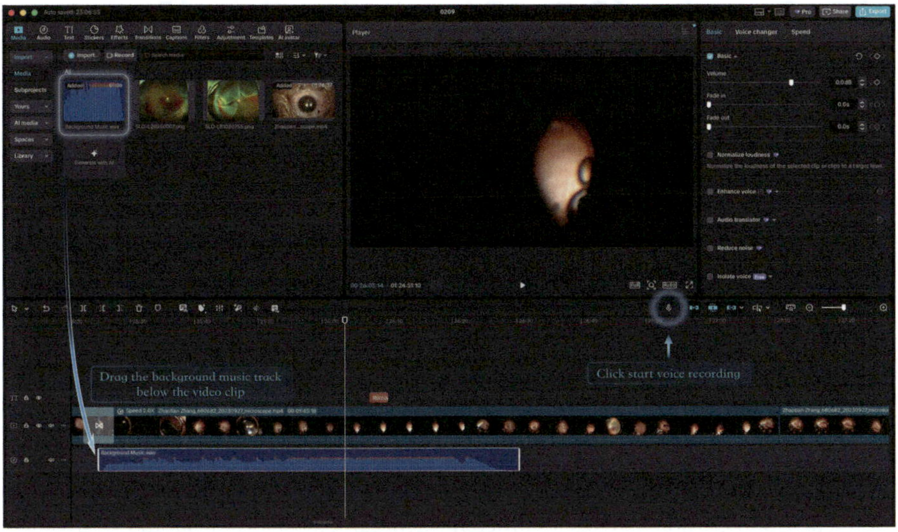

Fig. 13.10 Drag audio from Area A below the video segment in Area D; adjust audio effects (e.g., volume, fade-in/fade-out time) in Area C; click the "Record" button in the upper left corner of Area D to record narration

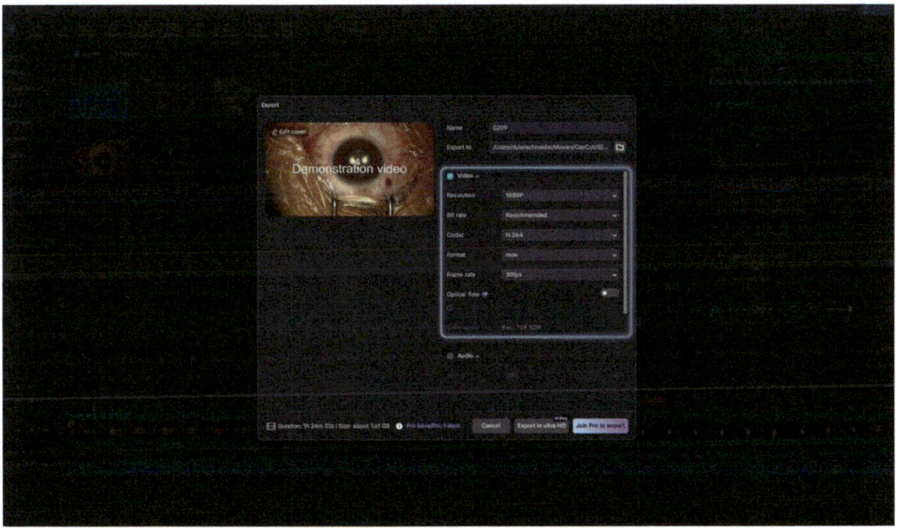

Fig. 13.11 Parameters in the red box include resolution, bitrate, codec, format, frame rate, etc.

(9) Saving the Video

After previewing the video and confirming it meets expectations, click the "Export" button in the upper right corner of the software interface. Enter the video parameters and save the file to the hard drive (Fig. 13.11).

13.7 Protection of Patient Privacy and Intellectual Property

With the rise of online platforms, the internet has become an important channel for surgical video dissemination. While we can access various multimedia resources online to enhance the professionalism and interest of surgical videos, this also brings risks such as patient privacy leaks and intellectual property infringement.

When creating videos involving specific patients, blur or remove their personal identification information. If the patient's face must be included, cover key areas (e.g., eyes) to prevent identification.

Multimedia files may involve intellectual property in the following aspects:

1. Fonts: Avoid unauthorized fonts—this issue has received increasing attention in online works in recent years.
2. Background music: Most online music is protected by intellectual property rights—avoid infringement when selecting music.
3. Video clips: Editors sometimes insert guiding or interesting video clips into surgical videos, which carries significant infringement risks and should be avoided.

13.8 Showcase Your Art Works

Surgical videos can be presented through multiple channels, mainly including the following:

1. Case presentations: The most common method. Surgical videos are usually inserted into slides and presented with key case points. Note: Videos should be concise, with clear key points and no excessive artistic effects; they should align closely with the slide text.
2. Academic conferences: Due to their high academic value and interest, surgical videos have become increasingly attractive in academic events at all levels. As overall production standards improve, requirements for case quality and editing techniques have also risen. In China, the influential "Zeiss Film Festival" of the Retina China Forum; internationally, the well-known "Film Festival" of the American Society of Retina Specialists (ASRS) are major platforms.
3. Professional journals: Surgical videos are published as electronic supplements with manuscripts to better describe case characteristics and surgical details. This increases the manuscript's information content and conveys more accurate and intuitive knowledge. Some professional journals accept video-focused submissions—for example, RETINA has a "Surgical Technique" section dedicated to new surgical techniques and methods.
4. Online platforms: In recent years, surgical videos are often shared as short videos on major social media platforms. However, due to the lack of strict peer review and screening, the content quality varies greatly, and the information conveyed is often single—there is significant room for improvement.

13.9 Summary

"A picture is worth a thousand words, but a well-edited video tells the soul of a story." This chapter provides a comprehensive framework for the fundamental concepts and technical workflows of surgical video production.

To excel in this digital medium, editors must move beyond simple documentation and strive for professional excellence through the following pillars: (1) Mastering the intricate functionalities of professional editing software to ensure a polished final product; (2) Prioritizing originality and academic rigor to maintain the integrity of clinical evidence; (3) Strategically aligning the narrative structure with specific presentation scenarios and target audiences; and (4) Leveraging creative storytelling to transform technical maneuvers into engaging educational experiences.

By synthesizing these elements, surgeons can share compelling cases with the global community, foster the exchange of innovative surgical methodologies, and ultimately enhance the vitality and depth of academic discourse in the field of vitreoretinal surgery.

Part III

Vitrectomy in Europe

14 General Introduction to Vitreoretinal Surgery in Europe

14.1 Education of Vitreoretinal (VR) Surgery

Cataract surgery is two dimensional and VR surgery is three dimensional. What does this mean? In cataract surgery as well as in VR surgery surgical performance is one key factor. But in VR surgery the assessment of a retinal case is a second key factor. A wrong assessment in VR surgery can easily result in a failed surgery. You must think twice before surgery. I have seen so many complications because VR surgeons pushed the vitreous cutter into the eye without reflecting the underlying pathology and then realizing that they cannot cope.

In cataract surgery the assessment is easy because the nucleus is clearly visible. But in VR surgery, the pathology may be hidden behind a vitreous bleeding or a dense cataract. In cataract surgery the timing is of minor importance. In VR surgery the timing is of major importance. In the case of a retinal detachment or a florid PDR, the approach and timing are of essential importance. Vitreoretinal surgery is 25% thinking and 75% surgery.

In Europe we start surgical education with cataract surgery. Then some cataract surgeons continue with vitrectomy. For vitrectomies the beginner starts with silicone oil removal and core vitrectomies. The next step is membrane removal and easy retinal detachments. The following steps are buckle/vitrectomy and easy diabetic vitrectomies.

The next step is a big step and requires mastering PVR detachments and tractional diabetic retinopathies. These pathologies require the bimanual peeling technique with a chandelier light.

14.2 Easy and Difficult Vitrectomy

In my working career, I have worked in three University hospitals and seen many different vitrectomy schools. And I have seen many complications. The cause of these complications is only partially due to poor surgical quality but especially due

Z. Zhang, U. Spandau, *Vitreoretinal Surgery*,
https://doi.org/10.1007/978-3-032-25271-5_14

to wrong surgical approach and technique. Which pathologies have most frequently a complication? PVR detachments and tractional diabetic retinopathy. These pathologies I consider and classify as difficult vitrectomies, whereas (almost) everything else are an easy vitrectomy. The exceptions are rare cases such as pediatric cases and trauma cases.

Peeling vitrectomies are easy vitrectomies, focal detachments are easy vitrectomies, and diabetic vitreous hemorrhage with complete PVD is an easy vitrectomy. In contrast, PVR detachments with stiff retina and preretinal and/or subretinal membranes are difficult vitrectomies. Diabetic eyes of young patients who never visited an ophthalmologist, which were never scatter laser treated and have vitreoretinal tractions, are difficult vitrectomies.

The latter pathologies should only be operated by experienced surgeons, and I can very much recommend to visit excellent vitrectomy clinics to observe and experience their surgical approach and quality.

In general, I recommend to visit excellent vitrectomy hospitals. You must experience excellent vitrectomy surgery and know the standard for high quality vitrectomy surgery. How do you otherwise know if a failed eye was your mistake or fate. Personally, I consider a failed eye as a personal mistake until the opposite is proved. This means that I search for surgical mistakes, wrong approaches, and wrong indication. As a surgeon you always make mistakes, but it is very important to avoid the same mistake a second time.

14.3 Cataract Surgery and Vitrectomy

The easiest eye for vitrectomy is a pseudophakic eye. Why? Firstly, the view to fundus is perfect. Secondly, the anterior vitreous can be completely removed and there is no risk of damaging the posterior lens capsule. This is especially important in vitreous bleedings. The anterior bloody vitreous can be completely removed, and there is no optical obstacle to core vitrectomy. In contrast, in a phakic eye, you can barely see the retina because the anterior bloody vitreous cannot be removed. The removal of anterior vitreous is also important in retinal detachments. It reduces the risk for redetachments. Thirdly, the peripheral vitreous and anterior hyaloid can be completely removed in a pseudophakic eye. All this is not possible in a phakic eye.

In peeling vitrectomies, we remove the lens in patients over 60 years of age. In retinal detachments we remove the lens in patients over 50 years of age, and in diabetics we remove the lens in patients over 40–45 years of age.

When should the cataract surgery be performed? Before, combined or after vitrectomy? The simple answer is before. Why? Cataract surgery is easiest before vitrectomy because the vitreous supports the nucleus. If cataract surgery is performed before vitrectomy, then the IOL is stable in a fibrotized lens capsule when performing vitrectomy. Combined phaco/vitrectomy is the second-best choice. The advantage is that the patient undergoes only one surgery. The disadvantage is that the anterior chamber is unstable during vitrectomy. If you insert the trocar cannulas, the anterior chamber collapses, and an IOL dislocation is possible due to gas tamponade or impression of sclera. Everybody who has already operated on cataracts in a vitrectomized eye has experienced how difficult surgery is and how much the risk for complication rises. The cataract is harder and the anterior chamber very deep.

Time interval between cataract and vitrectomy: One week time interval between cataract surgery and vitrectomy is sufficient.

In Conclusion For planned vitrectomies we send the patient to a cataract surgeon for lens removal and then perform vitrectomy in a pseudophakic eye. In emergency vitrectomies we perform combined phaco/vitrectomy. In diabetics we combine cataract surgery and anti-VEGF injection. The vitrectomy is usually performed 1 month later.

In the following chapters, I will show step-by-step how to perform an easy and difficult vitrectomy for retinal detachment and diabetic retinopathy.

All videos for my surgery can be found on my YouTube channel: Please find my playlists:

The playlist for detachment surgery is https://youtube.com/playlist?list=PL0dKYclPD7yMn861X0g-aHCS6KZ5NcH1N&si=_jtQa_sWVJL1PMe3.

The playlist for diabetic surgery is https://youtube.com/playlist?list=PL0dKYclPD7yM9qRjBoF1HMwtxFfbf2T6A&si=VIFMlS6XzusriySr.

Combined Phaco/Vitrectomy

15

A rhegmatogenous retinal detachment (RRD) with multiple breaks is a surgery for experienced surgeons, as there is a significant complication profile. The beginner should start with a localized detachment (one to two quadrant detachment and a single break), as this is usually easier to manage.

Regarding surgery, we recommend two things, which simplify vitrectomy very much: phacoemulsification and usage of a chandelier light. We recommend performing a phacoemulsification in all patients older than 50 years because the anterior vitreous and the vitreous base can be removed completely. See our treatment algorithm (Fig. 15.1). Secondly, we recommend the usage of a chandelier light because it facilitates every step of the vitrectomy. A complete removal of the anterior vitreous is only possible after the removal of the natural lens. Visualization and removal of the vitreous base is easier with chandelier light. The retinal breaks are located in the periphery and need to be indented with the scleral depressor: Nobody indents as well as your second hand.

PFCL or no PFCL?

Some vitreoretinal clinics use PFCL as a routine; others don't. PFCL is an excellent tool for vitreoretinal surgery and we recommend using it, if necessary. We use PFCL in large, macula-off detachments, and we work without PFCL in focal, macula-on detachments. In giant tears we always use PFCL due to the risk of slippage.

25G or 27G?

27G is superior to 25G in myopic eyes. 27G sclerotomies require no suture. Myopic eyes tend to leak and 27G sclerotomies have only minimal leakage. Minimal leakage results also in improved gas tamponade. The disadvantage of 27G is the soft instruments. In normal eyes a 25G cutter is therefore recommended. Another advantage is that passive aspiration with the fluid needle is more efficient with 25G than with 27G.

Z. Zhang, U. Spandau, *Vitreoretinal Surgery*,
https://doi.org/10.1007/978-3-032-25271-5_15

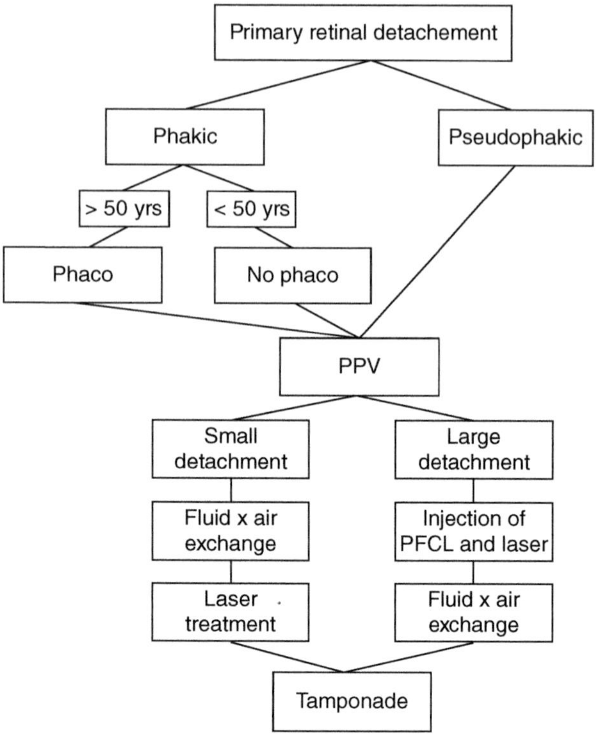

Fig. 15.1 Our treatment algorithm for retinal detachment surgery

Anesthesia

We always use peribulbar anesthesia. General anesthesia is not necessary.

15.1 The Surgery

Instruments

1. 25/27 gauge three-port trocar system
2. Chandelier light
3. 120D lens
4. Endodiathermy
5. Endolaser
6. Backflush instrument
7. Scleral depressor

Dye
Possibly: Triamcinolone to stain the vitreous

Tamponade
Intraoperative: PFCL
Postoperative: 20% SF_6 and 15% C_2F_6

15.2 Main Surgical Steps

1. 25G/27G three-port system with chandelier light
2. Phacoemulsification with IOL
3. Core vitrectomy and posterior vitreous detachment
4. Marking of breaks with endodiathermy
5. Injection of PFCL up to the posterior edge of the break and drainage of subretinal fluid
6. Vitrectomy of the break flap and the peripheral vitreous
7. PFCL injection up to ora serrata
8. Laser photocoagulation around breaks
9. Trimming of the vitreous base (shaving)
10. Fluid/air exchange
11. Drainage of subretinal fluid
12. Complete laser coagulation
13. Gas tamponade
14. Removal of trocars

15.3 The Surgery Step-by-Step (Figs. 15.2, 15.3, 15.4, 15.5, and 15.16)

15.3.1 25G/27G Three-Port System with Chandelier Light (Fig. 15.2)

Insert the trocars at the usual locations 3.5 mm behind the limbus. Visualize the location of the infusion cannula in order to avoid a choroidal detachment. Then insert the chandelier light inferonasally 3.5 mm behind the limbus.

15.3.2 Phacoemulsification

The IOL can be implanted in this step or later when all the breaks are treated (step 10). The advantage of early IOL implantation is that one works with a stable anterior segment and the IOL implantation is usually easier at this stage compared to the end of the surgery. The disadvantage is that the edge of the IOL may interfere with the view of the retinal periphery and the vitreous base.

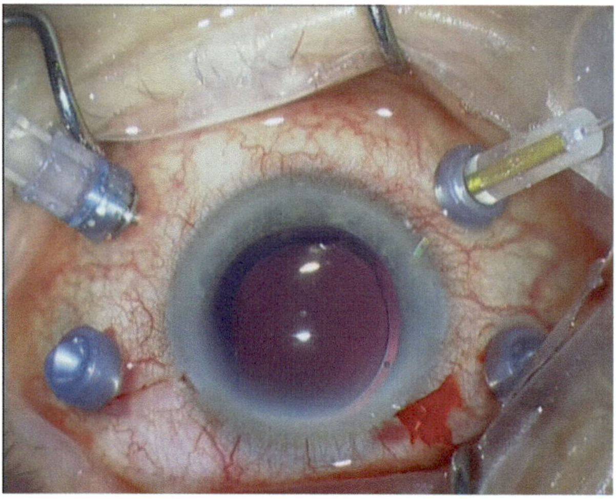

Fig. 15.2 Our regular setup for retinal detachment. Three-port vitrectomy and one chandelier light at the inferotemporal position

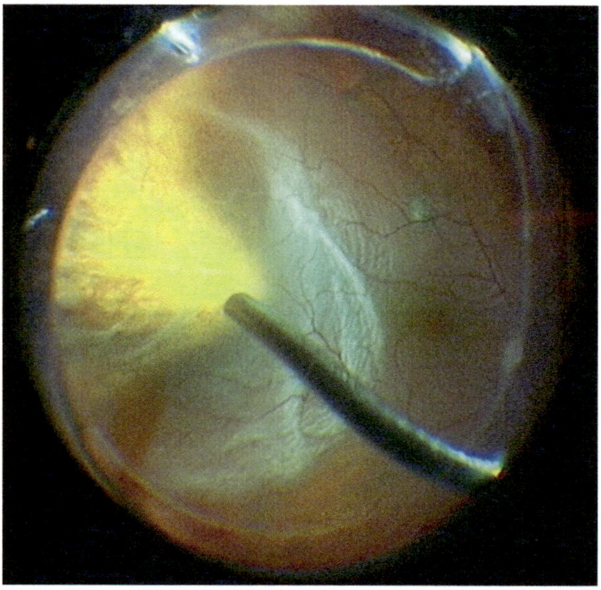

Fig. 15.3 The retinal break is hard to visualize

Surgical Pearls No. 71

Phaco or no phaco: If a cataract is present, then remove it during the same surgery. Why? The vitrectomy and the gas tamponade will increase the lens opacification resulting in a bad view to retina. The risk that you miss a recurrent detachment is high especially if it is inferior.

Surgical Pearls No. 72

Corneal suture: In the case of an unstable anterior chamber, place a single 10-0 nylon suture at the end of the phaco and IOL. This avoids accidental opening of the corneal wound during indentation, which may lead to flattening of the anterior

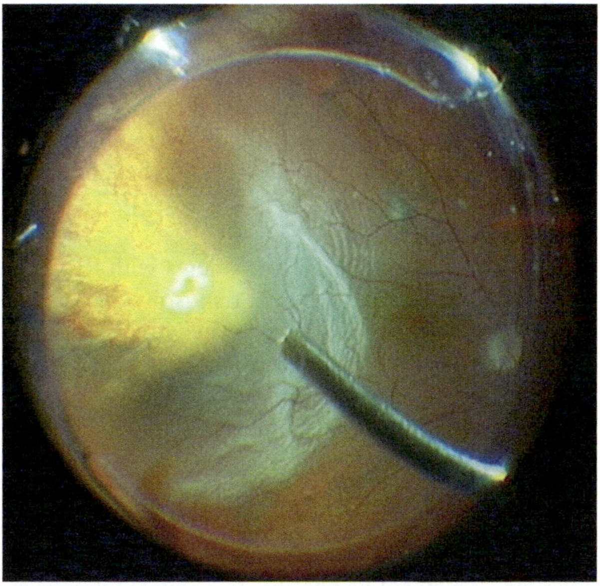

Fig. 15.4 After diathermy of the retinal edges the retinal break is easy to visualize

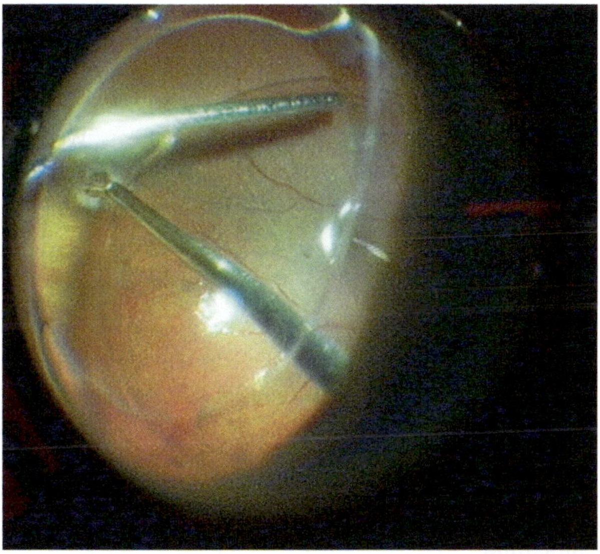

Fig. 15.5 Injection of PFCL and at the same time aspiration of subretinal fluid from the retinal break

chamber and even dislocation of the IOL. The suture can be removed once the vitrectomy has been completed.

Surgical Pearls No. 73

Corneal lubrication: A major problem during vitrectomy, especially in combined surgeries with duration of over 1 h, is corneal epithelial edema. With generous application of methylcellulose (Celoftal, Alcon), the cornea remains clear for the complete surgery.

15.3.3 Core Vitrectomy and Posterior Vitreous Detachment

Perform a core vitrectomy and identify the posterior vitreous face to verify that a PVD is present. If the vitreous is still attached, perform induction of a PVD. Then continue with vitrectomy, and search for retinal breaks. Carefully remove the vitreous close to the retina in the area of detached, fluttering retina.

Surgical Pearls No. 74
PVD in RRD: In about 15% of patients with RRD, the vitreous is still attached at the posterior pole. One group at risk is myopic patients below the age of 50 years with multiple small round breaks. The vitreous may be very adherent to the retina in such cases and trying to induce a PVD can lead to multiple iatrogenic breaks. These cases usually do very well with scleral buckling surgery. If in doubt, check the status of vitreous attachment/detachment with preoperative ultrasound before deciding to perform a vitrectomy.

Surgical Pearls No. 75
Triamcinolone and RRD: Many cases of RRD are caused by strong vitreoretinal adhesion. It may not be possible to separate vitreous and retina simply by engaging the vitreous with the vitreous cutter and pulling it off the retina—you may enlarge preexisting breaks or induce iatrogenic breaks in some cases. If you find very strong vitreoretinal adhesions, it is advisable to "stop pulling" and start "shaving" the vitreous of the retina. This is facilitated by staining the adherent vitreous with triamcinolone. When staining the vitreous with triamcinolone, use minimal amounts and direct the injection to the area of interest. We dilute triamcinolone 1:4 with BSS. Injecting too much triamcinolone may interfere with your view, and it can be cumbersome to remove this later on in the procedure.

15.3.4 Mark the Breaks with Endodiathermy (Figs. 15.3 and 15.4)

The key concept of all retinal detachment surgeries is to identify and treat all retinal breaks. Perform a thorough internal search for breaks following Lincoff's rules that point to the most likely areas of retinal breaks. If you fail to identify and treat a retinal break in detached retina, failure and retinal redetachment following vitrectomy are guaranteed. Mark the edges of the break with endodiathermy. A break, which is not marked, is hard to identify when it is attached to the underlying retinal pigment epithelium.

Surgical Pearls No. 76
Unseen breaks and Schlieren phenomenon: Inject PFCL slowly and watch for the "Schlieren phenomenon." In particular, in long-standing RRD, the subretinal fluid appears like a muddy stream when entering the vitreous cavity. This "Schlieren phenomenon" may point to the location of the retinal break at the entry site of the Schlieren in cases of "unseen breaks".

15.3.5 Injection of PFCL to Posterior Edge of Break and Drainage of Subretinal Fluid

The PFCL has three tasks in detachment surgery:

1. Stabilization of the mobile retina
2. Removal of the subretinal fluid
3. Elevation of the peripheral vitreous

The PFCL pushes the subretinal fluid from the central pole toward the periphery and presses it through the retinal break into the vitreous cavity. First, the PFCL is injected up to the posterior edge of the most central break, while we observe how the subretinal fluid is forced through the break into the vitreous cavity. You can accelerate this step by aspirating subretinal fluid actively with the Charles flute needle (Figs. 15.5 and 15.6). The PFCL also has the effect that the mobile retina is attached, and a vitrectomy in the vicinity of the detached retina is less dangerous (Fig. 15.7).

Surgical Pearls No. 77
PFCL is quite expensive. In more complicated cases, it may be necessary to perform multiple manipulations under PFCL, occasionally removing and then again adding PFCL at a later stage. If PFCL needs to be removed, you can easily aspirate it back into the injection syringe for reinjection at a later stage of the procedure.

15.3.6 Vitrectomy of the Tear Flap and the Peripheral Vitreous

After ensuring the presence and completion of a PVD, the next step is to perform a trimming of the vitreous base. Start within the area of the break(s) and also remove

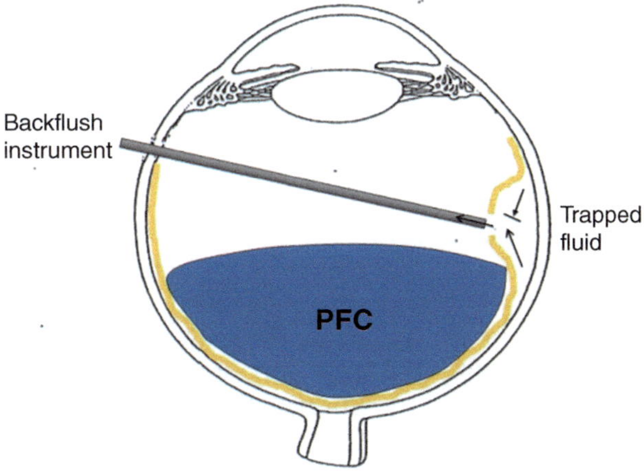

Fig. 15.6 Aspiration of subretinal fluid from retinal break. Note that only the posterior subretinal fluid can be removed and not the anterior located fluid. The latter will be removed later

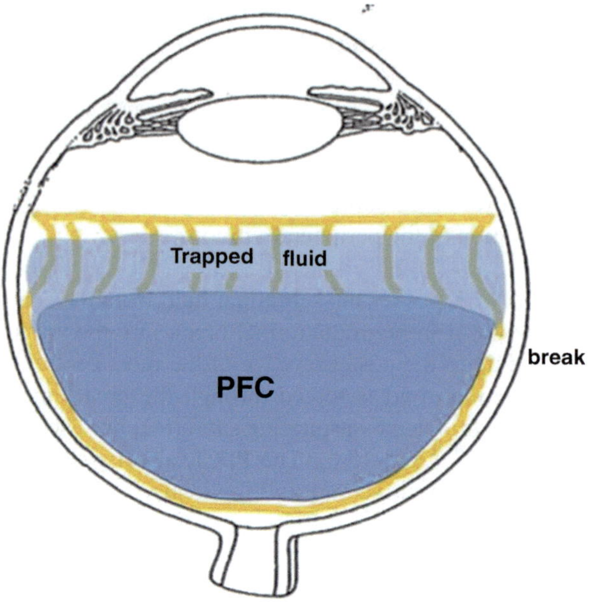

Fig. 15.7 Inject PFCL to the ora serrata. Note the trapped fluid anterior to the break

the flap, as the vitreous traction on the flap caused the detachment. The scleral depressor in the second hand is a great help when indenting the retina.

15.3.7 PFCL Injection Up to Ora Serrata

Depending on the anterior/posterior location of the break, there is more or less subretinal fluid anterior to the break (trapped fluid) (Figs. 15.7 and 15.8). If a break is located at the ora serrata, you can drain the residual subretinal fluid with a complete PFCL fill. However, if the break is located between the equator and ora serrata, then a complete drainage of subretinal fluid is not possible. The subretinal fluid is trapped between the break and the ora serrata (Figs. 15.7 and 15.8). In the first case, you can proceed with laser photocoagulation. In the latter case, a complete laser coagulation is not possible because the retinal break is partially detached. You can perform a partial laser photocoagulation and complete the laser after the fluid/air exchange in step 10.

Surgical Pearls No. 78

Iatrogenic break: If the retinal break and the bullous detachment are far apart from each other, it is difficult to drain the subretinal fluid from the break. In the first case, one can try to massage the subretinal fluid with a scleral depressor to the break. Or perform an iatrogenic break in the area of trapped fluid. Mark the inferior retina close to the ora serrata with endodiathermy. Then cut a hole with the vitreous cutter (setting: approximately 300 cuts/min) by suctioning the retina and then cutting it

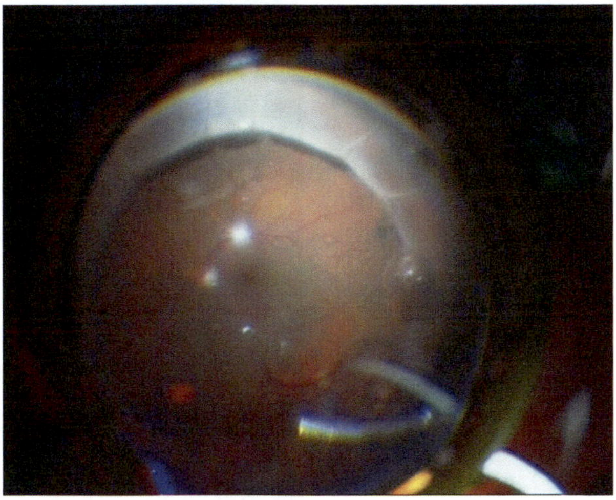

Fig. 15.8: Much trapped fluid anterior to the retinal break is visible

cautiously. Drain the subretinal fluid from this break. Another alternative is the aspiration of the subretinal fluid with a 41G cannula.

15.3.8 Laser Therapy of Breaks (Fig. 15.9)

Apply three rows of laser burns around the breaks. The settings depend on the laser device.

It is possible that subretinal fluid has accumulated anterior to the break (the so-called trapped fluid) which makes it difficult to apply a laser onto the anterior part of the break. Try to indent the break with the scleral depressor, so that the subretinal fluid is pushed away. Apply white laser burns. A good alternative is to freeze the break with a cryoprobe. If you do not succeed due to excess trapped fluid, then complete the laser treatment in a later step.

Surgical Pearls No. 79

Laser: Be careful with your laser energy. Only a mild whitening of the RPE is necessary. A 200-msec duration is sufficient; 300 msec is too much; you may create a laser necrosis. Burns which are too strong will weaken the retina and are a predilection site for the formation of new retinal breaks. They may also cause contraction of the choroid or even choroidal hemorrhages. A typical beginner's mistake is to perform too much laser or cryotherapy as an extra safety measure that then may turn out to have exactly the opposite effect.

Surgical Pearls No. 80

Laser cerclage: A circumferential 360° laser is not recommended. It is essential to identify and treat all retinal breaks. A circumferential laser has the big disadvantage that in the case of a redetachment the breaks are difficult to find within the patches of chorioretinal atrophy.

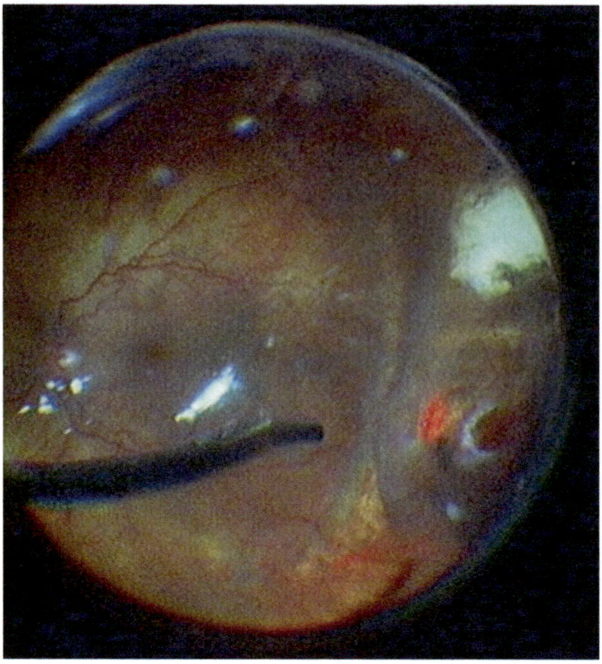

Fig. 15.9 Laser treat the complete break after removal of subretinal fluid

Surgical Pearls No. 81
Laser necrosis: Another complication of laser is a retinal necrosis. Too high laser intensity may cause a necrosis of the retina and small, difficult-to-find holes. These tears occur often at the outer edge of the laser treatment. The same applies for cryopexy.

15.3.9 Trimming of Vitreous Base (Shaving) (Figs. 15.10 and 15.11)

If it has not been performed before, a thorough vitrectomy of the vitreous base has to be performed at this stage using the scleral depressor. This procedure is also called "shaving." PFCL lifts the vitreous up and enables a secure and thorough trimming of the vitreous base. In those areas, where PFCL does not rest on the retina, there is vitreous which has to be removed. Indent the sclera and move the vitreous cutter along the meniscus of the PFCL. Hereby you can maneuver the vitreous cutter very close to the retina because the heavy liquid presses against the retina.

Surgical Pearls No. 82
Trimming of vitreous base: There are various ways to trim the vitreous base: (a) bimanual technique using a scleral indentor, (b) removal under coaxial light (only with microscope illumination) by using a cotton wool swab or a scleral depressor to

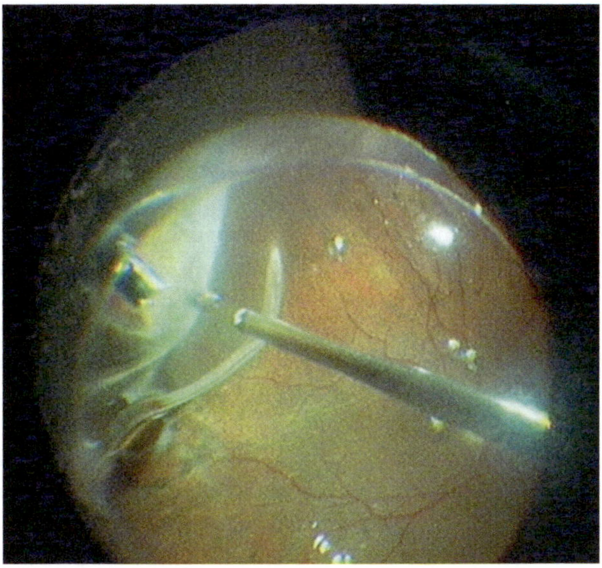

Fig. 15.10 Observe the "empty space" between retina and PFCL. The empty space is vitreous

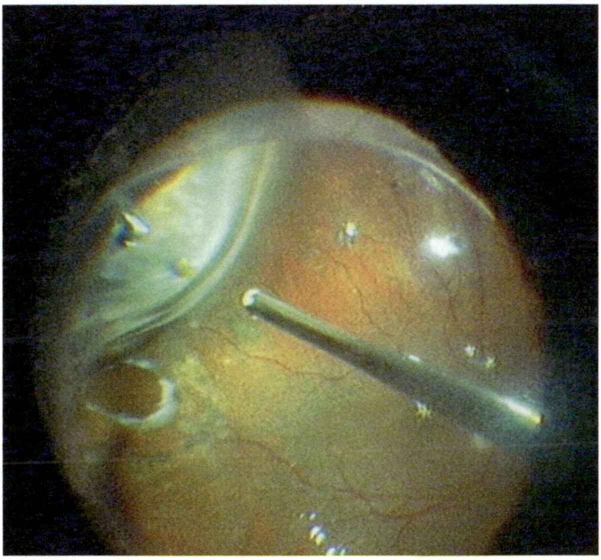

Fig. 15.11 Remove the peripheral vitreous and the PFCL will attach onto the retina

indent the sclera, or (c) using the light fiber as an external scleral depressor (this gives you a focused beam of light transsclerally to illuminate the vitreous base).

15.3.10 Fluid Against Air Exchange

If the shaving is finished, a PFCL x air exchange is performed. Before we perform this procedure, we have a look at Diagram 15.1, to get a better sense of the situation in the vitreous cavity. Before the PFCL x air exchange, the vitreous cavity is filled with PFCL and on top of it is a layer of water. During the PFCL x air exchange, there is an anterior phase of air, a middle phase of water, and a posterior phase of PFCL. After the PFCL x air exchange, only air is in the eye, which is then replaced by gas. Postoperatively, water will accumulate again under the gas phase. Consequently, the gas does not effectively tamponade the lower pole.

The PFCL x air exchange is certainly the most difficult and most important maneuver in the whole detachment surgery, mainly because visibility under air is bad. Therefore, it is essential to understand the characteristics of PFCL and air. PFCL and air "work" as antagonists. Air exerts a pressure in the eye from peripheral (anterior) to central (posterior) but PFCL vice versa from posterior to anterior.

PFCL presses most of the subretinal fluid from the central pole to the periphery through the retinal break into the vitreous cavity, but a part of it flows beyond the break up to the ora serrata, where it cannot be aspirated ("trapped fluid") (Figs. 15.7 and 15.8). This "trapped fluid" can, however, be removed with air: The air attaches the retina beginning in the periphery and ending at the central pole and thereby pushes the "trapped fluid" in the direction of the break (Figs. 15.12 and 15.13).

15.3.11 Drainage of Subretinal Fluid

How do we proceed in practice? Before you switch to air, hold the flute tip in the middle of the break. If necessary, take the scleral depressor to help. If several breaks are present, start with the most peripherally located break, and then move to the next more central break (Fig. 15.14). Now, the scrub nurse switches the three-way tap from BSS to air. In the beginning, disturbing air bubbles arise and the view

Intraoperatively			Postoperatively
PFCL x air exchange			
Before	During	After	
BSS	Air	Gas	Gas
	BSS		
PFCL	PFCL		Aqueous

Diagram 15.1 Diagram of the location of fluids during the PFCL x air exchange

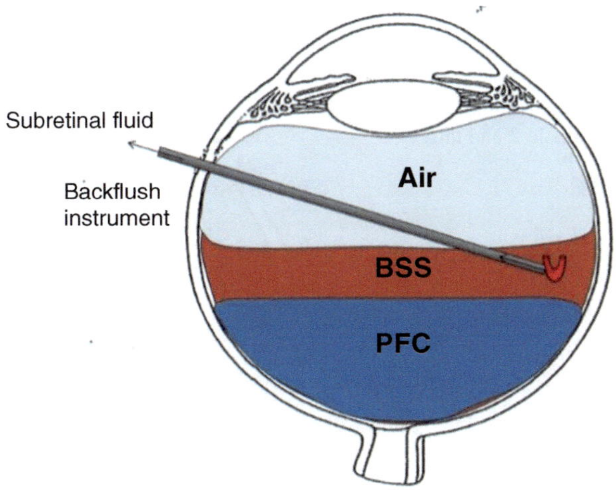

Fig. 15.12 Sandwich tamponade with air and PFCL. Aspirate first BSS and then PFCL until the PFCL meniscus reaches the posterior edge of the hole

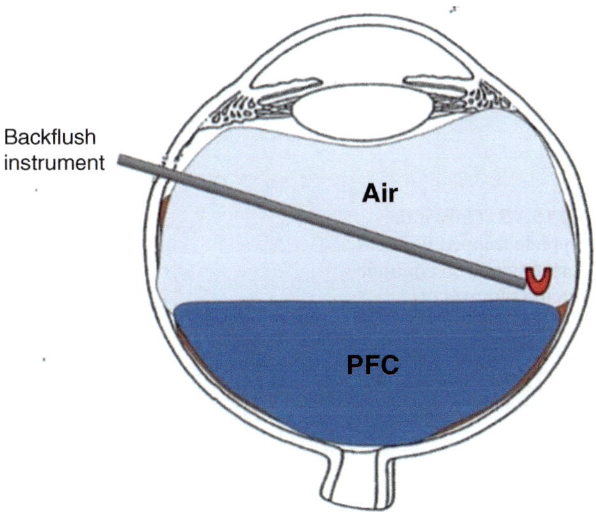

Fig. 15.13 If the PFCL has reached the inferior edge of the retinal break, then aspirate the subretinal fluid anterior to the retinal break. Then you can continue to remove the residual PFCL

deteriorates. Remain calm and turn the front lens with the BIOM-focus wheel up. The visibility will gradually improve.

In the beginning the break is covered with PFCL. After a short time, the PFCL is suctioned to the posterior edge of the break. Now the air presses the subretinal fluid in the direction of the break. The subretinal fluid is trapped between anterior located air and posterior located PFCL, the so-called sandwich tamponade. Now you aspirate the subretinal fluid through the break and at the same time the BSS phase between air and PFCL (Figs. 15.12, 15.13, and 15.15).

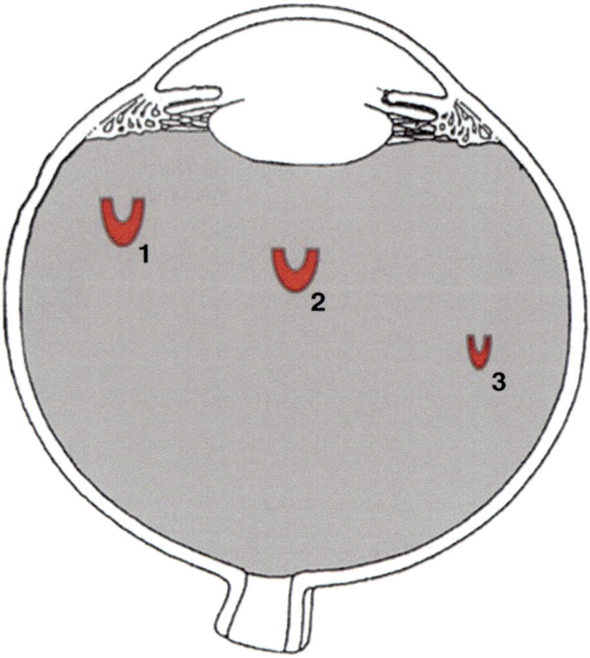

Fig. 15.14 If several holes are present then start to remove subretinal fluid from hole 1 and continue with hole 2 and then 3

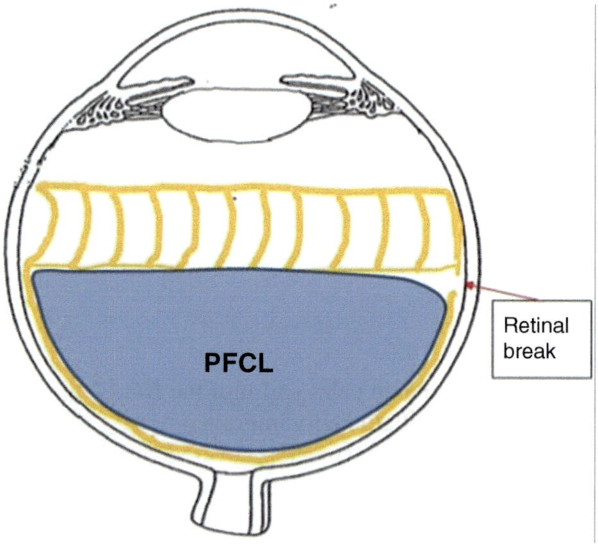

Fig. 15.15 Only if the complete trapped fluid is removed can you continue with the removal of PFCL. Otherwise the trapped fluid will flow toward the posterior pole and detach the macula

Only when the "trapped fluid" and the BSS in the vitreous cavity are completely aspirated can you continue to aspirate PFCL beyond the posterior edge of the break. This is very important because the subretinal fluid, which you do not aspirate, will continue to flow beyond the break in the direction of the optic disc.

If the "trapped fluid" is completely removed, you switch with the flute needle alternately between the PFCL bubble in order to reduce it and the break in order to aspirate fluid here. Try to aspirate without indenting the break. But sometimes you can only reach the break with the flute needle if you indent it with the scleral depressor. But you should not indent the break itself, but the retina on either side of the break. By indenting the break, you close it and prevent the aspiration of subretinal fluid. This procedure is usually not easy and requires patience.

The remaining PFCL is aspirated by holding the flute tip directly in front of the optic disc. Make sure that the PFCL is completely removed and that neither the retina nor the optic disc are affected.

If after complete removal of PFCL residual subretinal fluid remains in the central pole, then you may either inject PFCL again up to the break and aspirate the fluid or—if it is only a small amount—leave it. The subretinal fluid will be absorbed on the first postoperative day.

Surgical Pearls No. 83
Air test for detachment: When the retina is completely attached under air, you have drained the subretinal fluid completely. Air presses the entire subretinal fluid from the periphery to the optic disc, where it is easy to spot. This is only partly true for PFCL because PFCL pushes the subretinal fluid from the posterior pole to the periphery, where the "trapped fluid" is hard to detect.

Surgical Pearls No. 84
Active aspiration: In 25G/27G the aspiration of subretinal fluid is easier and more effective with active (than passive) aspiration. If you do not want to use PFCL, e.g., because only a focal retinal detachment is present, then you should absolutely aspirate subretinal fluid with active aspiration.

Surgical Pearls No. 85
Removal of PFCL: Two pearls for PFCL removal: (1) When using a flute needle with silicone tip, the risk of retinal or optic disc touch is much lower. (2) If you are not sure whether you aspirated the entire PFCL, instill a little water into the air-filled vitreous cavity (with a brief water x air exchange), and then completely remove the residual PFCL/water puddle.

15.3.12 Complete Laser Coagulation (Fig. 15.16)

If necessary, complete now the laser therapy around the retinal break in the air-filled eye.

15.3.13 Tamponade

Concerning the use of tamponade, there are significant differences between vitreoretinal units at national and international level. The trend nowadays is to use SF_6 in a primary detachment and longer-acting gases and silicone oils for redetachments.

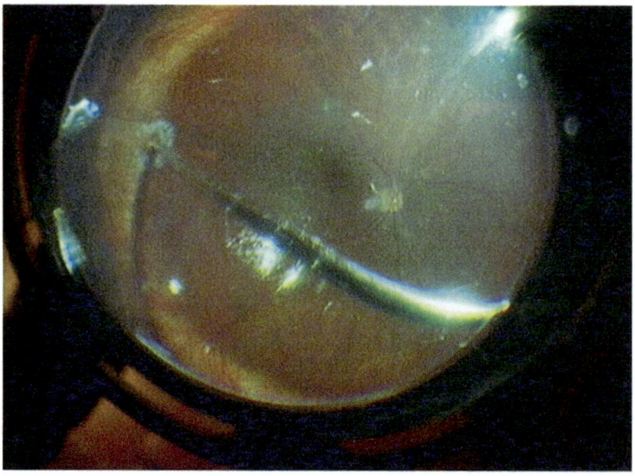

Fig. 15.16 Complete laser photocoagulation if necessary

We differentiate between detached breaks and attached breaks. The choice of tamponade depends only on the detached breaks. If all detached breaks are located above the 3 o'clock–9 o'clock meridian, we use SF_6. If one detached hole is located below the 3 o'clock–9 o'clock meridian, we use C_2F_6. If the detached break is located at 6 o'clock, we would use Densiron 68 or perform episcleral buckling. An alternative is of course C_3F_8.

Surgical Pearls No. 86

1. 27G and air tamponade: 27G sclerotomies leak very little. In the case of a superior detachment with a break between 11 o'clock and 1 o'clock, we use often only air as tamponade. There is an excellent tamponade present for 7–10 days, and laser treatment is effective after 3–4 days.

Why does it matter? Especially professionally active patients will appreciate to regain their visual acuity after 1 week. In comparison, C_3F_8 makes an eye blind and the patient earthbound for 2 months.

2. Gas tamponade: air against gas exchange

If the retina and the breaks are fully attached, you can flick the BIOM out and insufflate the diluted gas. The gas container is connected to the three-way tap, the scrub nurse injects the gas, and the surgeon decompresses the globe with use of a flute instrument. The globe should remain normotensive.

Surgical Pearls No. 87

Gas vs silicone oil: If the retina is attached under air in detachment surgery, then it will also be attached under gas, but that's not necessarily the case for silicone oil. Why? The surface tension pressure of the gas/water interface is the greatest and therefore is the most effective in closing retinal breaks (70 mN/N). So, when the retina is attached under air, then it is also attached under gas. The same statement is not true for silicone oil. Why? Because the surface tension of silicone oil/water with 50 mN/N is less than that of air/water. So, when the retina is attached under air, it might not be attached under silicone oil.

15.3.14 Removal of the Trocar Cannulas

Finally, the trocars are removed. Remove first the instrument trocars and at the end the infusion trocar. In the case of a gas tamponade, add some gas until the globe is normotensive. No suture is needed for either gas or silicone oil.

15.3.14.1 Postoperative Posture

In the case of macula-off detachment, we recommend 4–6 h face-down positioning in order to push the subfoveal fluid away. Then the face is positioned in a way that the apex of the gas bubble is located on the break.

In the case of macula-on detached, the patient is positioned straight away so that the apex of the gas bubble presses against the break.

15.3.14.2 Complications

1. *Posterior capsular defect*

This is a stupid complication during detachment surgery because the tamponade will press the IOL forwards and gas or silicone oil will flow into the anterior chamber. In the case of a gas tamponade, we would inject air into the anterior chamber to counterpress, and in the case of a silicone oil tamponade, we would perform an iridectomy and fill the anterior chamber with Healon GV.

2. *Slippage*

In cases of giant tears, the retina in the area of the break may slip/glide postoperatively toward the posterior pole (slippage). This is associated with the risk of developing retinal folds postoperatively which, in the worst of cases, may involve the macula. This phenomenon is caused by inadequate drainage of subretinal fluid during fluid-air exchange. To avoid slippage, perform a direct PFCL x silicone oil exchange.

15.3.14.3 How to Remove Submacular Fluid

An intravitreal gas tamponade in macula off detachments requires the complete removal of subretinal fluid. Otherwise a macular fold may develop.

Small amount of submacular fluid can be removed by postoperative face down posture for 3–6 h. But big amounts of submacular fluid have an increased risk of macular folds.

Patients with silicone oil tamponade have never macular folds even in case of submacular fluid. A gas tamponade, however, may cause a macular fold because the gas has a high surface tension pressure and creates a retinal fold when pressing the submacular fold away. Why? The surface tension pressure of silicone oil is lower than that of gas.

What to do in case of much residual submacular fluid?

1. Create a posterior retinotomy and aspirate the submacular fluid (Fig. 15.17).
2. Use a silicone oil tamponade.

Summary Residual submacular fluid is a common problem when performing vitrectomy for retinal detachment. There are several solutions for this problem. We recommend the solutions 3 and 4: Posterior retinotomy or silicone oil tamponade.

15.3.14.4 Tips for PFCL Injections

We inject PFCL bimanually; one hand holds the PFCL syringe and the other hand holds the Charles flute needle. Hold the tip of the PFCL cannula in the middle of the vitreous cavity, and inject a little bit. If air bubbles escape, then aspirate them at once with the flute needle. Then start to inject the PFCL at the posterior pole, and keep the tip of the cannula always in the PFCL bubble in order to prevent small bubbles (Fig. 15.18). These small bubbles will fusion after some time with the large bubble. Be cautious where the PFCL cannula is aiming to. Aim never toward the macula or a retinal break (Fig. 15.19). The PFCL bubble becomes bigger and

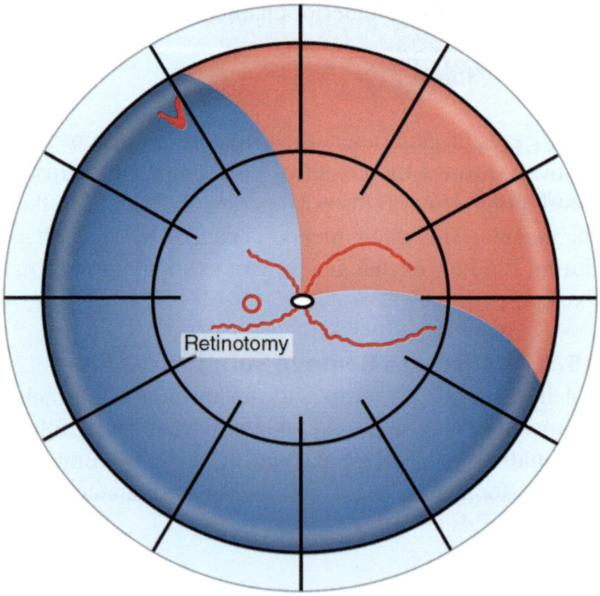

Fig. 15.17 A central retinotomy is created to remove the submacular fluid

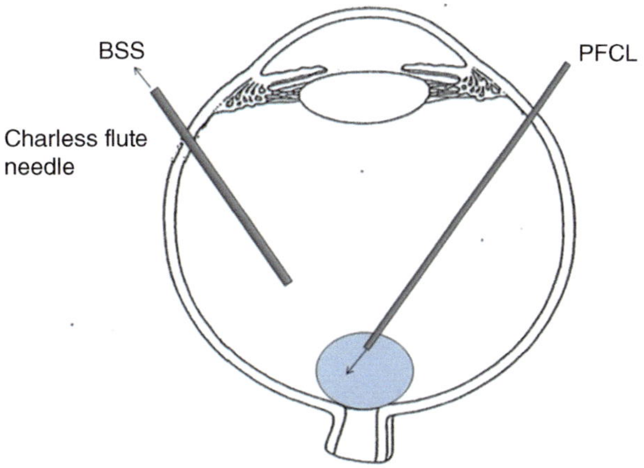

Fig. 15.18 Work bimanual. Start with a small PFCL bubble

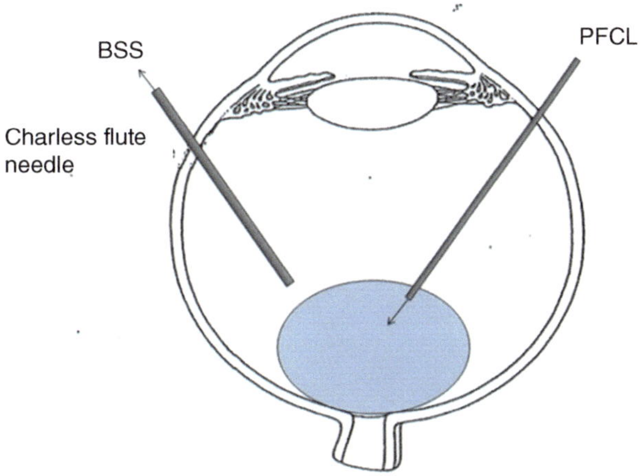

Fig. 15.19 Retract the injection needle slowly as the bubble is growing. But keep the tip constantly in the PFCL bubble to prevent emulsification

bigger; pull the PFCL cannula slowly backwards but the tip remains constantly inside the bubble (Fig. 15.20).

15.3.14.5 Fractionized PFCL Injection

What does fractionized injection of PFCL mean?

The PFCL is not injected at once but in fractions (Fig. 15.21). Inject first PFCL to the posterior edge of the retinal break. Then continue vitrectomy. Inject then PFCL up to the ora serrata. Continue with vitrectomy. Fractionized PFCL injection helps to drain subretinal fluid, stabilize the retina, and remove the vitreous base.

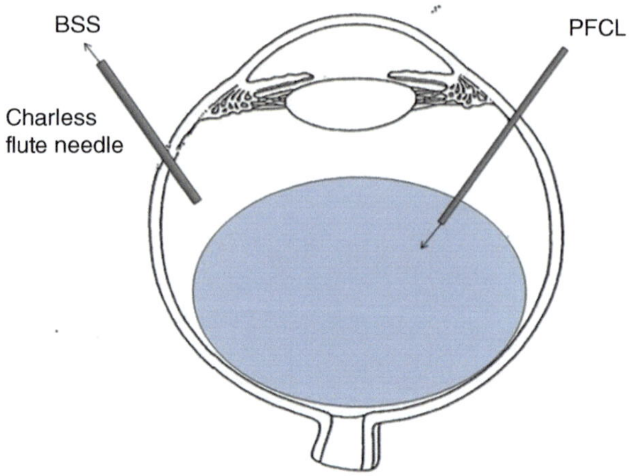

Fig. 15.20 Do not inject the PFCL toward the macula or a retinal break

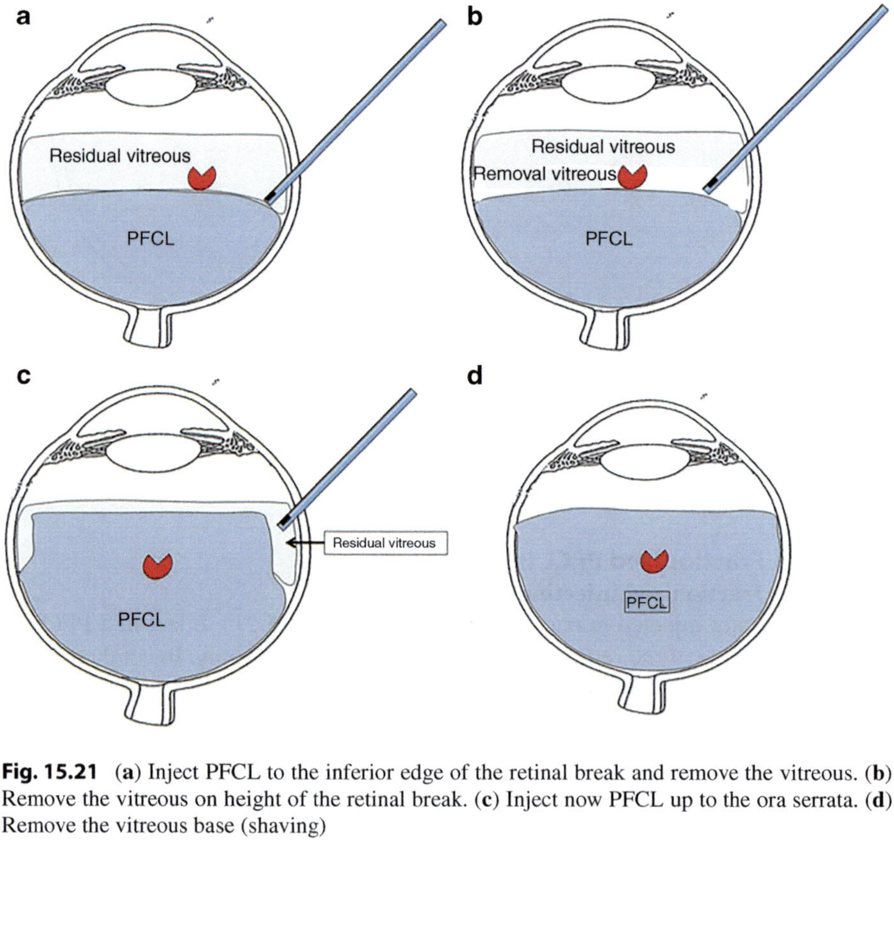

Fig. 15.21 (**a**) Inject PFCL to the inferior edge of the retinal break and remove the vitreous. (**b**) Remove the vitreous on height of the retinal break. (**c**) Inject now PFCL up to the ora serrata. (**d**) Remove the vitreous base (shaving)

15.3.15 FAQ

How do you deal with what type of detachment?
The general recommendations are that in young phakic patients, one should perform a buckling surgery if possible. In old and pseudophakic patients, a PPV is recommended. In pseudophakia with multiple breaks, we always perform a PPV; this is often named "primary vitrectomy for retinal detachment."

There is a strong tendency toward a combined phaco/vitrectomy for RRD in all phakic patients of 50 years or above. Phacoemulsification greatly facilitates the trimming of the vitreous base that is necessary in retinal detachment.

Must I change the position of the trocars according to the location of the detachment?
No. The trocars are always located at the same positions. You can however make small deviations according to the location of the break, i.e., to reach the break more easily. For example, if the retinal break is located at 12 o'clock, then place the trocars more toward 3 and 9 o'clock. This way you can reach the 12 o'clock break easier.

What do you do if a macular hole is present?
Always check for the presence of a macular hole. This is present in 0.5% of all retinal detachments and if you don't consider it, chances are that you will miss it. Check either during the preoperative examination or during the surgery. This is important for prognostication and your surgery, as you may be able to perform an ILM-peeling during the vitrectomy in order to increase the chances of a postoperative hole closure. To correctly identify a macular hole in cases of macula-off, RRD is difficult as the thinned retina at the fovea may be mistaken for a macular hole by the inexperienced examiner.

Should I perform an ILM peeling under PFCL?
If the macula is attached, then perform an ILM-peeling in a water-filled eye. If the macula is detached, then ILM peeling is difficult. Stain first the ILM and create a small opening in the ILM. Then inject a small PFCL bubble, search for the small ILM opening, and peel the ILM.

How do I remove the subretinal fluid in case of a big retinal detachment?
You remove the complete fluid with air, PFCL, and a scleral depressor (Fig. 15.22). The anterior subretinal fluid is removed with air. The posterior-located subretinal fluid is removed with PFCL. The horizontal-located subretinal fluid is removed with a scleral depressor. Massage the fluid toward the retinal break.

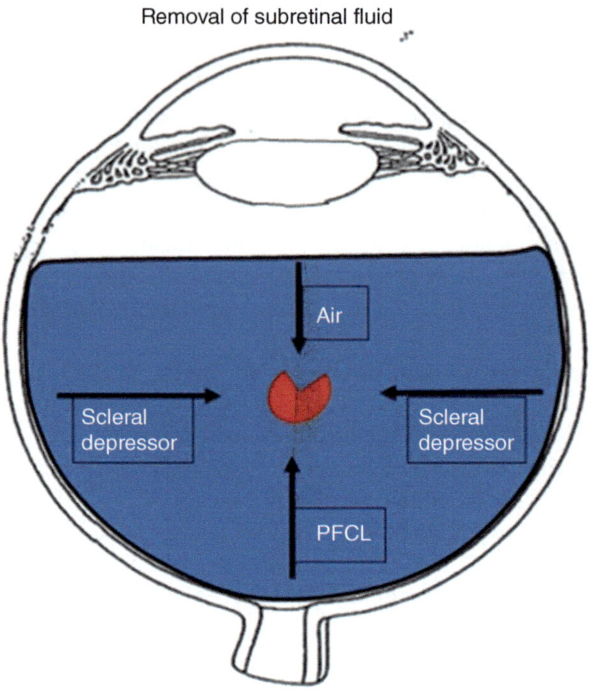

Fig. 15.22 A total retinal detachment with one retinal break. The anterior subretinal fluid is removed with air. The posterior-located subretinal fluid is removed with PFCL. The horizontal-located subretinal fluid is removed with a scleral depressor

Encircling Band, Vitrectomy, Retinotomy, and C_3F_8 (Stockholm Technique) 16

This technique is the standard surgical technique for retinal detachments at the University hospital in Stockholm, Sweden. The typical patient has its natural lens and is myopic with lattice. All types of detachments including an inferior detachment can be operated with this technique (Figs. 16.1 and 16.2). The surgery is performed with encircling band, vitrectomy and C_3F_8 tamponade. The encircling band is 3.5 mm wide (Labtician, Canada).

A second feature of this technique is that in most cases a phacoemulsification is not performed. Only in the case of a dense nucleus a phacoemulsification is performed.

Another feature is that the subretinal fluid is removed with a posterior retinotomy. (Remark: The subretinal fluid can either be removed with PFCL from a peripheral rupture or with air from a central rupture. The central retinal rupture is iatrogenic and called posterior retinotomy.) However, this depends on the surgeon's preference, and removal of subretinal fluid with PFCL is also possible.

Anesthesia We always use general anesthesia because the placement of the encircling band causes pain.

Z. Zhang, U. Spandau, *Vitreoretinal Surgery*,
https://doi.org/10.1007/978-3-032-25271-5_16

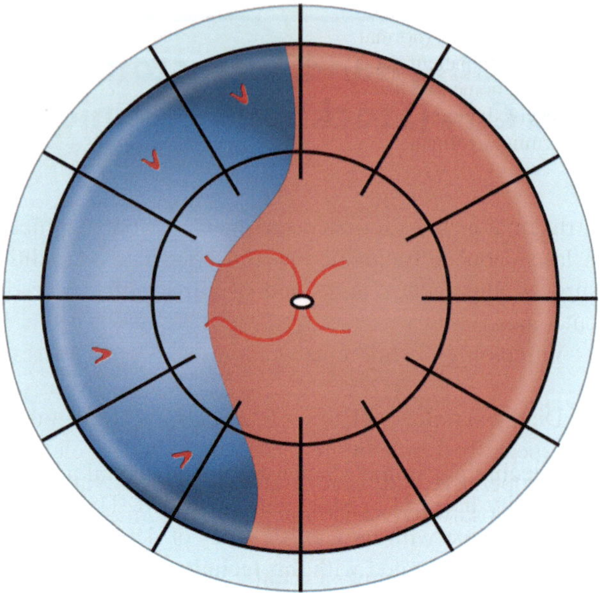

Fig. 16.1 All types of retinal detachments can be operated with this method

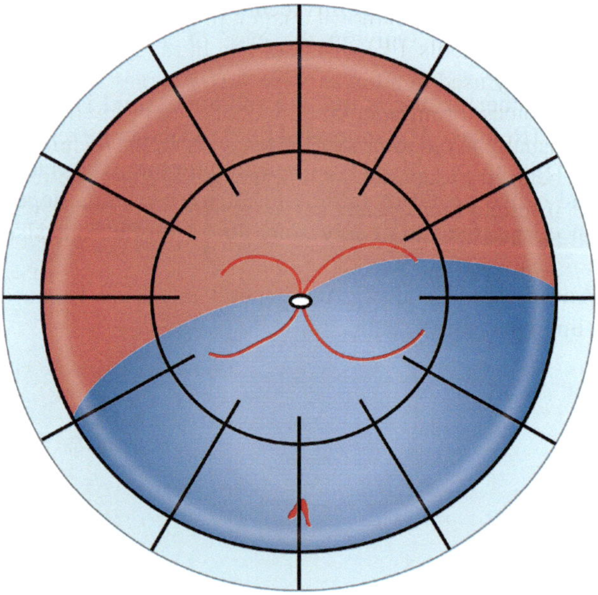

Fig. 16.2 Even an inferior detachment with a break at 6 o'clock can be operated with this technique. But the break must be located on the impression of the encircling band because the gas cannot tamponade this break

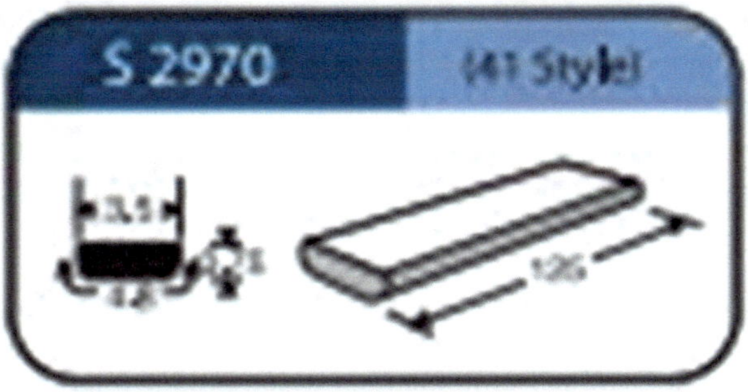

Fig. 16.3 3.5-mm encircling band from Labtician (S2970), Canada

16.1 Surgery

Instruments

1. 25G or 27G four-port vitrectomy with chandelier light
2. Retinal detachment tray
3. 3.5-mm encircling band (Labtician, Canada) (Fig. 16.3)

16.2 Main Surgical Steps

1. Four holding sutures
2. Encircling band
3. Insertion of trocars and chandelier light
4. Maybe: phaco + IOL
5. Core and peripheral vitrectomy
6. Marking of breaks with endodiathermy
7. Posterior retinotomy
8. BSS against air exchange
9. Laser treatment
10. C_3F_8 tamponade
11. Close the conjunctiva

16.3 Every Step in Detail

1. Four holding sutures
2. Encircling band

Open the conjunctiva along the limbus 360° with Westcott scissors, dissect the Tenon capsule from the sclera with a strabismus scissors, and place four holding silk 3-0 sutures on all straight muscles. Place the encircling band under all four straight muscles, and then fixate the band with a Mersilene 5-0 suture in each quadrant. The band should be located on the equator. You can measure this location; it is the axial length divided by two (AXL/2).

3. Insertion of trocars and chandelier light
4. Maybe: phaco + IOL
5. Core and peripheral vitrectomy

Then insert the trocars and a chandelier light. Start with a core vitrectomy. Be cautious with the natural lens. Then continue with a peripheral vitrectomy. Also perform limited vitreous base shaving with scleral indentation; thorough vitreous base shaving is not required.

6. Marking of breaks with endodiathermy
7. Posterior retinotomy

Mark the retinal breaks with endodiathermy. Decide whether you want to continue with or without PFCL. If you choose to continue without PFCL, you need to remove the subretinal fluid with a central retinotomy. The retinotomy is located outside the temporal arcade at the site of the maximal amount of subretinal fluid (Fig. 16.4).

8. BSS against air exchange
9. Laser treatment
10. C_3F_8 tamponade
11. Close the conjunctiva

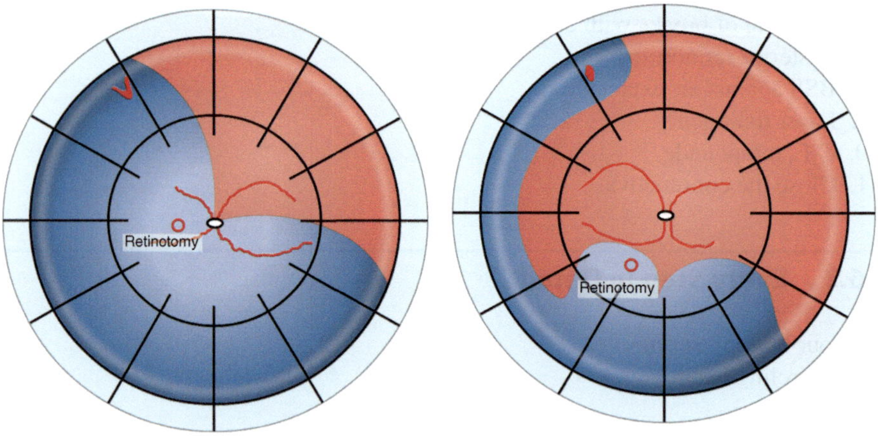

Fig. 16.4 Depending on the shape of the detachment you need to create a retinotomy. The retinotomy is located outside the temporal arcade at the site of the maximal amount of subretinal fluid

The next step is a BSS against air exchange. Remove the peripheral subretinal fluid first from the peripheral break, and then the central subretinal break from the (posterior) retinotomy. Continue with laser photocoagulation. Laser three rows of laser around the retinal ruptures. Then continue with the PFCL against air exchange. This is the most difficult step because visualization is poor. Remark: The best visualization system for an air-filled eye is the Resight system from Zeiss. We use a 14% C_3F_8 tamponade. Finalize surgery and close the conjunctiva with Vicryl 8-0.

16.4 FAQ

Q: How is the risk for macular folds?
A: The risk for slippage is small with this technique.

Q: Choice of gas tamponade
A: We recommend a long-lasting gas such as C_2F_6 or C_3F_8 for this technique because both gases cover the peripheral breaks as well the retinotomy well. SF_6 may not be sufficient to cover the retinotomy.

Q: What are the pros and cons of no phacoemulsification?
A: Pros are reduced postoperative inflammation. Cons are that the anterior vitreous is not removed and that the visualization of the fundus is much reduced in the post-operative follow-up. This is especially true for the first postoperative week and improves at the second postoperative week.

Easy Diabetic Retinopathy 17

17.1 Introduction

The difficulty of a diabetic retinopathy depends on the status of a PVD. If a PVD is present then the vitrectomy is easy. If a PVD is not present and if tractional membranes are present, then vitrectomy is difficult.

The grade of surgical difficulty depends on the severity of the diabetic retinopathy. We differentiate between *easy* and *difficult* proliferative diabetic retinopathy:

Easy PDR A complete PVD with vitreous hemorrhage is present. The retina is treated with scatter laser (Fig. 17.1).

The surgical planning of the diabetic eye is very important; this is especially the case in active proliferative diabetic retinopathies. What is the right timing for a vitrectomy? Do not operate too early; if the eye is not pretreated with PRP or anti-VEGF injections and the diabetes is poorly controlled, then the vitrectomy becomes VERY difficult (see Fig. 17.2).

We therefore favor a stepwise procedure, i.e., we operate the eye in several sessions: First, phacoemulsification combined with an anti-VEGF injection and 4 weeks later a vitrectomy. The vitrectomy is much easier, if the eye is pretreated with phacoemulsification and Avastin. The posterior hyaloid is easier to open, less intraoperative bleeding will occur, the membranes are easier to remove, and so forth. And the postoperative healing is of course faster.

A cautionary note regarding the *timing* of phaco and *Avastin treatment*: The effect of Avastin lasts 6 weeks. After 4–6 weeks, a laser treatment with/without vitrectomy should be scheduled. Alternatively, repeat an Avastin injection. Otherwise, the proliferative vessels will reopen and the PDR will reoccur after 2–3 months.

The more active the retinopathy, the more stepwise we operate:

In an *easy PDR*, we operate in two sessions: (1) Phacoemulsification and intravitreal anti-VEGF and 4 weeks later (2) vitrectomy (Fig. 17.2).

Z. Zhang, U. Spandau, *Vitreoretinal Surgery*,
https://doi.org/10.1007/978-3-032-25271-5_17

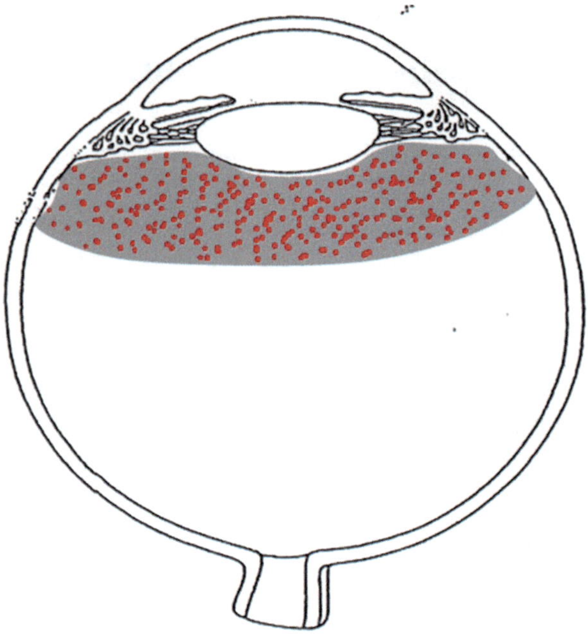

Fig. 17.1 A mild (surgically easy) PDR with vitreous hemorrhage. Note that a complete PVD is present. Fibrovascular membranes are usually not present because the posterior hyaloid is detached

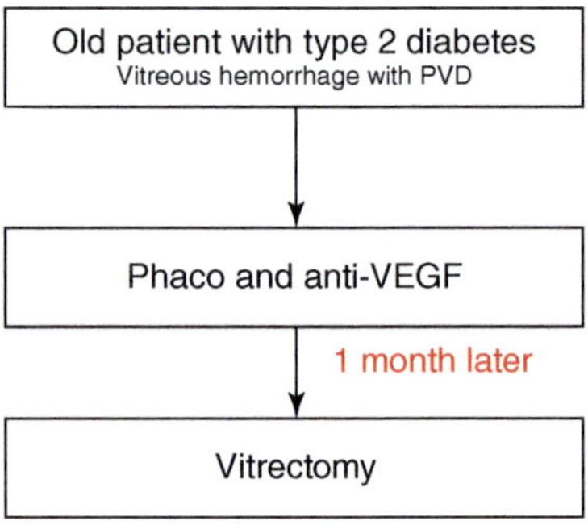

Fig. 17.2 Our treatment algorithm for surgical planning of a PDR for an easy diabetic vitrectomy

17.2 Combined Phacoemulsification and Anti-VEGF Treatment

A diabetic vitrectomy is easier if the eye is pretreated with anti-VEGF 1–4 weeks prior to the vitrectomy. If you have an opacified lens and the patient is older than 50 years, then also perform cataract surgery before the vitrectomy. It only takes 10 minutes of extra surgical time. Especially in advanced diabetic retinopathy cases, avoid anterior segment inflammation with iris rubeosis. A diabetic eye, which is pretreated with anti-VEGF and cataract surgery, is much easier to vitrectomize.

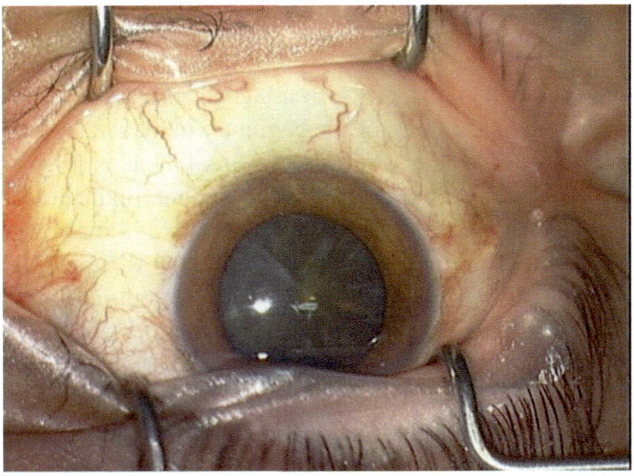

Fig. 17.3 A diabetic eye with vitreous hemorrhage. We apply a stepwise technique: First, a combined phacoemulsification with intravitreal Avastin and 1 month later, if still necessary, a vitrectomy

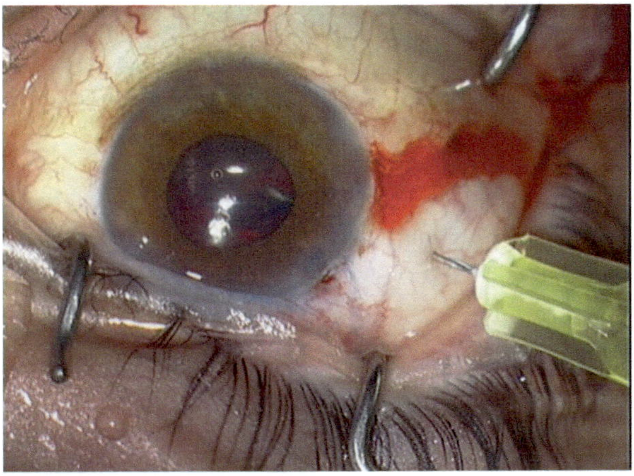

Fig. 17.4 After implantation of the IOL and before removal of the viscoelastics, an intravitreal injection of Avastin (0.1ml) is performed

Perform a phacoemulsification as usual. Inject the IOL and place it into the capsular bag. Before removing the viscoelastics, perform an intravitreal injection with an anti-VEGF medication. Inject 0.1 to 0.2 ml. Then remove the viscoelastics and hydrate the incisions (Figs. 17.3 and 17.4).

Surgical Pearls No. 95
If a patient has a *bilateral PDR* and you decide to vitrectomize one eye, then do not forget the other eye. Treat the other eye in the same session (or shortly after) with phaco + IOL + Avastin or at least only Avastin. It easily happens that the clinical focus lies on the vitrectomized eye and the other eye (often the better eye) gets worse.

17.3 Vitrectomy

A vitreous hemorrhage with attached retina and no associated major vitreoretinal pathology is suitable for the beginner. In most cases, a PVD is present and the hemorrhage fills out the vitreous gel behind the lens (Fig. 17.5). In the presence of vitreous hemorrhage, a previous history of panretinal photocoagulation usually facilitates the surgery, because it is associated with a higher rate of posterior vitreous detachment and promotes retinal adhesion to the RPE and choroid. He/she learns to work with the vitreous cutter and apply a PRP, but does not need to perform any significant manipulations of the retina.

The main problem with this procedure is that there is no view of the fundus. The procedure is even harder when the natural lens is still present, due to the risk of injuring the posterior capsule. In the learning phase, perform only PPV's in pseudophakic eyes.

Practice the application of panretinal laser photocoagulation (PRP) very well using a chandelier light. On the one hand, hold the scleral depressor and indent the sclera and retina, and on the other hand, hold the laser probe and apply a PRP up to the ora serrata. This surgery can be performed under local anesthesia. We use mostly 27G for these cases.

Surgical Pearls No. 96

B-scan: In cases with vitreous hemorrhage, always perform a detailed preoperative ultrasound examination. Try to determine the state of the posterior vitreous face (attached, partially attached or detached) and the retina.

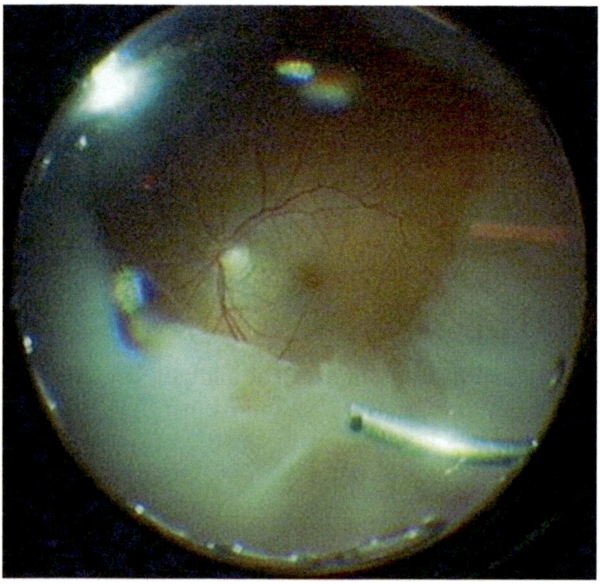

Fig. 17.5 A dense vitreous hemorrhage with attached retina behind the vitreous

Instruments

1. 27G three-port trocar system with or without chandelier illumination
2. 120D lens
3. Vitreous cutter
4. Backflush instrument
5. Scleral depressor

Tamponade
Air, SF_6

Individual Steps

1. Three-port trocar system with or without chandelier illumination
2. Core vitrectomy
3. Peripheral vitrectomy
4. PRP
5. Tamponade and intravitreal anti-VEGF treatment
6. Removal of the trocar cannulas

17.3.1 The Surgery Step-by-Step

1. Three-port trocar system with or without chandelier illumination
2. Core vitrectomy

The vitreous hemorrhage reduces the illumination of the light fiber, because the light cone is hidden by blood. Therefore, the surgeon should first make a core vitrectomy. Keep the vitreous cutter behind the IOL and remove all vitreous gel. It might be easier to work first without BIOM and use the microscope only as you would in cataract surgery. If the visibility is not improved, then try only to aspirate the liquefied blood. Try next to cut a break in the posterior hyaloid in order to obtain a view of the fundus. It is important to identify the retinal vessels to make sure that the surgeon is in the right plane (and not in the subretinal space). If successful, continue the vitrectomy from the break into the posterior hyaloid.

Surgical Pearls No. 97
Blocked infusion: The hemorrhagic vitreous blocks sometimes the infusion. Check the infusion trocar before vitrectomy, and if in doubt then cut the hemorrhagic vitreous around the infusion trocar.

Surgical Pearls No. 98
Removal of anterior hyaloid: In the case of a hemorrhage directly behind the lens, it may be necessary to remove the anterior hyaloid. This is an easy procedure in pseudophakic patients but a lens threatening procedure in phakic patients. We

perform two techniques: Work at the edge of the lens (i.e., behind the zonules) in order to avoid a lens touch. (1) With help of a serrated jaws forceps, grab the anterior hyaloid/vitreous and pull it towards the center of the globe. Work from both sides. (2) With the help of a vitreous cutter, suck the anterior hyaloid/vitreous (only aspiration), and pull the vitreous cutter toward the center of the globe. Cut the vitreous there. Work from both sides.

3. Peripheral Vitrectomy

Proceed to trim the vitreous base. Do not trim the vitreous base completely because the risk of causing damage to the retina is higher than the benefits. If the posterior vitreous body is not detached, then a PVD should be performed now. If the etiology of the bleeding is, for example, a bleeding vessel, treat it now with laser, diathermy, or cryo.

Surgical Pearls No. 99

How should epiretinal blood be removed? (1) Aspirate epiretinal blood by sweeping with a silicone tip flute needle over the retina. (2) By pressing several times on the side opening/tubing of the backflush instrument, water is ejected from the tip of the flute needle and blows the epiretinal blood upward. The blood can then be easily aspirated at the same time with the vitreous cutter. (3) Clotted blood can be grasped with an ILM forceps and be removed with the vitreous cutter.

4. Panretinal Photocoagulation (PRP)

We recommend completing a PRP intraoperatively in all cases of vitrectomy for proliferative diabetic retinopathy. This is the best opportunity to complete the PRP, as rebleeding into the vitreous cavity is a common problem following vitrectomy, which will have a negative influence on performing additional PRP after the vitrectomy. Use the scleral depressor and apply a dense PRP up to the ora serrata (Fig. 17.6). For PRP we recommend the following laser parameters: power: 100–150

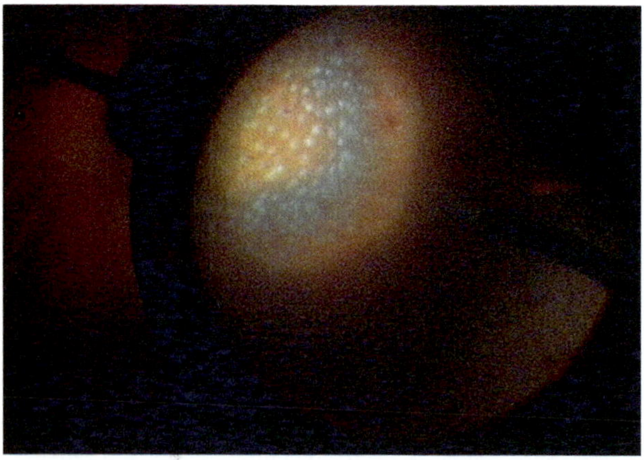

Fig. 17.6 Perform a PRP up to the ora serrata

m我; duration: 200 ms; and interval: 200–300 ms at an OcularLight GL Company Iridex. These values are dependent on the device and the pigmentation of the fundus.

After endolaser photocoagulation check if a new hemorrhage occurred at the central pole, and treat it before you move on to the tamponade.

Surgical Pearls No. 100

Small pupil: If the pupil constricts during surgery, inject 0.01% Adrenalin into the anterior chamber. The pupil enlarges within seconds. If the small pupil is caused by posterior synechiae, use stretching instruments such as a push-pull or insert iris hooks to enlarge the pupil.

5. Tamponade and Intravitreal Anti-VEGF Treatment

An air or gas tamponade is recommended to avoid a rebleeding into the vitreous cavity. Inject 0.2 ml bevacizumab at the end of the procedure to inhibit proliferative vessels.

6. Removal of Trocar Cannulas

The trocars are removed, as described above. In cases of a 25G trocar and silicone oil tamponade, suture the sclerotomy.

Postoperative Tamponade and Posture

For a mild PDR, we use in the most cases air and sometimes SF_6.

17.3.2 Complications

Important Air does not expand at sea level. But patients with an air tamponade are not allowed to fly because air expands with increasing altitude. The air pressure in the plane corresponds to an air pressure at 2500 m above sea level. Travel to higher elevations should also be avoided.

Recurrent Vitreous Hemorrhage After a vitrectomy for a vitreous hemorrhage, bleeding may reoccur after surgery. If the recurrence is associated with a hyphema, then check if the patient takes anticoagulants, i.e., aspirin. The patient should stop taking blood thinning medication for approximately 1 month. In most cases the hyphema resolves. Do not reoperate on the patient before the hyphema has resolved.

17.4 FAQ

Do you peel the ILM in diabetic retinopathy?

No, never. The only exception would be a very difficult case complicated by PVR. There are no double-blind studies published which justify the prophylactic removal of physiologic tissue such as ILM.

Part IV

Difficult Vitrectomy in Europe

Usage of a Chandelier Light 18

Surgery for retinal detachment means bimanual vitrectomy and the usage of a chandelier light. Bimanual vitrectomy is an essential part of modern minimal incision vitreoretinal surgery (MIVS). By inserting a stationary chandelier light in the sclera (four-port vitrectomy, Fig. 18.1), the surgeon has two active hands. To operate with two active hands is a new and exciting method of surgery. For example, in retinal detachment surgery, you can indent the sclera with one hand and vitrectomize the vitreous base with the other hand. In diabetic retinopathy, you can apply laser photocoagulation up to the ora serrata with the help of a scleral depressor. You can remove membranes with two different instruments and also apply counteraction and so on.

For optimal use of a chandelier light, three requirements have to be met:

1. Inferonasal insertion enabling a good rotation of the globe
2. A rigid cable allowing the light source to be aimed in all directions in the vitreous cavity
3. Strong light source for optimal illumination

The chandelier light is best positioned inferonasally, because here its location does not affect the rotation of the eye. The 12 o'clock or 6 o'clock insertion sites disturb the rotation of the globe, and the light fiber is easily dislocated when the globe is rotated upward or downward. The rigid cable allows the light fiber to be bent and therefore allows the light to be directed in different directions within the vitreous cavity. The light source of modern vitrectomy machines (Constellation, Stellaris, Eva) is sufficient for optimal illumination of chandelier light. The light source of old vitrectomy machines (Accurus) is *not* sufficient for optimal illumination of chandelier light. In the latter case, an external light source (Photon or Xenon) is required for a sufficient illumination of the vitreous cavity.

Z. Zhang, U. Spandau, *Vitreoretinal Surgery*,
https://doi.org/10.1007/978-3-032-25271-5_18

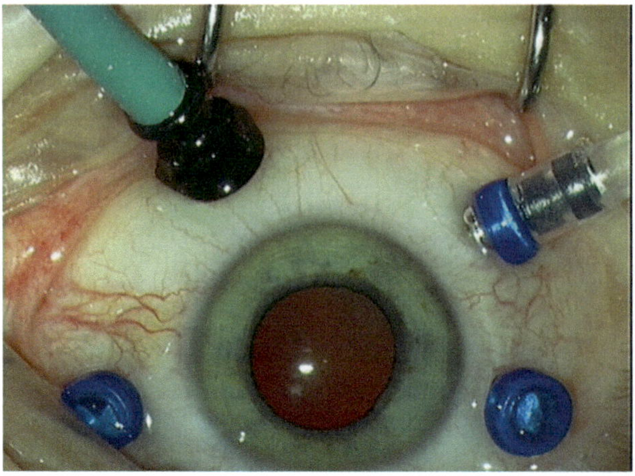

Fig. 18.1 An eye with four-port vitrectomy. In addition to the known three-port system, a chandelier-light fibre was firmly inserted into the sclera (top left)

Table 18.1 Features of different types of chandelier lights

Chandelier light	ALCON [a]	DORC[b]	Synergetics[c]
Light source	Photon	Xenon	Photon
Illumination	Good	Good	Very good
Rigid cable	Yes	No	Yes
Maneuverability	Average	Reduced	Good
Method of insertion	Trocar	Trocar	Sclera
Difficulty of insertion	Simple	Simple	Average

ALCON[a]: Chandelier Accurus 8065751574; DORC[b]: 23-gauge Chandelier light 3269.EB06; Synergetics[c]: 25-Gauge Awh Chandelier 56.20.25

18.1 Insertion of Chandelier Light

If you have never used a chandelier light before, then start with one which can easily be inserted. The 25-gauge chandelier light from ALCON and the 23-gauge chandelier light from DORC are relatively unproblematic to use (see Table 18.1) as the light fiber can be placed inside a normal one-step trocar (Figs. 18.2 and 18.3).

The chandelier light from Synergetics is trickier to be put in place but on the other hand provides an excellent panoramic illumination of the vitreous cavity. Rotate the globe with a swab in a superotemporal direction so that there is space for the insertion of the chandelier light inferonasally. With the sclerotomy needle supplied by the manufacturer one first performs a transconjunctival sclerotomy 3.5 mm posterior to the limbus with a perpendicular (not lamellar) path. The chandelier light is then inserted into the sclerotomy. This procedure requires some practice. The Synergetics chandelier light requires an external photon light source. By bending the rigid cable of the chandelier light, you can manipulate the light source. Sometimes you need to tape the cable to the drape.

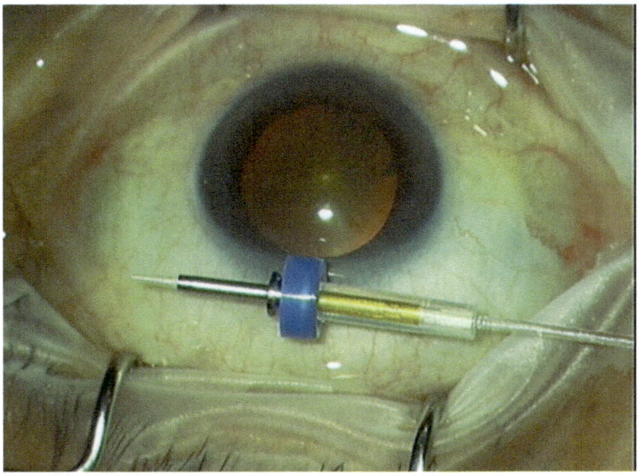

Fig. 18.2 A 23-gauge chandelier light from DORC, which is very easy to insert because it is placed in a trocar. Similar chandelier lights are available from Alcon and Synergetics

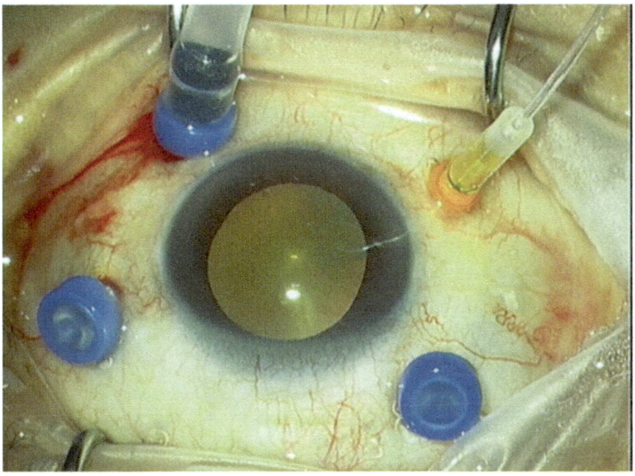

Fig. 18.3 Same 23-gauge chandelier light. Place a 23-gauge trocar inferonasally. Then insert the light fiber into an ALCON or DORC trocar (with or without valve). DORC: 23-gauge Chandelier light 3269.EB06

Surgical Pearls No. 65
Chandelier Light

1. The insertion of the chandelier light is easier using your hands than with the trocar forceps. But you must exert a relatively strong pressure to insert the tip of the chandelier through the sclera. If you fail, you can expand the sclerotomy with a 23-gauge cannula/needle. The insertion is easier, but the chandelier sits a little loosely in the sclerotomy.
2. Conjunctival chemosis or hemorrhage may make it difficult to identify the sclerotomy. In such cases, open the conjunctiva focally with scissors and forceps in order to visualize the sclerotomy.

The following surgeries in bimanual technique are listed in increasing levels of difficulty. The most demanding surgeries are PVR detachment and proliferative diabetic retinopathy. In these pathologies, a bimanual peeling facilitates surgery immensely and is warmly recommended.

Vitrectomy for Difficult Retinal Detachment (PVR)

19

19.1 Introduction

The term *proliferative vitreoretinopathy* was provided in 1989 by the *Silicone Oil Study group* (1). The name is derived from *proliferation* of the *retinal pigment epithelial* and *glial cells* and *vitreoretinopathy* to include the tissues which are affected, namely the *vitreous* and the *retina* (Fig. 19.1).

The *current management* is the surgical relief of vitreal, preretinal, and subretinal tractions. The final aim is the reestablishment of retinal attachment and visual function.

The *principles of management* are (1) closure of all retinal breaks, (2) relief of traction, and (3) long-term retinal stabilization. The following Table 19.1 shows the principles and surgical procedures for PVR detachment.

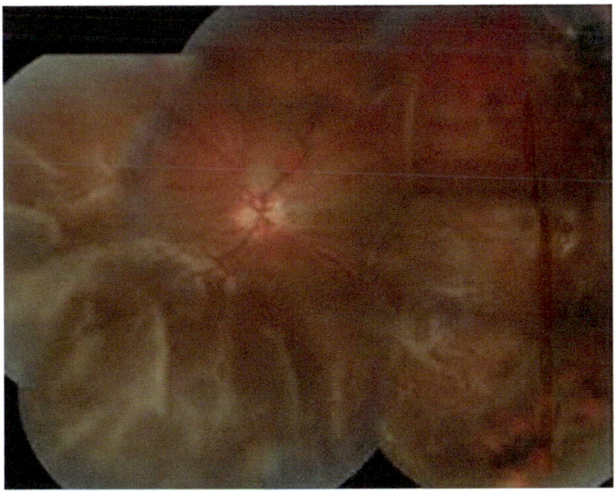

Fig. 19.1 PVR detachment stage C3

Z. Zhang, U. Spandau, *Vitreoretinal Surgery*,
https://doi.org/10.1007/978-3-032-25271-5_19

Table 19.1 Principles and surgical procedures for PVR detachment

Principle	Surgical procedure
Closure of all retinal breaks	Identification Closure
Relief of traction	Membrane dissection Retinotomy/retinectomy
Long-term retinal stabilization	Laser photocoagulation Scleral buckle Intraocular tamponade

Regarding the *timing of surgery* an *early* surgical treatment is favorable because it limits photoreceptor loss and improves a favorable visual outcome. A delayed surgical treatment (after 6 weeks) is unfavorable for the visual function but surgery is easier; the proliferative membranes become "mature" and are therefore surgically easier to remove.

Indication Feasible pathologies for this surgery are the *first* surgery of PVR detachments grade C2, C3, and D.

19.2 Instruments for PVR Detachment

Membrane Removal
Trypan blue
27G endgripping forceps
27G DORC wide-grip forceps (1286.WRD04)
Knob spatula or
Membrane pic
Atkinson cannula
Straight scissors

19.3 The Surgery Step-by-Step

1. Encircling band (cerclage)
2. Phacoemulsification and IOL implantation
3. Pars plana vitrectomy
4. Vitreous staining with triamcinolone
5. Vitreous base shaving
6. Staining of membranes with Trypan blue
7. Removal of epiretinal membranes
8. Removal of subretinal membranes
9. 180° retinotomy
10. Instillation of PFCL

11. Laser photocoagulation
12. Prepare the anterior chamber
13. Tamponade

19.4 Every Surgical Step in Detail

19.4.1 Encircling Band (cerclage)

Introduction An encircling band relieves traction at the vitreous base. It facilitates also the closure of peripheral retinal breaks. And finally, an encircling band supports the vitreous base during anterior dissection. An encircling band is used less and less nowadays. We place an encircling band in PVR stage C3 and in PVR redetachments.

The surgery of an encircling band is described in detail in Sect. 12.1.

19.4.2 Phacoemulsification and IOL Implantation

For vitrectomy of PVR detachment, we recommend regardless of the age a phacoemulsification with IOL implantation in the bag. The lens removal allows the visualization of the vitreous base and assessment of anterior PVR, and it allows more importantly the surgical access to the vitreous base. We avoid a (pars plana) lensectomy because the lens capsule is absent which serves otherwise as a scaffold between the posterior and anterior chamber. For example, in the case of a silicone oil tamponade, the oil may prolapse into the anterior chamber and cause anterior chamber complications.

Surgical Pearls No. 88
Management of miotic pupil: A miotic pupil may be a major obstacle for PVR surgery because the pathology is often located in the periphery. In many cases an intracameral injection of Adrenaline (1:10) is sufficient. Adrenaline may also be given during surgery. If posterior synechiae are present, then a synechiolysis is recommended. This can be achieved through iris stretching. Insert two Sinskey hooks through the paracenteses and stretch the pupil (Fig. 19.2). Alternatively, iris retractors with four-point fixation or a Malyugin ring can be implanted (Figs. 19.3 and 19.4).

19.4.3 Pars Plana Vitrectomy

A main step in pars plana vitrectomy is the *removal of the core vitreous* resulting in relief of transvitreal traction.

We use a standard three-port PPV with 25G trocars. We use 25G and not 23G because smaller trocars require smaller instruments, and this results in less

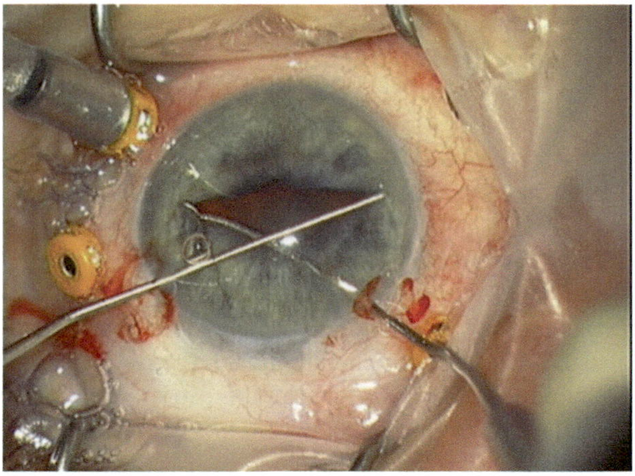

Fig. 19.2 Iris stretching with Sinskey hooks

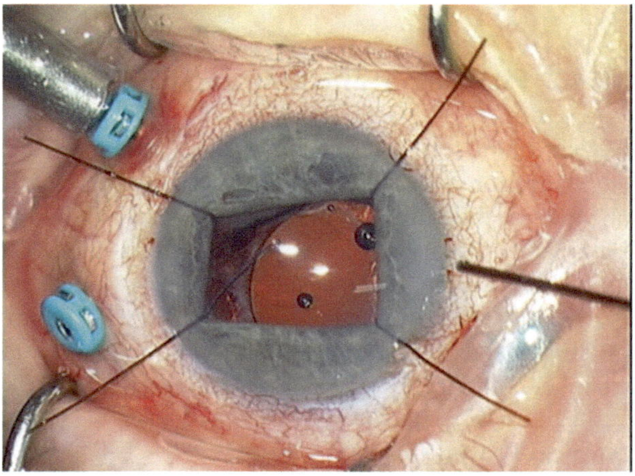

Fig. 19.3 Iris retractors

traumatic surgery and less leakage from the trocars. In the case of pseudophakia, the sclerotomies are placed 3.5 mm behind the limbus and in the case of a natural lens 4.0 mm. Insert the infusion line in a quadrant without anterior traction. Otherwise the infusion will be located subretinally. In complicated vitrectomies, we insert always a chandelier light (four-port PPV) which allows for bimanual dissection of membranes, bimanual injection of PFCL, and injection of silicone oil under view to the retina.

A vital point for successful and complication free vitrectomy is a good visualization. *Wide-angle viewing systems* have a viewing field of 60° to 130°. They allow for anterior dissection and limit the need of scleral indentation. The visualization in an air-filled eye is improved. The stereopsis is however reduced. The *conventional contact lens system* has a viewing field of only 20° to 30° and requires scleral indentation. We use the Resight Biom system from Zeiss together with a Zeiss Lumera microscope.

Fig. 19.4 Malyugin ring

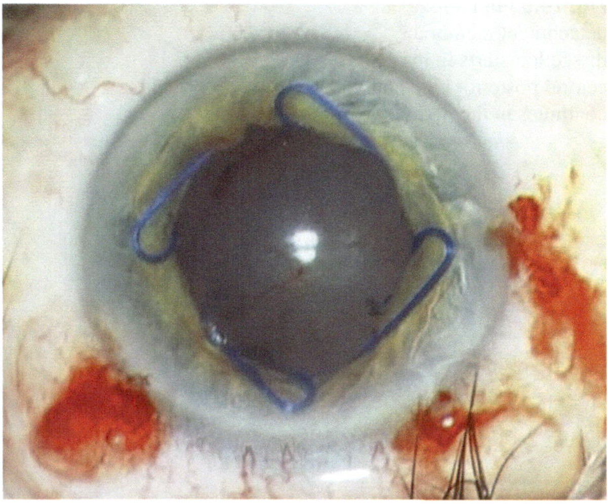

19.4.4 Vitreous Staining with Triamcinolone

19.4.5 Vitreous Base Shaving

A *posterior vitreous detachment (PVD)* is usually present in idiopathic PVR. In contrast, a PVD is not present in diabetic and traumatic PVR. Induce the PVD as far anteriorly to the vitreous base as possible. The vitreous in PVR is inflamed and therefore a thorough removal is important. We recommend the staining of the vitreous with triamcinolone to assess if a PVD is present and to allow a meticulous shaving of the vitreous base. "Shaving" means that the vitreous cortex is removed to the surface of the peripheral retina. The settings of the vitreous cutter are a high clip rate (5000–7500 cuts/min) and a low aspiration rate (200 mmHg). Crucial for a successful shaving is a wide-angle viewing system and scleral indentation. Ideally the scleral indentation is performed bimanually under illumination of a chandelier light.

19.4.6 Membrane Dissection

In general: The removal of preretinal membranes results in relief of preretinal traction. *All* epiretinal membranes must be removed. Even in the case of retinotomy, remove all membranes up to the retinotomy edges. If you leave epiretinal membranes, then they will continue to proliferate and cause a tractive detachment. In contrast, remove subretinal proliferation *only* if the posterior retina is not flattened under PFCL. Begin with the removal of the membranes located at the posterior pole and continue with membrane dissection in the peripheral retina (Fig. 19.5).

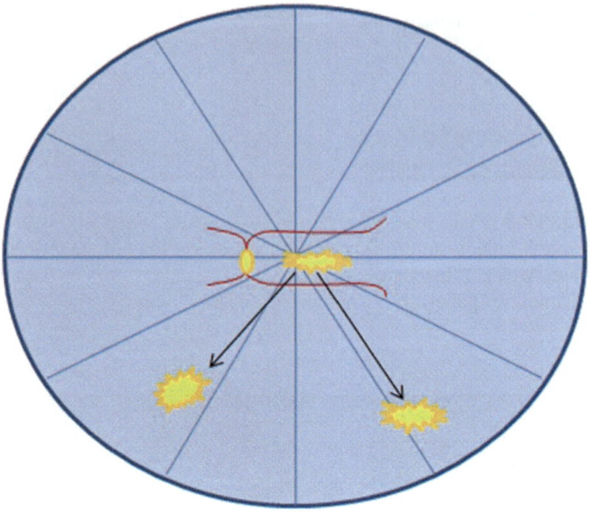

Fig. 19.5 In PVR detachment membrane dissection starts in the central posterior pole and continues in the periphery

Technique of Membrane Staining We refill the dye into a regular 3cc syringe because the dye can be ejected in more controlled manner (Figs. 19.6 and 19.7). In PVR detachments the membranes are located centrally and peripherally. It is easy to stain central membranes in a BSS-filled eye because the dye falls down on the posterior pole. This maneuver is, however, difficult for peripherally located membranes.

We stain, therefore, in an air-filled eye. In an air-filled eye, the contact between membrane and dye is longer and more concentrated before the dye falls down on the posterior pole. Perform a fluid x air exchange, and drop a few drops of the dye directly on the membranes (Figs. 19.8 and 19.9). Wait 30 s, aspirate first the dye from the posterior pole, and then continue with an air x fluid exchange. With this method, a higher concentration of the dye is achieved and therefore a better staining of the membranes.

Technique of Membrane Removal The peeling of PVR membranes is technically very difficult. It requires patience, good visualization, and good instruments. Centrally located membranes can be removed with one hand, but peripherally located membranes require bimanual peeling. Our setup is a four-port PPV with three trocars and one chandelier light.

19.4.7 Removal of Epiretinal Membranes (Fig. 19.10)

A successful membrane removal depends to a large amount on the instrument, even if you are an experienced vitreoretinal surgeon. You need good delamination instruments and good forceps. Test therefore many different peeling forceps to find the one which suits you best.

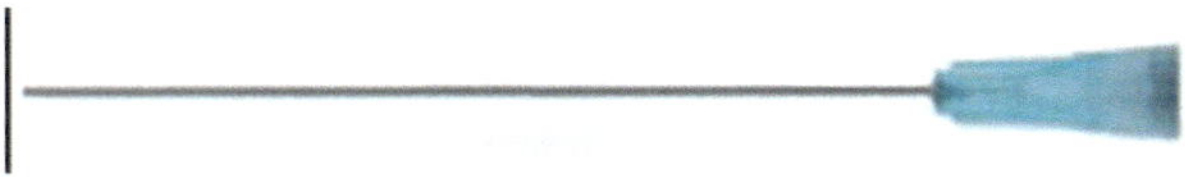

Fig. 19.6 A Charles flute needle

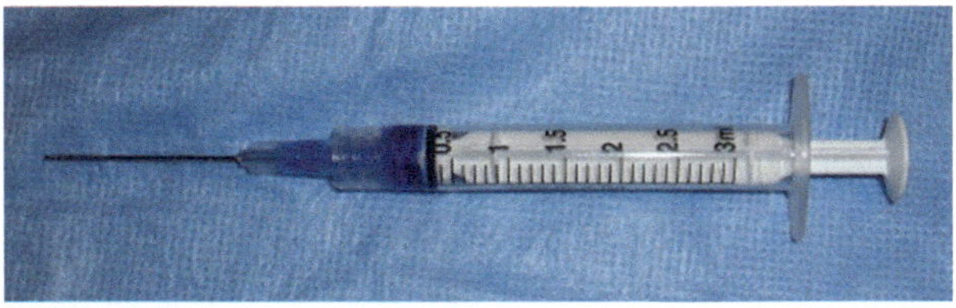

Fig. 19.7 A 3cc syringe filled with Trypan blue is easier to use than an original syringe

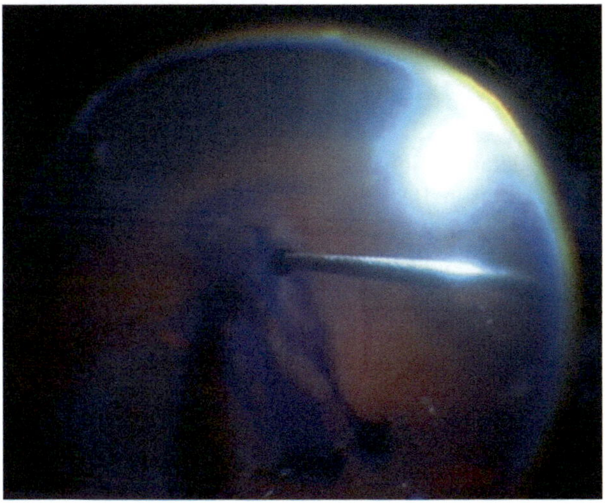

Fig. 19.8 The dye is dropped on the membrane

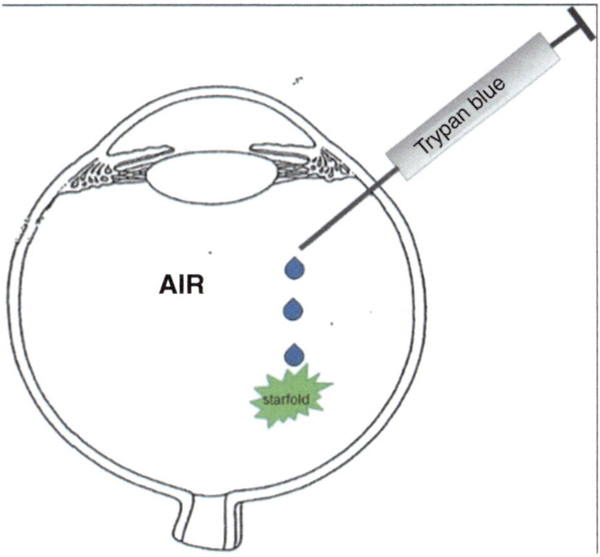

Fig. 19.9 The vitreous cavity is filled with air. This method increases the concentration of the dye and enables the staining of peripheral membranes

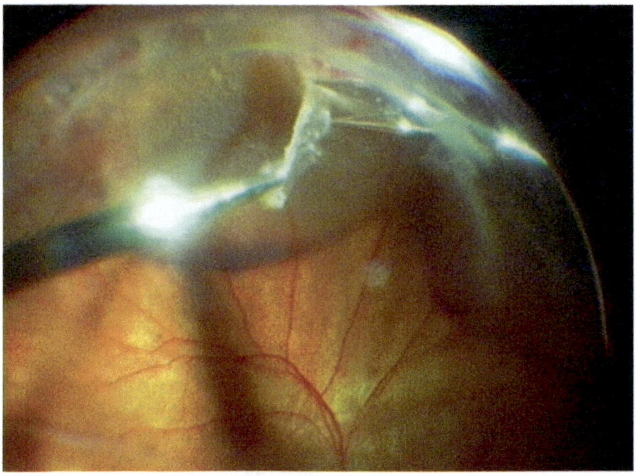

Fig. 19.10 Removal of peripheral membranes with endgripping forceps and straight scissors

For delamination of the membrane, we use a 25G or 27G blunt retrobulbar cannula (Atkinson, Beaver Visitec). Alternatively, you can use a membrane pic (DORC). For dissection of membranes, three different forceps from DORC are available. In our experience the 27G endgripping forceps (DORC) is suitable for every tissue from ILM to thick membranes. Membranes with strong adhesions require stronger forceps such as the serrated jaws forceps or a strong endgripping forceps. Vitreoretinal tractions can be cut with straight 25G microscissors (Fig. 19.10) (DORC, NL, and Eye Tech, UK) and curved 27G microscissors (DORC).

The most difficult surgical maneuver for removal of PVR membranes is the delamination of the membranes from the retina. This maneuver is even more difficult in the eyes after a silicone oil tamponade. After a silicone oil tamponade, the membranes are even more adherent to the retina. Delaminate the membrane with an Atkinson cannula, and create an opening between membrane and the retina. Then lift the membrane here with a forceps, and move at the same time the delamination cannula or alternatively a 25G knob spatula (Eye Tech, UK) backward and forward through the opening.

The peripheral membranes are very difficult to remove because the retina is detached and because the membranes are difficult to reach with the instruments. Instill PFCL to stabilize the posterior retina and facilitate membrane removal. In addition, perfluorocarbon liquids (PFCLs) draw the vitreous base more posteriorly. This effect facilitates anterior dissection and reduces the chances of retina or vitreous incarceration in a sclerotomy site. Furthermore, it facilitates drainage of subretinal fluid through anterior retinal breaks. *Important:* All breaks must be *freed of traction* before they come in contact with the PFCL. Otherwise there is a risk that the PFCL tracks subretinally.

Subretinal proliferations are present in nearly half of the cases of PVR but rarely prevent retinal reattachment. *Must all proliferations be removed? No, only the significant ones.* A significant subretinal membrane is one that will preclude flattening of the retina unless it is removed. Their significance becomes obvious when PFCL is instilled. Remove a subretinal proliferation *only* if the posterior retina is not flattened under PFCL. A special case of a subretinal proliferation is a "napkin ring." A napkin ring is a tight annular band near the optic disc. Its removal requires a 360° retinotomy. See chapter "Traumatic PVR."

19.4.8 Removal of Subretinal Proliferations

Before removing subretinal membranes, perform a complete posterior and anterior epiretinal dissection.

The complete surgery is shown step-by-step in Sect. 12.2.

19.4.9 Retinotomy

Introduction

If despite meticulous transvitreal, epiretinal, and subretinal dissection, the retina remains foreshortened preventing an attachment of the retina with the retinal pigment epithelium; the surgeon should perform a retinotomy or retinectomy in order to relax the retina. *Retinotomy* involves incising the retina, whereas *retinectomy* involves excising the retina. The peripheral retina is cut parallel to the ora serrata (180°, 270°, or 360°), and the retinotomy edges are treated with laser photocoagulation in order to reattach the retina. See Diagram 1.

Retinotomy could be performed in a *radial* fashion, but most commonly it is done *circumferentially*, parallel to the ora serrata. Most PVR cases can be managed without retinotomy/retinectomy. We almost never use it in the first surgery, except for the penetrating injuries with PVR and incarceration of the retina in the penetrating wound. *The circumferential retinotomy* in repeated surgery for idiopathic PVR detachment is performed in the area with persistent contraction of the retina usually affecting the two lower quadrants, due to the physical property of the 1000 cSts silicone oil that is regularly used for the first surgery. This silicone oil is lighter than water and therefore is leaving some space filled with aqueous inferiorly thus tamponing better the upper two quadrants where recurrent detachment almost never occurs.

The relaxing retinotomy consists of three main surgical steps:

1. Ora parallel diathermy
2. Retinotomy
3. Removal of anterior retina (retinectomy)

The most common problem with the retinotomy is underestimation of the necessary size of the tissue to be removed so that contraction persists. The most common size of retinotomy is 180° tapered to the two lower quadrants and extending from 3 over 6 to 9 o'clock. A 360° retinotomy is seldom and may be required in penetrating injuries with incarceration of the retina and PVR stage D. It is usually followed by some distortion of the retina after reattachment and requires relocation of the retina using the flute needle with silicone tip in order to reestablish its normal anatomical position. The complete surgery is shown step-by-step in Sect. 12.3.

19.4.10 Instillation of PFCL

As next step, we perform an *attachment test*: Fig. 19.11. For an attachment test, you can use PFCL or air. PFCL attaches the retina with its gravity. Air attaches the retina with its surface tension pressure. If the retina is attached under PFCL, then perform a PFCL against air exchange and check if the retina is also attached under air. If this is the case, then the retina will also be attached under a gas tamponade. But the retina is not necessarily attached under a silicone oil tamponade because the surface tension pressure of silicone oil is lower than the surface tension pressure of air.

Injection of PFCL We inject PFCL bimanually; one hand holds the PFCL syringe and the other hand holds the Charles flute needle. Hold the tip of the PFCL cannula in the middle of the vitreous cavity and inject a little bit. Then start to inject the PFCL at the posterior pole, and keep the tip of the cannula always in the PFCL bubble in order to prevent small bubbles (Fig. 19.12). Aim never toward the macula or a retinal break. The PFCL bubble becomes bigger and bigger; pull the PFCL cannula slowly backwards but the tip remains constantly inside the bubble.

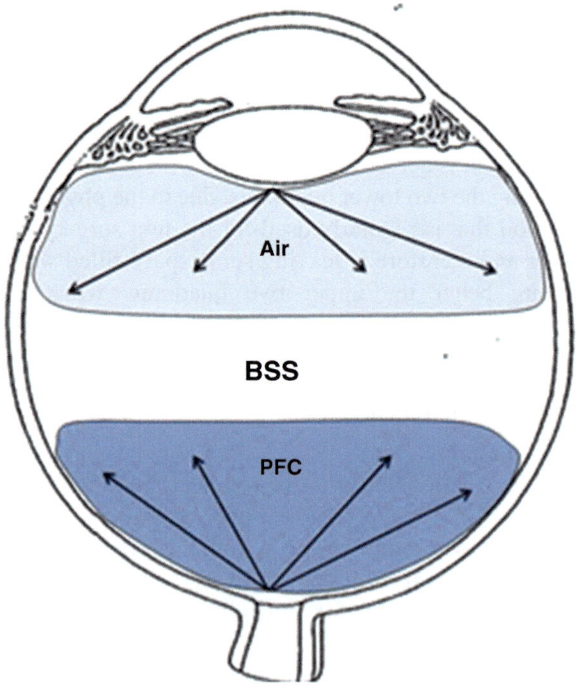

Fig. 19.11 Opposite mechanisms of action of PFCL and air in a BSS-filled eye. Air fills the globe from anterior to posterior. PFC fills the globe from posterior to anterior

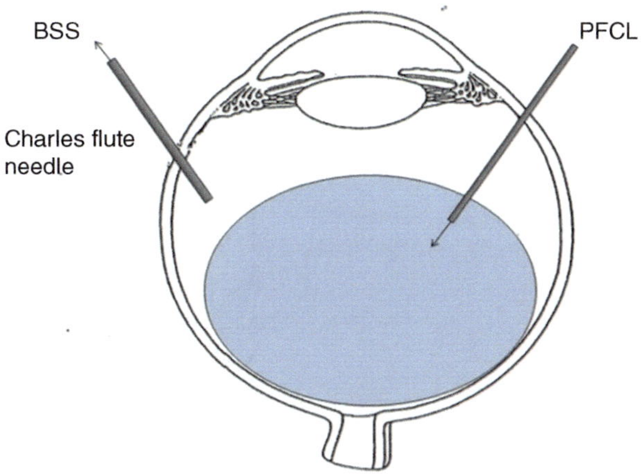

Fig. 19.12 Work bimanual. The left hand releases BSS with a backflush instrument and the right hand injects PFCL

19.4.11 Laser Photocoagulation

The aim of laser photocoagulation is a long-term stabilization of the reattached retina. Laser photocoagulation causes less RPE cell dispersion than cryotherapy and consequently less PVR. In addition, laser photocoagulation induces no disruption of the blood-aqueous barrier.

Technique of Laser Photocoagulation
Laser photocoagulation can be performed in the PFCL-filled eye or in the air-filled eye. Apply the laser effects confluently surrounding all retinal breaks. Our laser power for retinal breaks with an argon laser (Iridex, CA) is power: 100–300 mW; duration: *200* msec; and interval: 300 msec.

Surgical Pearls No. 89
Laser cerclage ≠ encircling band (Fig. 19.13). Both, an encircling band and a laser cerclage, create a barrier for tears located anterior to the barrier. In addition, an encircling band creates an indentation of the retina which results in a relaxation of the shortened retina. A laser cerclage, however, does not create an indentation and can therefore not help in relaxing a shortened retina. This is important for PVR detachments with intraretinal PVR and a shortened retina.

Surgical Pearls No. 90
Cryopexy versus laser photocoagulation: Cryopexy creates PVR; this is especially the case if the posterior hyaloid is detached. In vitrectomy for retinal detachment surgery, laser photocoagulation is recommended because it induces less PVR.

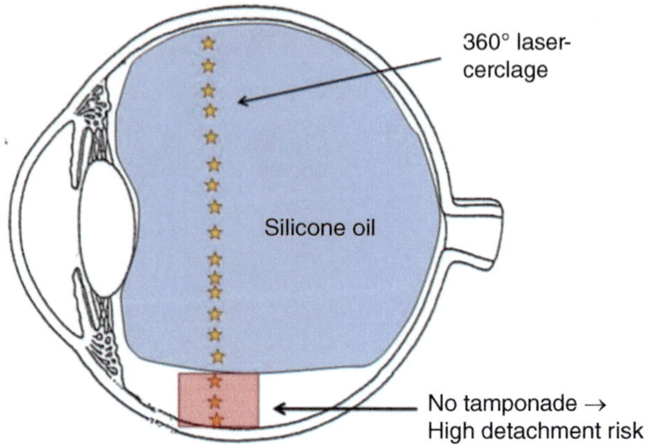

Fig. 19.13 In the case of a 360° laser cerclage, there is a risk of a laser necrosis at the inferior pole due to a lack of tamponade

19.4.12 Prepare the Anterior Chamber

Before finalizing surgery with the intraocular tamponade, *the anterior segment must be prepared* (Figs. 19.14 and 19.15). In the case of 1000 or 5000 cSts silicone oil, an inferior Ando iridectomy is performed to enable a flow of aqueous from the inferiorly located aqueous phase in the posterior chamber to the anterior chamber. In the case of a Densiron 68 tamponade, a superior iridectomy is performed to enable the flow of aqueous from the superior located aqueous phase in the posterior chamber to the anterior chamber. Not in all cases an iridectomy must be performed. In a normal pseudophakia situation, an iridectomy is not necessary. An iridectomy is however necessary in aphakia, in 360° posterior synechiae and in partial zonular lysis. In the aphakic eye, the inferior peripheral iridectomy prevents a pupil block by the anterior surface of silicone oil. Face-down positioning for the first 24 h is necessary to ensure the reformation of the anterior chamber.

In addition, you can inject methylcellulose into the anterior chamber to prevent an immediate postoperative flow from silicone oil into the anterior chamber. The methylcellulose causes no IOP increase in case of a silicone oil tamponade.

19.4.13 Tamponade

PFCL Removal and Tamponade

For gas tamponades, a PFCL x air exchange is routine. For silicone oil tamponades two surgical techniques exist: (1) a PFCL against silicone oil exchange and (2) a PFCL against air and then an air against silicone oil exchange. We use a PFCL against silicone oil exchange in traumatic retinal detachments. Otherwise, we use always a PFCL against air exchange.

Slippage is a complication which occurs in giant tears or retinotomies. If subretinal fluid is present at the posterior pole and the eye is filled with gas and the patient

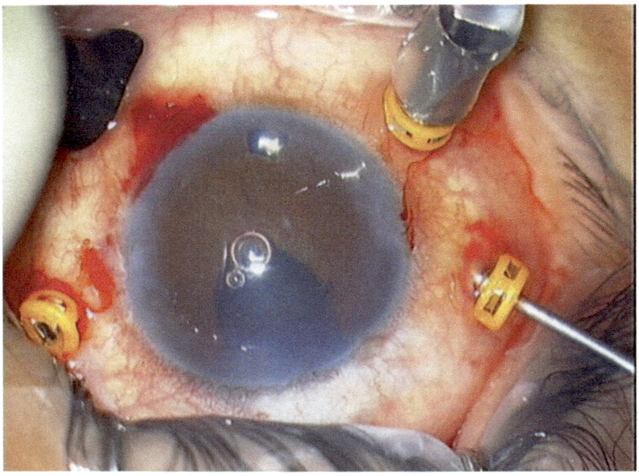

Fig. 19.14 Ando iridectomy with vitreous cutter

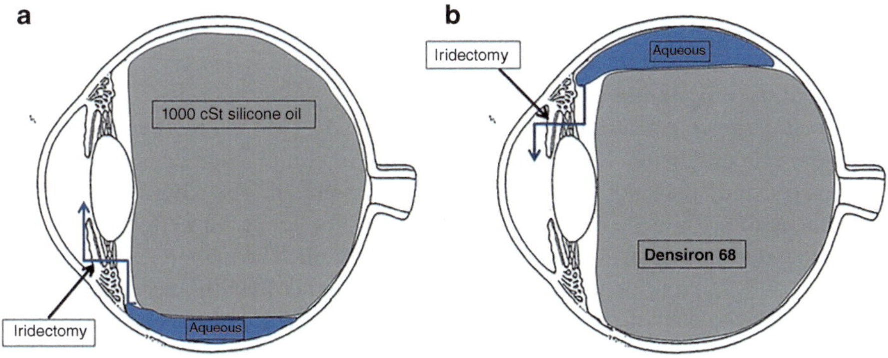

Fig. 19.15 An inferior (**a**) or superior (**b**) iridectomy depending on the silicone oil

is located face down, then a slippage at the posterior pole with macular folds may occur. To avoid the slippage, use PFCL and perform a thorough aspiration of fluid at the giant tear edges and avoid face down positioning directly after surgery. In silicone oil, slippage with macular folds does not occur. The reason for this is that the surface tension pressure of silicone oil is too low to press away the fluid at the posterior pole; the fluid is resorbed by the pigment epithelium and the retina slowly reattaches.

PFCL Against Silicone Oil Exchange: (Fig. 19.16) For this step a chandelier light is not required. If you exchange PFCL against silicone oil, one hand aspirates the PFCL, and the other hand holds the light fiber while the silicone oil is injected with the infusion line.

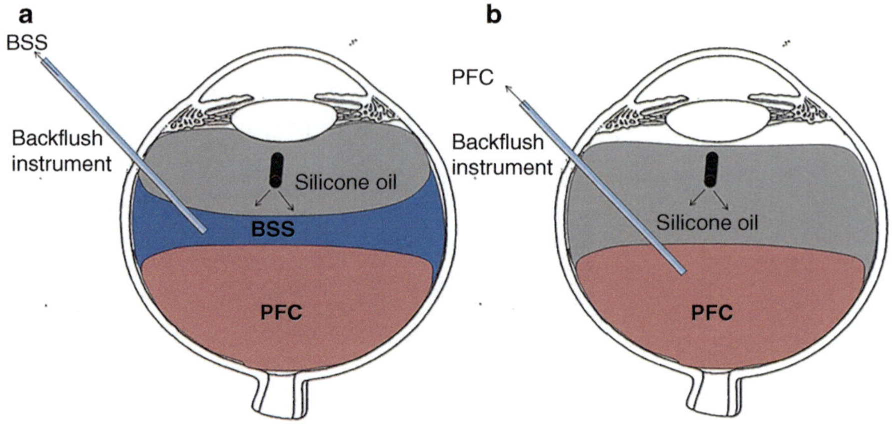

Fig. 19.16 *PFCL against silicone oil exchange*: In a first step (**a**), silicone oil is injected and fills the eye from anterior to posterior. Aspirate first the BSS phase. After the removal of BSS (**b**), hold the flute needle into the PFCL phase and remove it

Intraocular Tamponade

Gas or silicone oil: According to the silicone oil study, C_3F_8 is superior (higher reattachment rate and better visual outcome) to SF_6 in complicated detachments. The silicone oil study does not compare C_3F_8 with silicone oil. The advantages and disadvantages of C_3F_8 are listed in Table 19.2 and of silicone oil in Table 19.3. For complicated retinal detachments, we prefer silicone oil. The main reason is that the recurrent detachment risk in complicated RD's is higher than in easy detachments. And a recurrent detachment under silicone oil is better than a recurrent detachment under gas. Why? A recurrent detachment under gas develops fast into a PVR detachment. A recurrent detachment under silicone oil develops slowly. Under gas an immediate surgery is required. Under silicone oil you can postpone and plan surgery.

Gas Tamponade Gas has two great advantages over silicone oil. The surface tension pressure of gas is much higher than for silicone oil which enables a more effective sealing of retinal holes. Secondly, the gas is a temporary tamponade. Long-term damages of gas are therefore not existent compared to silicone oil.

Injection of gas: SF_6, C_2F_6, and C_3F_8 are heavier than air because of their fluorine atoms. The gases sink therefore to the ground whereas the lighter air stays above. Hold the Charles flute needle behind the lens to aspirate the air, and the gases can fill the vitreous cavity from posterior to anterior (Figs. 19.17 and 19.18).

Surgical Pearls No. 91

Shake the 50cc *gas syringe* before injection because the gas sinks to the bottom of the syringe resulting in a wrong concentration of the gas in the eye.

Table 19.2 The pros and cons of C_3F_8

Advantages of C_3F_8	Disadvantages of C_3F_8
Disappears spontaneously	Only temporary tamponade
High surface tension pressure	Specific head positioning (not for children, disabled)
	Air travel must be postponed (risk of expansion)
	Vision is restricted (not for monocular patients)
	Cataractogenic

Table 19.3 The pros and cons of silicone oil

Advantages of silicone oil	Disadvantages
"Non-temporary" longer tamponade	Need for a second operation
Does not require positioning	Scaffold for reproliferation (?)
Earlier visualization (option for monocular patients)	Cataractogenic
Air-travel is possible	Low surface tension pressure
Lower risk of hypotony	

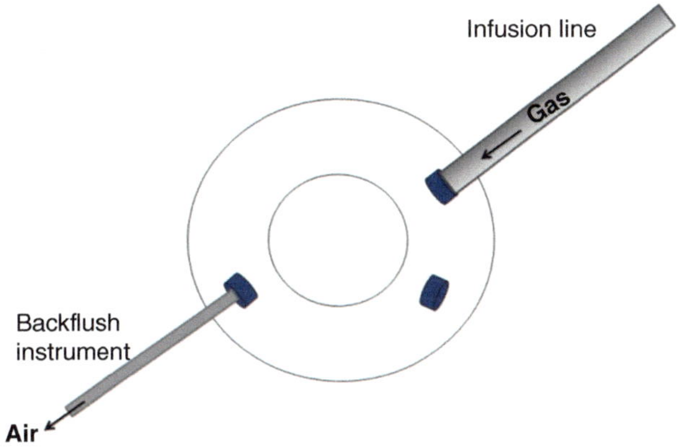

Fig. 19.17 The setup for a gas injection. The gas is injected through the infusion line and the flute needle evacuates the air

Silicone Oil Tamponade

Silicone oil is an excellent temporary tamponade but a very bad permanent tamponade. It causes high IOP, emulsifies, and the final result is an optic atrophy. Silicone oil should be avoided in fresh and primary detachments. Silicone oil is indicated in recurrent detachments, in complicated PVR detachments, and in diabetic tractive detachments. But even in these cases, try to remove the silicone oil after 3 months.

Silicone Oil Injection (Figs. 19.19, 19.20, and 19.21)

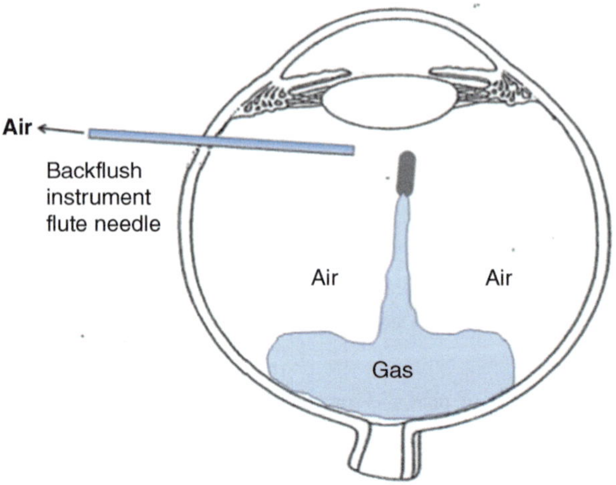

Fig. 19.18 The heavy gas fills the vitreous cavity from posterior to anterior and the flute needle aspirates the light air

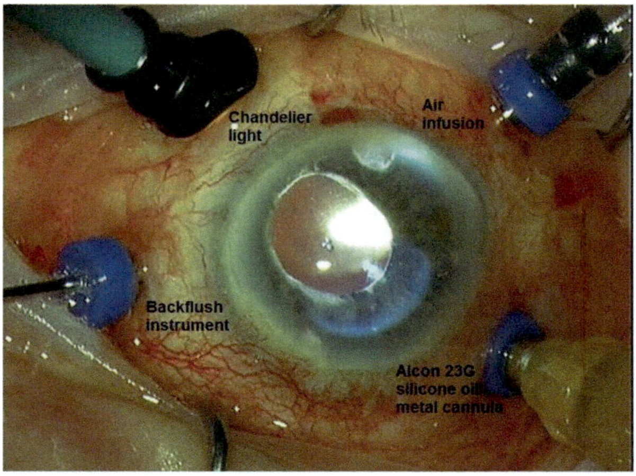

Fig. 19.19 Silicone oil injection *under* view to the retina. Note that a chandelier light is required

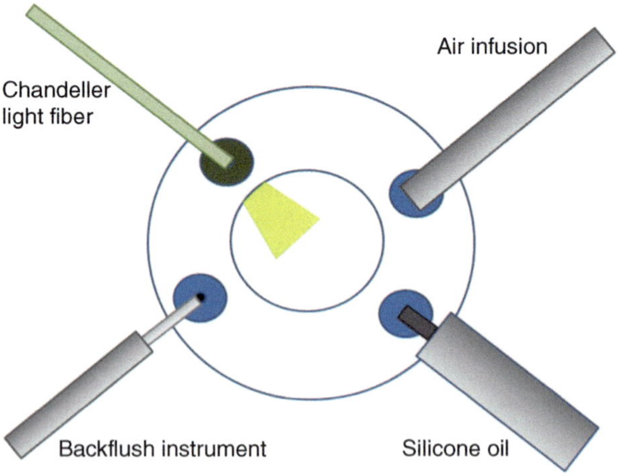

Fig. 19.20 Setup for oil injection with view to the retina

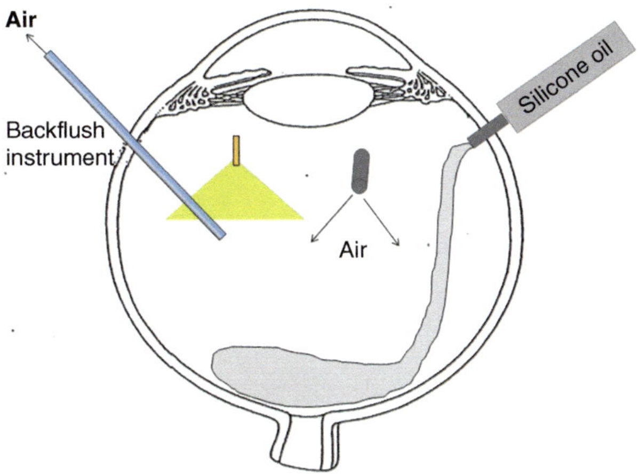

Fig. 19.21 You work bimanual in order to inject the silicone oil under view to the retina

Table 19.4 The duration of a silicone oil tamponade at the University of Uppsala

Duration of silicone oils	Normal case	Young patient	Trauma case (with low IOP)
1000/1300 cSts silicone oil	1.5–3 months	6–8 weeks	6 months to ∞
5000 cSts silicone oil	3 months to ∞	6–8 weeks	6 months to ∞
Densiron 68	1.5–3 months	6–8 weeks	Exchange to 5000 cSts silicone oil

1000 cSts or 5000 cSts Silicone Oil 5000 cSts induces less IOP increase and less emulsification. If you plan a long silicone oil tamponade (longer than 6 months), then use 5000 cSts silicone oil. If you plan a short duration (shorter than 6 months), then use 1000 cSts silicone oil. The duration of the silicone oil is listed in Table 19.4.

Surgical Pearls No. 92

Silicone oil overfill (Fig. 19.22): Cut the infusion line with a scissors so that the excessive silicone oil can escape. An IOP of approximately 10 mmHg is fine, or wait so long until no more oil escapes from the infusion line.

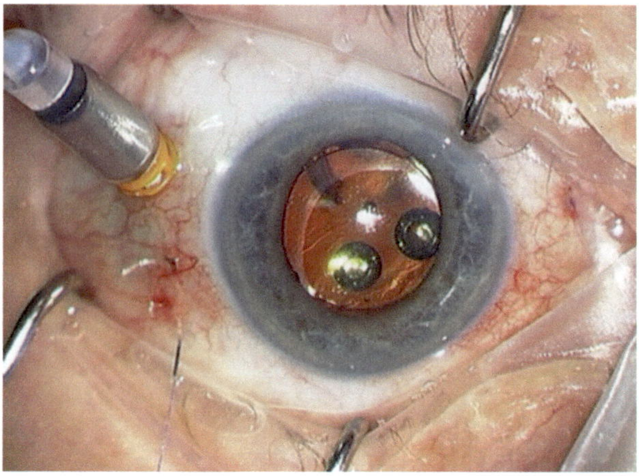

Fig. 19.22 Cut the infusion line after silicone oil injection so that excessive oil can flow out

Difficult Proliferative Diabetic Retinopathy

20

20.1 Introduction

The surgical planning of the diabetic eye is very important; this is especially the case in active proliferative diabetic retinopathies. What is the right timing for a vitrectomy? Do not operate too early; if the eye is not been pretreated with PRP or anti-VEGF injections and the diabetes is poorly controlled, then the vitrectomy becomes VERY difficult (see Fig. 20.1). Surgical trauma triggers the diabetic retinopathy and consequently the postoperative healing. It also increases the risk of recurrence of fibrovascular membranes. If you only operate on the cataract of an eye with active proliferative diabetic retinopathy, then the retinopathy will progress in most cases, and an iris rubeosis may occur. Therefore, combine a phacoemulsification always with an intravitreal anti-VEGF treatment in order to prevent a progression of the retinopathy and to quiet the retinopathy for the following vitrectomy.

We therefore favor a stepwise procedure, i.e., we operate the eye in several sessions: first, phacoemulsification combined with an anti-VEGF injection and 4 weeks later a vitrectomy. The vitrectomy is much easier, if the eye is pretreated with phacoemulsification and Avastin. The posterior hyaloid is easier to open, less intraoperative bleeding will occur, the membranes are easier to remove, and so forth. And the postoperative healing is of course faster.

Why a stepwise procedure? The difficulty of the vitrectomy depends on the severity of the PDR. A severe diabetic retinopathy requires a long traumatic surgery. The surgical trauma however aggravates the diabetic retinopathy, resulting in a vicious cycle. It is therefore vital to dry out the fibrovascular membranes BEFORE vitrectomy; i.e., remove the vascular component with laser and anti-VEGF.

The main rule is not to perform a vitrectomy in an untreated eye. Pretreat the eye first with PRP and anti-VEGF, keep a tight follow-up until the retinopathy is inactive, and then schedule surgery. Secondly, avoid a combined phaco/vitrectomy. Operate instead first a phaco with Avastin and 1–4 weeks later a vitrectomy.

Z. Zhang, U. Spandau, *Vitreoretinal Surgery*,
https://doi.org/10.1007/978-3-032-25271-5_20

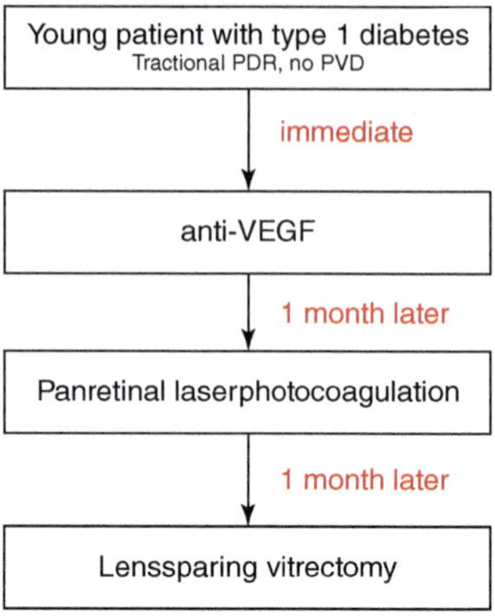

Fig. 20.1 Our treatment algorithm for surgical planning of a difficult diabetic vitrectomy

A cautionary note regarding the *timing* of phaco and *Avastin treatment*: The effect of Avastin lasts 6 weeks. After 4–6 weeks, a laser treatment with/without vitrectomy should be scheduled. Alternatively, repeat an Avastin injection. Otherwise, the proliferative vessels will reopen and the PDR will reoccur after 2–3 months.

In conclusion The grade of surgical difficulty depends on the severity of the diabetic retinopathy. We differentiate an *easy* and a *difficult* proliferative diabetic retinopathy:

Difficult PDR Only a partial PVD is present. Fibrovascular membranes are located at the posterior pole. A tractional retinal detachment is present. No or insufficient laser treatment has been performed (Fig. 20.2).

The more active the retinopathy, the more stepwise we operate:

In a *difficult PDR*, we operate in several sessions: In young type 1 diabetics,we inject anti-VEGF into both eyes within 1 week. One month later, if the vitreous is clear, we perform a laser photocoagulation. The laser photocoagulation is performed in general anesthesia with a laser helmet: the so-called laser indirect ophthalmoscopy (LIO). If the vitreous is not clear, we repeat anti-VEGF. A vitreous hemorrhage clears up after a maximum of four anti-VEGF injections. Then we perform a lens-sparing vitrectomy. In old patients, we start with phacoemulsification and intravitreal anti-VEGF and 3–4 weeks later 2) vitrectomy (Fig. 20.1).

Caution Do not forget the second eye while treating the first eye. We use to inject anti-VEGF in the second eye every time when operating the first eye. We have seen many times a second eye progress to a tractional PDR under treatment of the first eye.

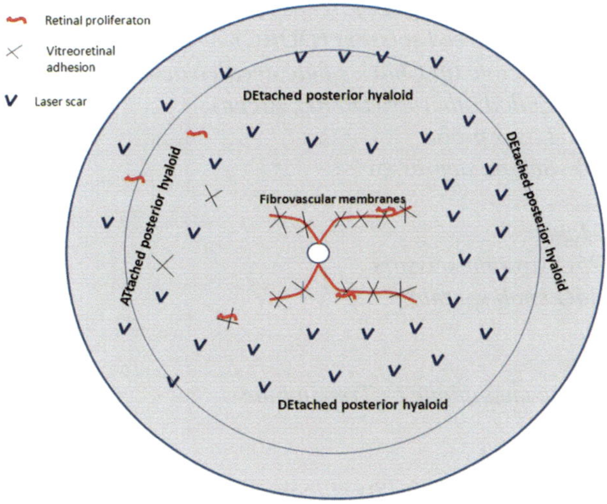

Fig. 20.2 Illustration of a difficult PDR. The retina is laser treated. Many retinal proliferations and vitreoretinal adhesions are present. The posterior hyaloid is attached in the posterior pole and partially detached in the periphery; the nasal posterior hyaloid is often attached

20.2 General Introduction

The *main surgical steps* in a severe PDR are as follows:

1. Posterior hyaloid rhexis
2. Bimanual removal of membranes

In most cases of severe PDR, you can use the periphery to disc (outside-in) technique. Start therefore with a posterior hyaloid rhexis.

The surgical time is approximately 90–150 minutes.

The eye should be pseudophakic, an exception is the young type I diabetic patient. In the latter case, we perform a lens-sparing vitrectomy. We usually work with a 27G trocar system. If extensive membranes are present, we use a hybrid 25G/27G system because the whole range of 25G peeling instruments is required. In the case of a long eye, we use 27G.

Surgical Pearls No. 101

BSS damages the phakic lens: In pseudophakic eyes BSS is used as irrigation fluid and in phakic eyes BSS Plus® (Alcon). BSS Plus® also contains glutathione, glucose, and sodium bicarbonate.

Instruments

1. *27G three-port trocar system with chandelier illumination*
2. *120D lens, for peeling: 60D lens*
3. *Vitreous cutter*
4. *Backflush instrument*

5. *27G endgripping forceps (DORC)*
6. *27G curved scissors (DORC)*
7. *Silicone tip Charles flute needle/vacuum cleaner*
8. *Endodiathermy (DORC, Alcon)*
9. *Laser probe*
10. *Scleral depressor*

Maybe:
25G straight scissors
25G knob spatula

Dye
- *Triamcinolone or Trypan blue*

Tamponade
- *20% SF_6, 1000 cSts silicone oil*

Individual Steps

1. *Three-port trocar system with chandelier illumination*
2. *Posterior hyaloid rhexis*
3. *Removal of tractional membranes*
4. *Instruments for removal of membranes*
   - Delamination of membranes with membrane pic, knob spatula, and vacuum cleaner
   - Dissection of membranes with curved scissors
   - Removal of dissected membranes with vitreous cutter
5. *Hemostasis*
   - Slight bleeding
   - Moderate bleeding
   - Strong bleeding
6. *Removal of attached posterior hyaloid in the periphery*
7. *PRP under BSS*
8. *Fluid against air exchange*
9. *Intravitreal Avastin*
10. *Internal tamponade*
    - Gas tamponade
    - Silicone oil tamponade
11. *Removal of trocars*

20.3 The Surgery Step-by-Step: Figs. 20.3, 20.4, 20.5, 20.6, 20.7, 20.8, 20.9, 20.10, 20.11, 20.12, 20.13, 20.14, 20.15, 20.16, 20.17, 20.18, 20.19, 20.20, 20.21, 20.22, 20.23, 20.24, 20.25, 20.26, 20.27, 20.28, 20.29, 20.30, and 20.31

20.3.1 Three-Port Trocar System with Chandelier Illumination

Insert first three trocars and then inferonasally the chandelier light. Continue with a core vitrectomy. We recommend 27G trocars (Fig. 20.3); an alternative is a hybrid system.

Surgical Pearls No. 102

Corneal lubrication: A major problem during vitrectomy, especially in combined surgeries with a duration of over 1 hour, is corneal epithelial edema. With the application of methylcellulose (Celoftal®, Alcon or Ocucoat®, Bausch&Lomb) on the cornea, the cornea can remain clear for many hours. A debridement of the epithelium is rarely necessary, but if needed use a broad blade (crescent knife).

20.3.2 Posterior Hyaloid Rhexis (Figs. 20.4 and 20.5)

The posterior vitreous is usually attached in eyes with fibrovascular membranes. An important aim of surgery is the induction of PVD. The induction of PVD is extremely challenging in eyes with ischemic retina because the posterior hyaloid is firmly attached to the retina. When inducing a PVD, the surgeon can easily make tears in the retina.

To avoid this damage, the surgeon should begin with a peripheral vitreous detachment. In most cases of proliferative diabetic retinopathy, a partial vitreous

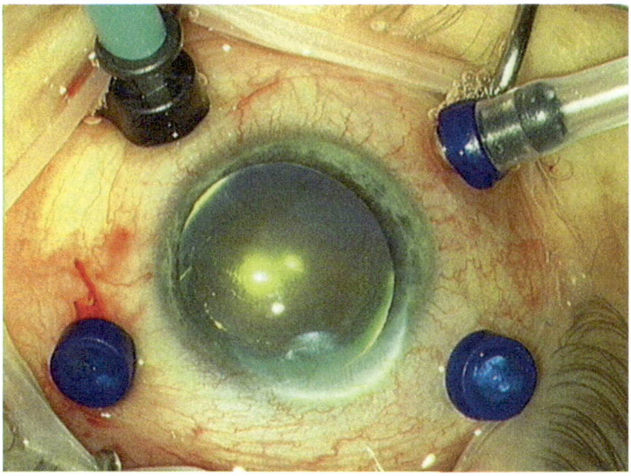

Fig. 20.3 A three-port vitrectomy with chandelier light is the best surgical setup for a difficult PDR; a chandelier light allows bimanual surgery and bimanual removal of membranes

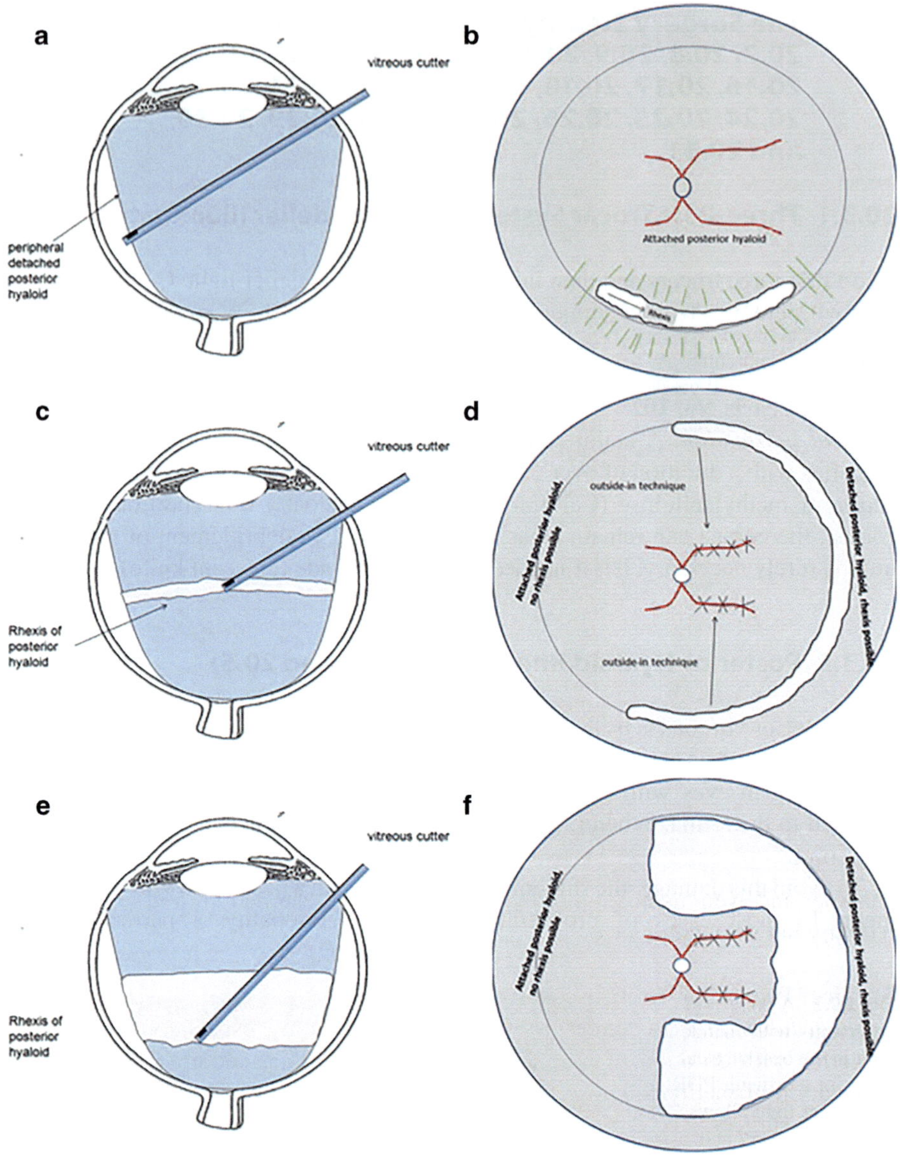

Fig. 20.4 (**a**, **b**) The first important step of diabetic vitrectomy: The posterior hyaloid rhexis. (**c**, **d**) Perform a rhexis of the detached posterior hyaloid on the height of the equator. (**e**, **f**) Then continue with the removal of the vitreous to the nasal and temporal arcades. The attached (nasal) hyaloid cannot be removed in this stage (**f**)

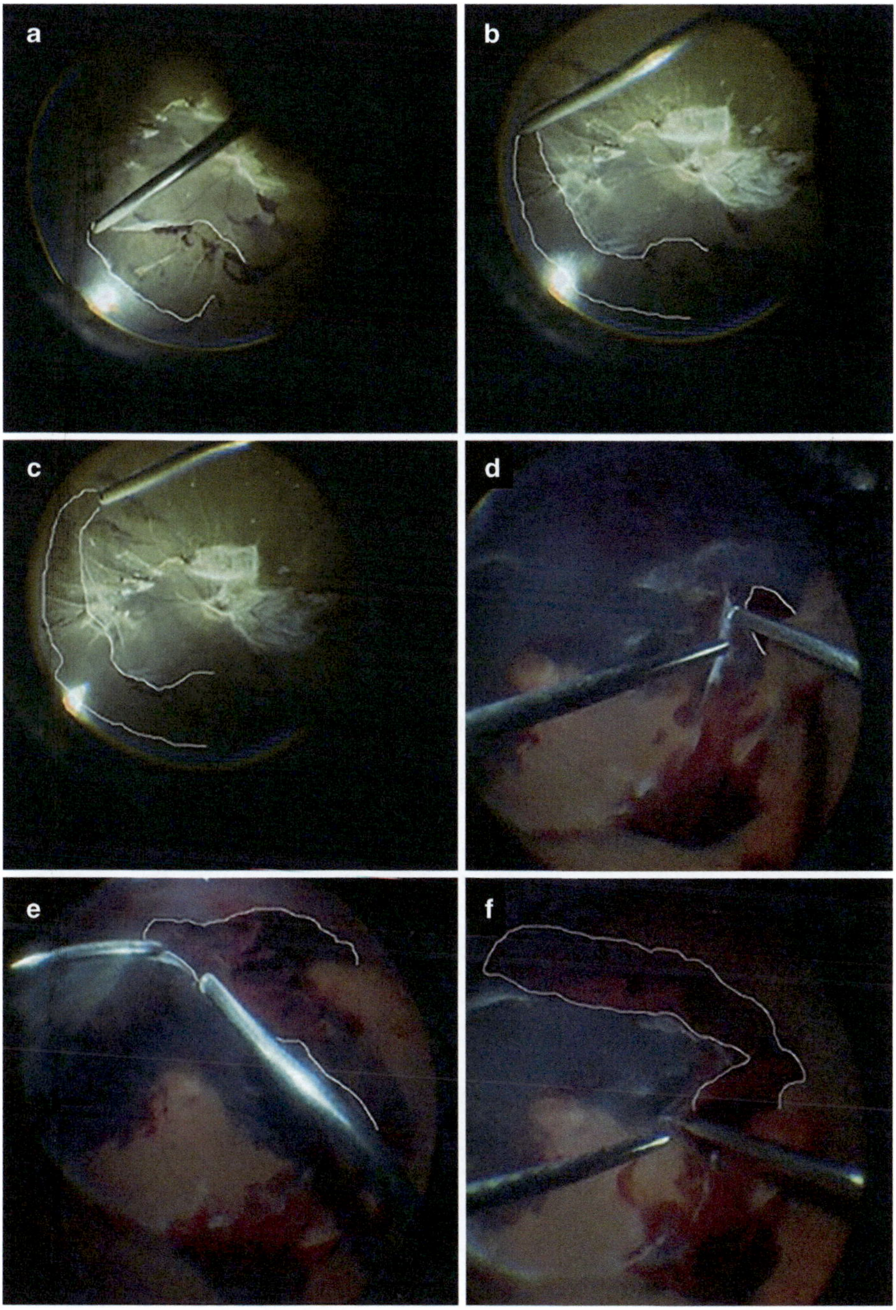

Fig. 20.5 (**a**) Posterior hyaloid rhexis without subhyaloidal hemorrhage. (**b**) Be careful not to damage the retina. (**c**) Perform a posterior hyaloid rhexis of the detached hyaloid. A rhexis of the attached hyaloid is not possible. (**d**) An opening of the posterior hyaloid with presence of subhyaloidal hemorrhage. (**e**) Use the vitreous cutter with a low cutting frequency such as 1000 cuts/min. (**f**) Open the posterior hyaloid as far as possible, i.e., try to perform a round rhexis as far as possible

detachment is present. This means that the vitreous is still attached centrally but partially detached in the mid-periphery. Try to find where the peripheral vitreous is detached. Create here an opening of the posterior hyaloid on the height of the equator. Then remove the vitreous along the posterior vitreous face (Figs. 20.4 and 20.5) on a constant level in a circular fashion (posterior hyaloid rhexis). Do not perform a posterior hyaloid rhexis in the area where the posterior hyaloid is attached.

Then carefully vitrectomize further from the periphery toward the beginning of the tractional membranes. Be careful that you do not exert any strain on the membranes. If the surgeon succeeds with the posterior hyaloid rhexis, he or she can continue removing the tractional membranes bimanually.

20.3.3 Removal of Tractional Membranes

The fibrovascular membranes are usually located along the vascular arcades. The membranes are removed together with the posterior hyaloid. The way to success is bimanual delamination (Fig. 20.6).

20.3.4 Instruments for the Removal of Proliferations

For lifting the membranes, both the 27G endgripping forceps and the backflush instrument are suitable. The forceps grasp the membrane and the flute needle elevates the membrane through aspiration force. For manipulation of the membrane, use the vacuum cleaner, the 27G retrobulbar cannula (Atkinson, Beaver Visitec), the curved scissors, and the vitreous cutter.

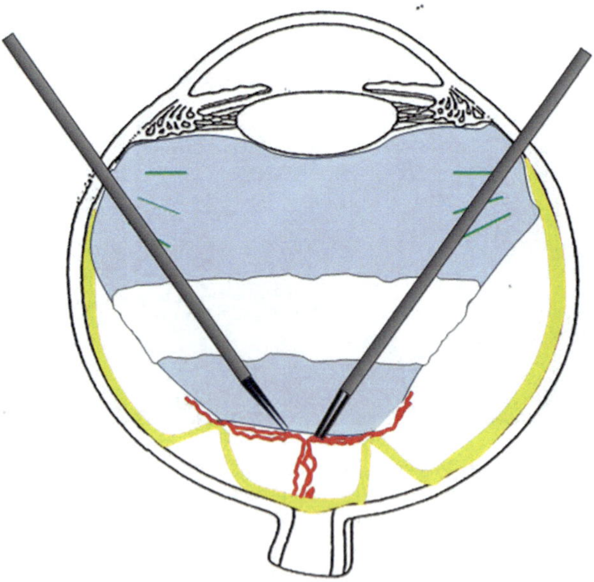

Fig. 20.6 The next and most difficult step is the bimanual removal of fibrovascular membranes

- *Delamination of Membranes with 27G Atkinson Cannula and 27G Vacuum Cleaner or 25G Knob Spatula*

This instrument is suitable for opening of the posterior hyaloid or delamination of flat membranes. The membrane can be lifted up with the blunt cannula and then removed with the microforceps (Figs. 20.7, 20.8, and 20.9).

Grasp the peripheral portion of the membrane with the Eckardt forceps or a backflush instrument in one hand and delaminate the membrane with the knob spatula (Figs. 20.10, 20.11, and 20.12) or the vacuum cleaner in the other hand (Figs. 20.13, 20.14, 20.15, and 20.16).

- *Dissection of Membranes with 27G Curved or 25G Straight Scissors*

The membranes are partially attached by "tissue bridges" to the retina. These bridges have to be identified by careful delamination and then be cut with the straight or curved scissors (Fig. 20.17). The vertical scissors can be used for horizontal tissue bridges. The tractional membranes are dissected and removed through a constant change of instruments between delamination and cauterization. If a bleeding occurs during this step, then perform a hemostasis.

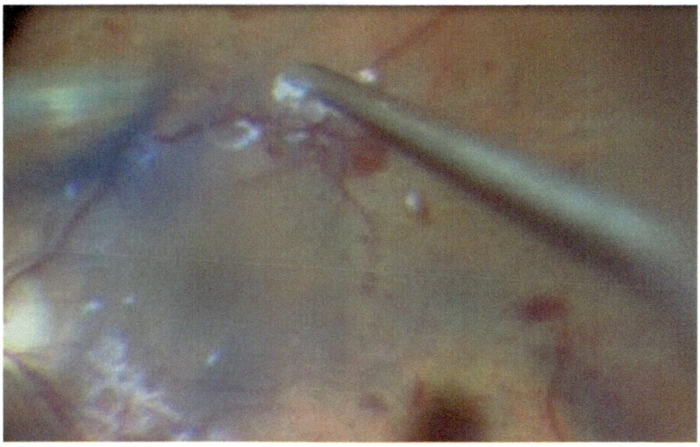

Fig. 20.7 Create an opening in the posterior hyaloid with the 27G blunt cannula (Atkinson, B&D)

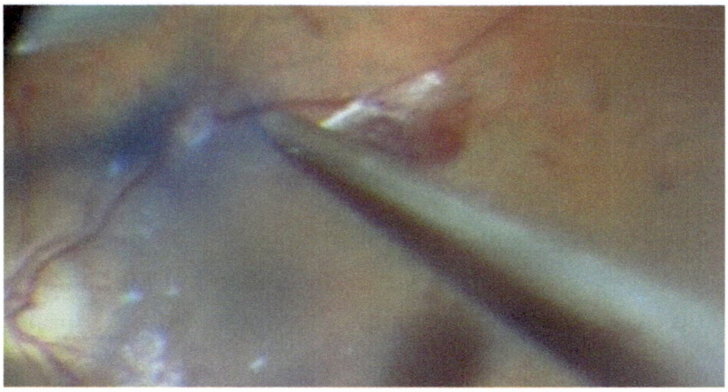

Fig. 20.8 Enlarge the opening in the posterior hyaloid

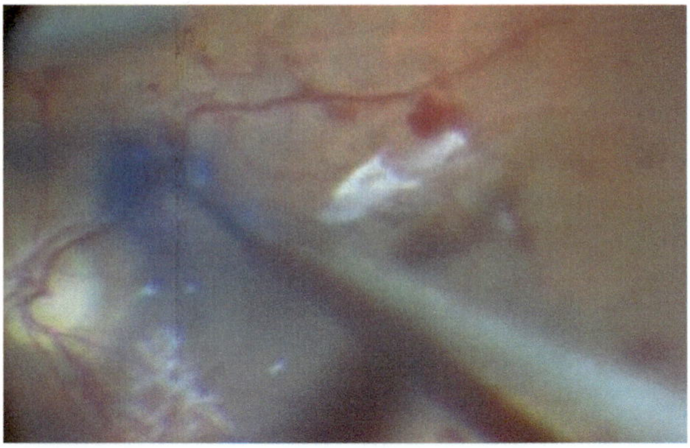

Fig. 20.9 The blunt cannula (25G and 27G) is a very convenient instrument for opening of the posterior hyaloid and for delamination of membranes

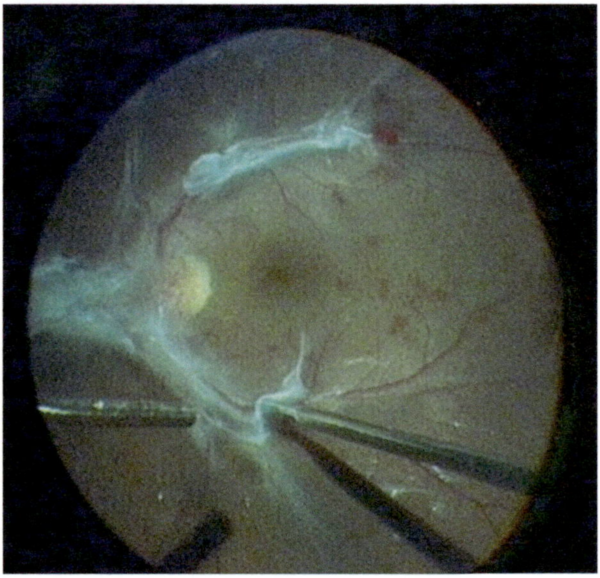

Fig. 20.10 Delaminate the membrane with a knob spatula or a vacuum cleaner

- *Removal of Dissected Membranes with Vitreous Cutter*

Grasp the membrane with intravitreal forceps, and hold it in the middle of the vitreous cavity. Then cut it with the vitreous cutter (1000–2000 cuts/min) (Figs. 20.18 and 20.19).

Surgical Pearls No. 103
Peeling and choroidal hemorrhage: Do not pull a membrane forwards to the lens—you may cause a choroidal hemorrhage. Pull the membrane parallel to the retina.

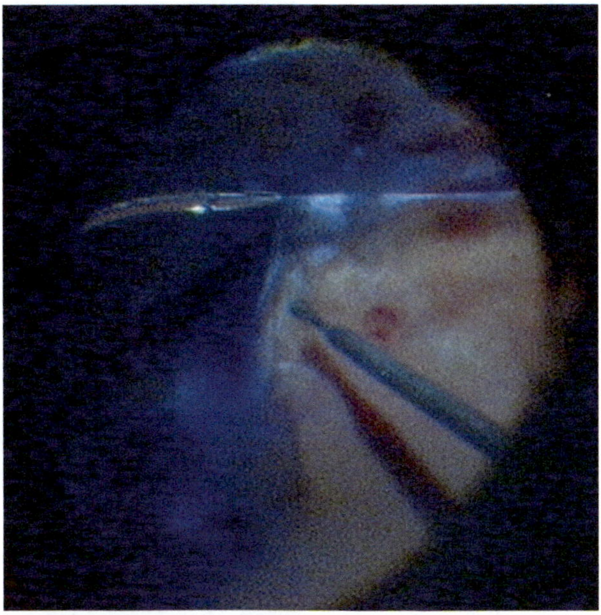

Fig. 20.11 If necessary stain the posterior hyaloid with trypan blue, and delaminate it from the retina

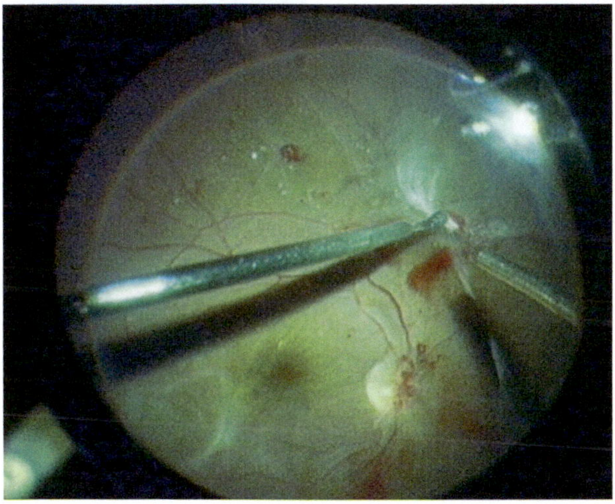

Fig. 20.12 Use a knob spatula or Charles flute needle with silicone tip or membrane pic for delamination

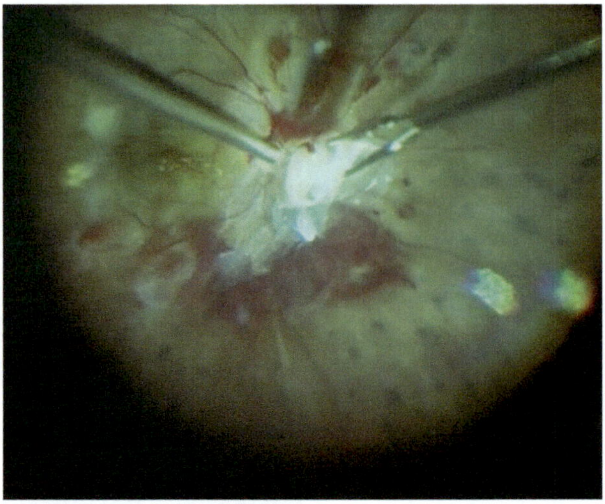

Fig. 20.13 You can also remove membranes with a silicone tip flute needle and a forceps

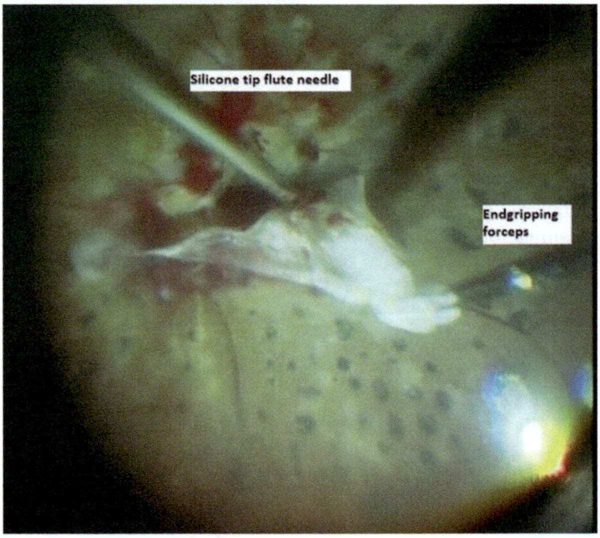

Fig. 20.14 Always pull the membrane parallel to the retina. Pulling vertically may cause a choroidal bleeding

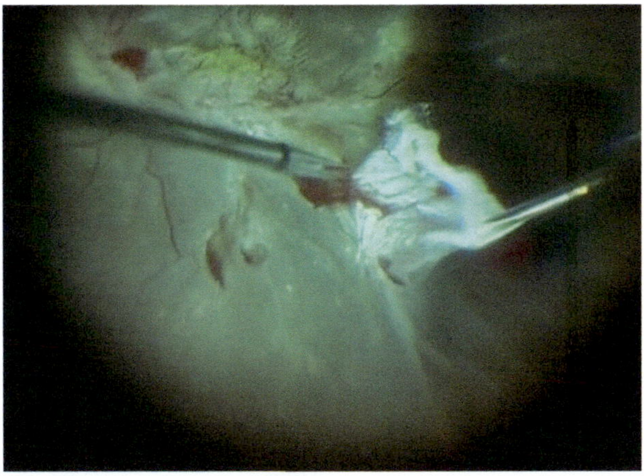

Fig. 20.15 For delamination of membranes, the knob spatula and the silicone tip flute needle are superior to the membrane pic

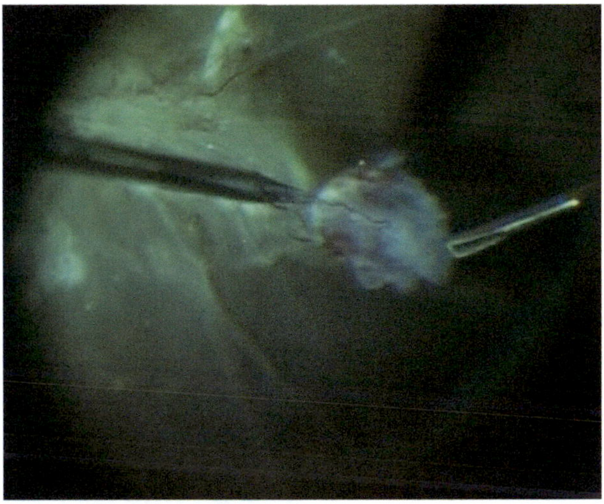

Fig. 20.16 The surgeon's right hand pulls the membrane parallel to the retina, and the left hand cuts the tissue bridges with the straight scissors

20.3.5 Hemostasis

There are different methods to stop intraoperative bleeding, depending on its severity:

- *Slight Bleeding*

Increase the intraocular pressure to approximately 40 mmHg.

Aspirate the blood with the left hand, and cauterize the bleeding source with endodiathermy or the laser probe in the right hand. Inside the arcades, we cauterize the bleeding sites with laser. Outside the arcades, we cauterize retinal bleeding sites with endodiathermy (Figs. 20.20 and 20.21). Start with relatively low energy, as too

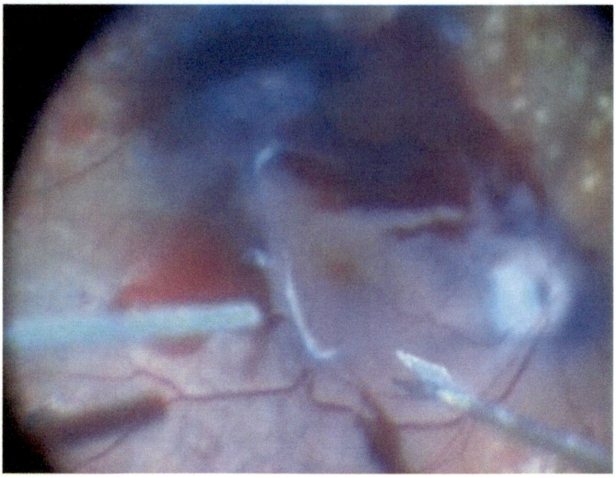

Fig. 20.17 The 27G curved microscissors allows precise cutting of vitreoretinal adhesions

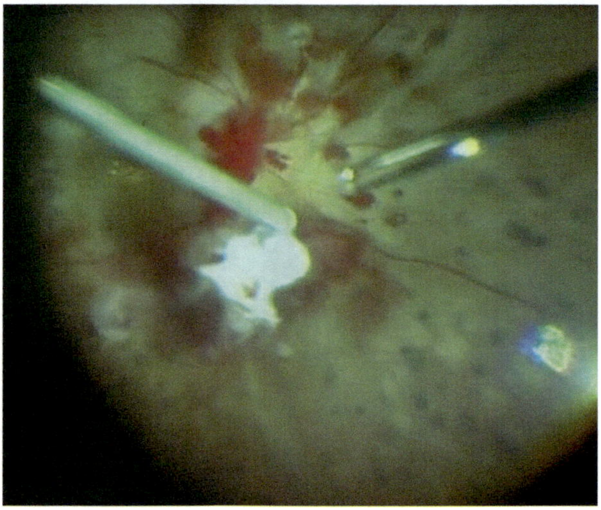

Fig. 20.18 Hold the membrane in the middle of the vitreous cavity, and cut the membrane

vigorous endodiathermy may create breaks in ischemic retinal tissue. Avoid diathermy on the disk; this may cause destruction of nerve fiber bundles. If the bleeding occurs within the temporal vascular arcades, then use a laser probe to cauterize the bleeding instead. Often you have to work bimanually.

- *Moderate Bleeding and Bleeding at the Optic Disc*

In the case of a strong bleeding source, hold the knob spatula or the vitreous cutter for about 1 minute onto the bleeding source (1 minute is longer than most people think).

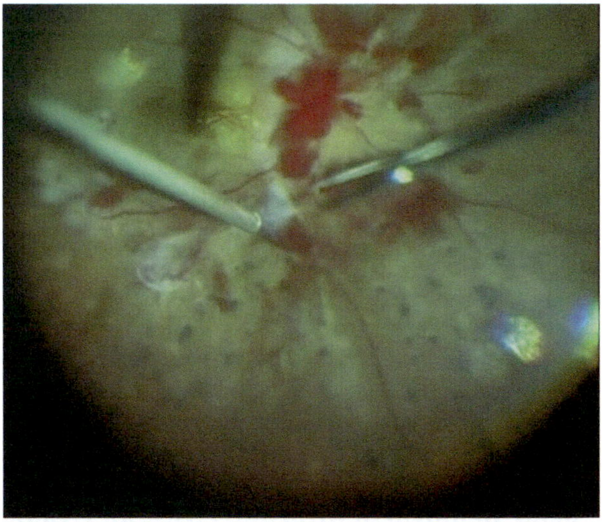

Fig. 20.19 The membrane is completely removed

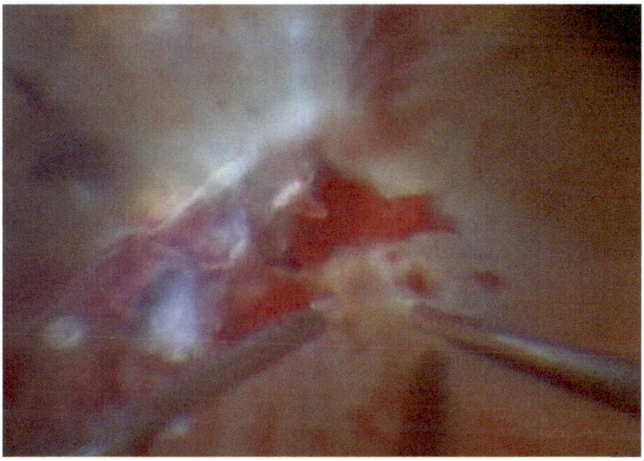

Fig. 20.20 Perform a meticulous hemostasis. We use endodiathermy outside the temporal arcades and laser inside the temporal arcades

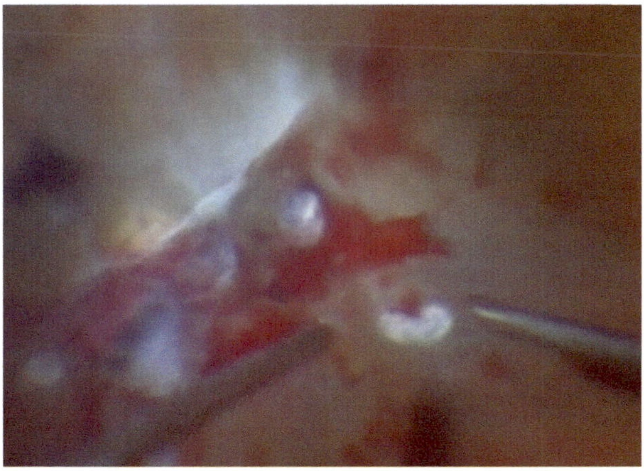

Fig. 20.21 Also hemostasis is performed bimanually. The surgeon's left hand holds the Charles flute needle and aspirates the blood. The right hand cauterizes the bleeding source

- *Severe Bleeding*

If the bleeding is so severe that there is no view of the fundus, and despite aspiration with the flute needle it does not clear up, then you should perform a fluid x air exchange. The bleeding will stop. Now try to cauterize the bleeding source with endodiathermy or compress it mechanically with the knob spatula. The vitrectomy can also be continued in an air-filled vitreous cavity. Another alternative is silicone oil. One can either work under silicone oil or end surgery with a silicone oil tamponade with Avastin.

Surgical Pearls No. 104

Intraoperative hemorrhage and adrenaline: If there is constant bleeding from several vessels under surgery, then add adrenaline to the BSS bottle. Adrenaline will constrict the vessels and reduce the bleeding.

20.3.6 Removal of Attached Posterior Hyaloid in the Periphery (Figs. 20.22, 20.23, and 20.24)

Trim the peripheral vitreous and the vitreous base with a bimanual technique. Indent the sclera with the sclera depressor and cut the vitreous with the vitreous cutter.

After the removal of the posterior hyaloid from the posterior pole, remove the residual attached posterior hyaloid in the periphery. Remember: The posterior hyaloid in the periphery is in the most cases only partially detached. The detached part with a posterior hyaloid rhexis was opened in the beginning. Now the attached part must be removed. This part is firmly attached to the retina (Fig. 20.22). Simply inducing a PVD with the vitreous cutter does not work because this creates retinal tears. The surgeon must delaminate the posterior hyaloid with a bimanual technique (Fig. 20.23). The posterior hyaloid has to be removed up to the vitreous base (Fig. 20.24).

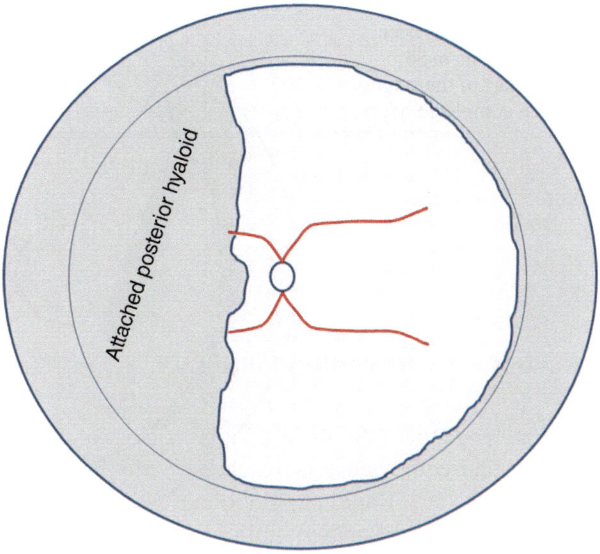

Fig. 20.22 In the initial steps a vitreous rhexis was performed, and the vitreous was removed to the arcades. Then the fibrovascular membranes together with the central posterior were removed. The final step is the removal of the attached posterior hyaloid in the periphery—often on the nasal side

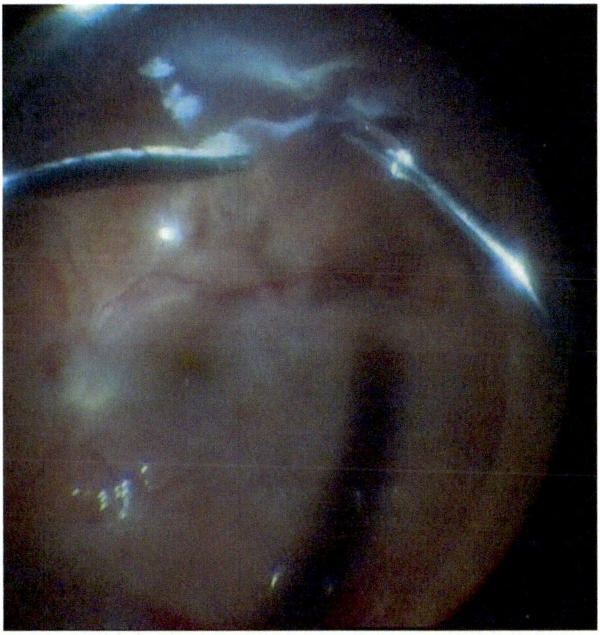

Fig. 20.23 Using bimanual technique—with an endgripping forceps and a knob spatula—the residual posterior hyaloid is removed from the disc to the ora serrata

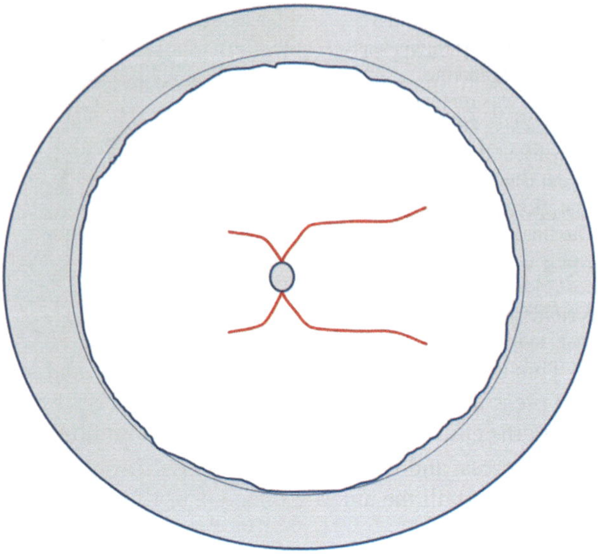

Fig. 20.24 Now a complete PVD has been performed. The most difficult part of the surgery has been completed

20.3.7 Panretinal Photocoagulation (PRP) Under BSS (Figs. 20.25 and 20.26)

The next step is a PRP. Perform a dense PRP from the arcades up to the ora serrata. By using the scleral depressor, the surgeon can laser treat up to the ora serrate.

After endolaser photocoagulation check if a new hemorrhage has occurred at the central pole, and treat it before moving on to the tamponade.

Surgical Pearls No. 105

Postoperative vitreous hemorrhages are the number one problem following vitrectomy for proliferative diabetic retinopathy. In order to lower the rate of this complication, be meticulous with hemostasis. Watch out for small oozing bleeding sites after PRP has been performed. Even small collections of blood point at continuous bleeding sites that should be treated before closing up.

20.3.8 Fluid Against Air Exchange (Figs. 20.27 and 20.28)

Perform a fluid against air exchange. In the case of 25G or 27G, use active aspiration with a backflush instrument or use the vitreous cutter.

Air bubbles behind IOL: During a fluid-air exchange, the water condenses at the posterior surface of the IOL in the area of the capsulotomy, thereby greatly impairing the view of the fundus. It can either be removed with a flute instrument or injection of viscoelastics onto the posterior surface of the IOL.

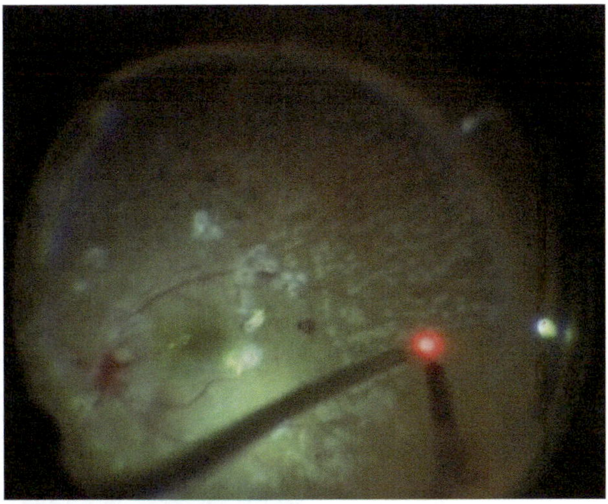

Fig. 20.25 Perform a dense PRP from the arcades to the ora serrata

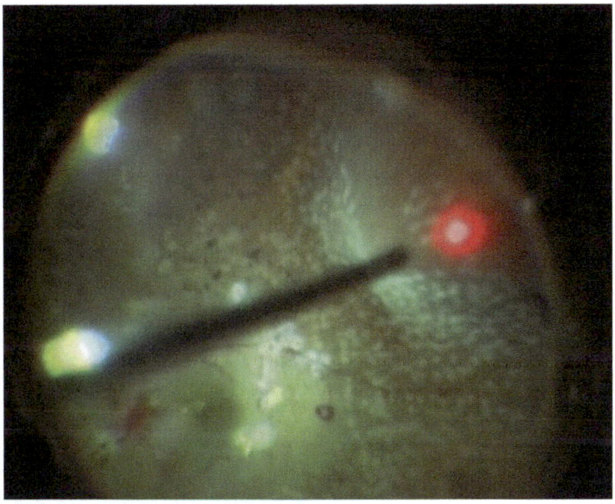

Fig. 20.26 Use preferably a curved laser probe in order to perform a laser treatment up to the ora serrata

20.3.9 Intravitreal Avastin

We always inject 0.2 ml of Avastin intravitreally at the end of a diabetic case. We use 0.2 ml and not 0.1 ml because the vitreous is removed.

20.3.10 Internal Postoperative Tamponade

In young type 1 diabetics, we prefer 15% C2F6 as postoperative tamponade because it causes less postoperative secondary glaucoma compared to silicone oil. Silicone oil may result in secondary glaucoma after silicone oil removal. We use silicone oil

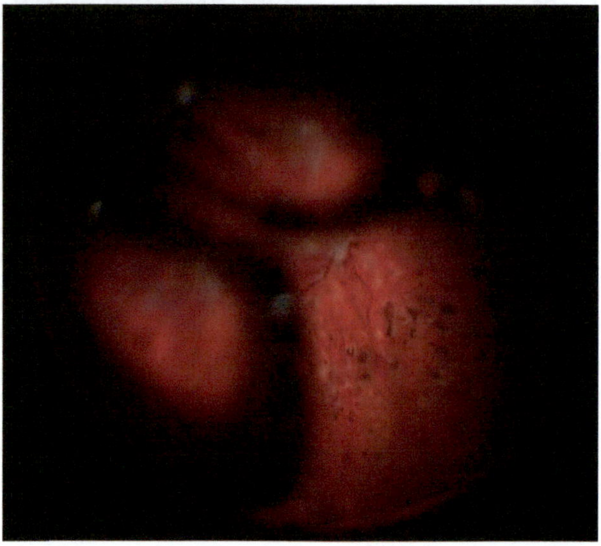

Fig. 20.27 We perform in almost all cases a fluid against air exchange. If the vitreous cavity is filled with PFCL, we perform a PFCL against air exchange and then the tamponade. In this case with a detached retina, we would use 1000 cSts silicone oil

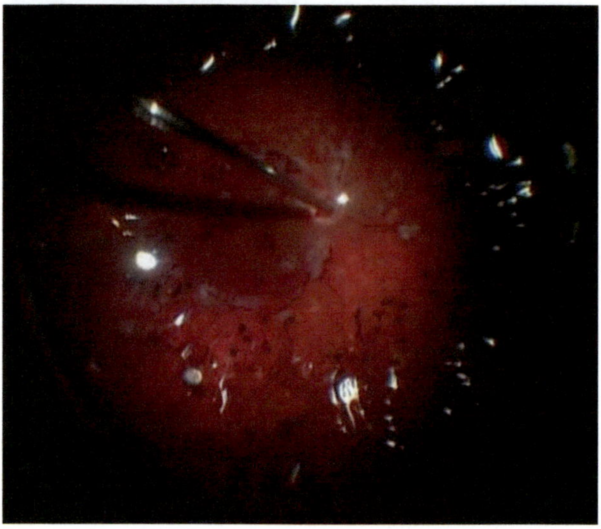

Fig. 20.28 For 23G we use a Charles flute needle with passive aspiration. For 25G and 27G, we use Charles flute needle with active aspiration

in difficult cases, extensive retinal bleeding, and in functionally only the eyes. In old type 2 diabetics, we use in the most cases only an air tamponade.

- *Silicone Oil Tamponade* (Figs. 20.29 and 20.30)

In the case of a silicone oil, we use in most cases 1000/1300 cSts silicone oil. Inject the silicone oil under BIOM view. In the case of overfill, cut the infusion line and excessive silicone oil will escape. Inject a 0.1–0.2 ml of Avastin bubble into the silicone oil bubble.

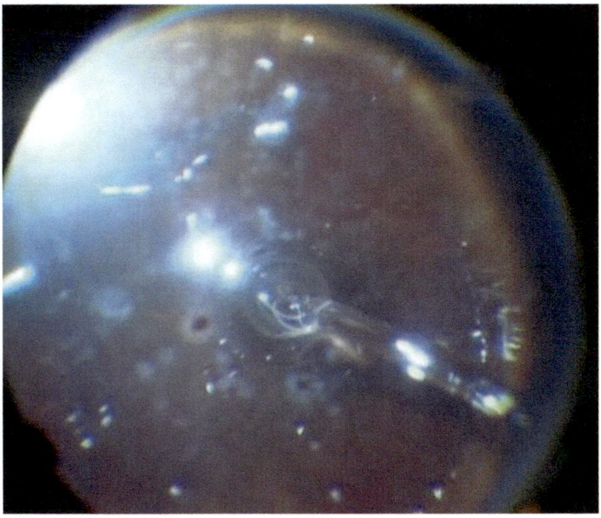

Fig. 20.29 Injection of 1000 cSts silicone oil into an air-filled vitreous cavity. If possible, try to perform an air against silicone oil exchange. It is technically much easier than a PFCL against silicone oil exchange

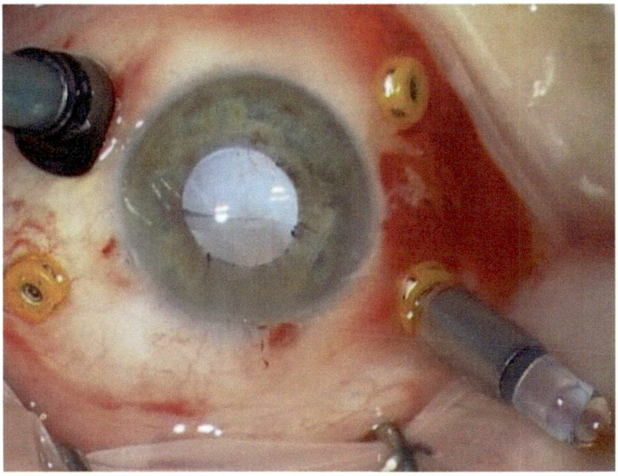

Fig. 20.30 The excessive silicone oil can escape and overfill is avoided. Then 0.2 ml of Avastin is injected into the silicone oil bubble

Surgical Pearls No. 106
Lens-sparing vitrectomy: In young diabetic patients, we experienced good results with a lens-sparing vitrectomy and then a C_2F_6 gas or 1000 cSts silicone oil tamponade. Even after 10–20 years, the lens hardly opacifies.

20.3.11 Removal of Trocars (Fig. 20.31)

If silicone oil is used, one should suture the sclerotomies, otherwise oil might flow under the conjunctiva. Suture 25G sclerotomies with Vicryl 8-0. 27G sclerotomies require usually no suture.

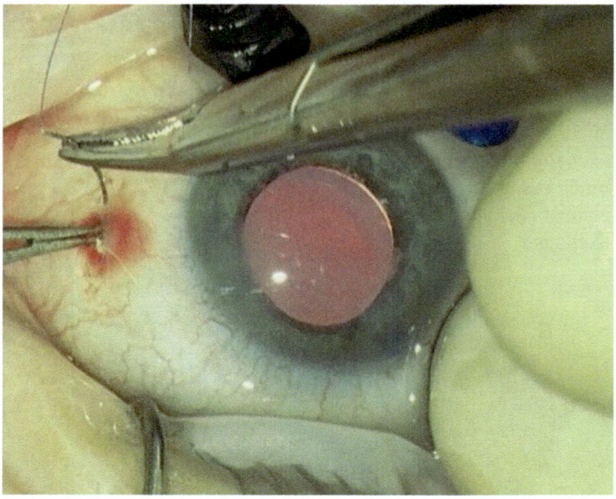

Fig. 20.31 The sclerotomies are sutured with Vicryl 8-0

20.4 Complications

1. *Injury of a retinal artery* during peeling. Fibrovascular membranes may hide the temporal arcade. Be careful with delamination here. Begin with blunt instruments such as a knob spatula or a vacuum cleaner. Prefer a curved scissors (27G curved scissors, DORC).
2. *Extensive bleeding*: (1) Try to cauterize the bleeding vessel. (2) Place the tip of the vitreous cutter or the knob spatula onto the bleeding vessel for 1 minute. (3) Perform a BSS against air exchange and try to cauterize the vessel. (4) Inject silicone oil and anti-VEGF, and close the case; reoperate when the bleeding has subsided.

20.5 FAQ

Which type of silicone oil you use?
We use routinely 1000/1300 cSts silicone oil. We remove the oil after 3 months. We see no advantage of using 5000 cSts oil in diabetic cases, even with tractional detachment.

What procedure do you recommend in the case of an eye with iris rubeosis, cataract, and vitreous hemorrhage?
Do not operate this eye before the iris rubeosis is treated and has disappeared. We would inject immediately 0.1 ml of Avastin. After 1 month, we would perform a combined phacoemulsification + IOL implantation + intravitreal 0.1 ml of Avastin. Again 1 month later we would perform a vitrectomy.

What procedure do you recommend in case of a young type 1 diabetic with PDR and poor compliance?

I would perform an immediate Avastin injection in both eyes. One month later I would schedule a laser coagulation (LIO) in general anesthesia (Figs. 20.32 and 20.33). And again 1 month later, I would perform a lens-sparing vitrectomy if necessary.

What procedure do you recommend in case of an old type 2 diabetic with vitreous hemorrhage secondary to diabetes?

I would schedule a phaco + Avastin. One month later I would perform a vitrectomy with laser, Avastin, and air tamponade.

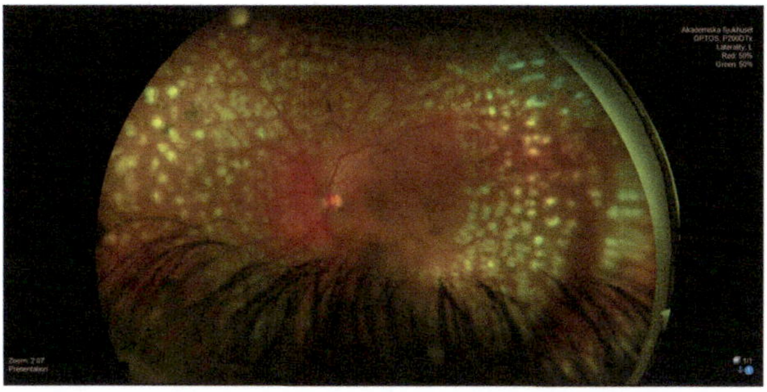

Fig. 20.32 The retina was treated from the temporal arcades to the ora serrata with 1879 laser effects

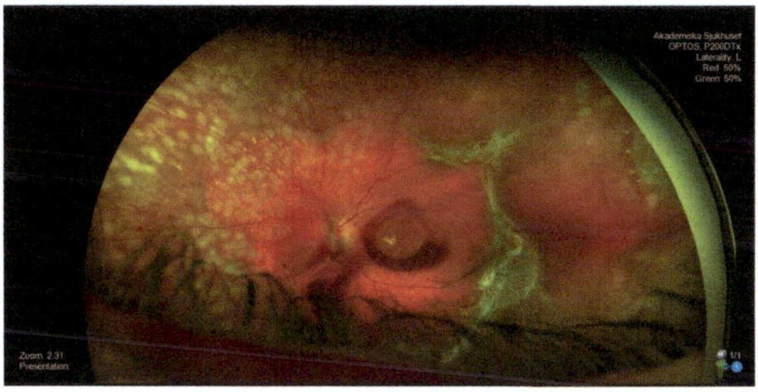

Fig. 20.33 This eye was treated with 1500 laser effects

Bibliography

1. Williamson TH. Vitreoretinal surgery. 3rd ed. Berlin Heidelberg: Springer; 2013.
2. Narendran V, Kothari AR. Principles and practice of vitreoretinal surgery. New Delhi: Jaypee Brothers Medical Publishers (P) Ltd; 2014.
3. Schachat AP. Ryan's retina. 6th ed. Amsterdam: Elsevier Inc; 2018.
4. Wang B, Toslak D, Alam MN, et al. Contact-free trans-pars-planar illumination enables snapshot fundus camera for nonmydriatic wide field photography [J]. Sci Rep. 2018;8(1):8768.
5. Fung AT, Galvin J, Tran T. Epiretinal membrane: a review [J]. Clin Experiment Ophthalmol. 2021;49(3):289–308.
6. Fu Z, Sun Y, Cakir B, et al. Targeting neurovascular interaction in retinal disorders [J]. Int J Mol Sci. 2020;21(4):1503.
7. Sodhi A, Leung LS, Do DV, et al. Recent trends in the management of rhegmatogenous retinal detachment [J]. Surv Ophthalmol. 2008;53(1):50–67.
8. Daruich A, Matet A, Moulin A, et al. Mechanisms of macular edema: beyond the surface [J]. Prog Retin Eye Res. 2018;63:20–68.
9. Gupta B, Wong R, Sivaprasad S, et al. Surgical and visual outcome following 20-gauge vitrectomy in proliferative diabetic retinopathy over a 10-year period, evidence for change in practice [J]. Eye (Lond). 2012;26(4):576–82.
10. Afrashi F, Erakgun T, Akkin C, et al. Conventional buckling surgery or primary vitrectomy with silicone oil tamponade in rhegmatogenous retinal detachment with multiple breaks [J]. Graefes Arch Clin Exp Ophthalmol. 2004;242(4):295–300.
11. Kuhn F, Aylward B. Rhegmatogenous retinal detachment: a reappraisal of its pathophysiology and treatment [J]. Ophthalmic Res. 2014;51(1):15–31.
12. Stalmans P, Benz MS, Gandorfer A, et al. Enzymatic vitreolysis with ocriplasmin for vitreomacular traction and macular holes [J]. N Engl J Med. 2012;367(7):606–15.
13. Snead MP, Mcninch AM, Poulson AV, et al. Stickler syndrome, ocular-only variants and a key diagnostic role for the ophthalmologist [J]. Eye (Lond). 2011;25(11):1389–400.
14. Sweitzer BJ. Preoperative medical testing and preparation for ophthalmic surgery [J]. Ophthalmol Clin N Am. 2006;19(2):163–77.
15. Dwyer T, Burns D, Nauth A, et al. Regional anesthesia and acute compartment syndrome: principles for practice [J]. Reg Anesth Pain Med. 2021;46(12):1091–9.
16. Steel DH, Charles S. Vitrectomy fluidics [J]. Ophthalmologica. 2011;226(Suppl 1):27–35.
17. Rizzo S, Genovesi-Ebert F, Belting C. The combined use of perfluorohexyloctane (F6H8) and silicone oil as an intraocular tamponade in the treatment of severe retinal detachment [J]. Graefes Arch Clin Exp Ophthalmol. 2006;244(6):709–16.
18. Stanescu-Segall D, Jackson TL. Vital staining with indocyanine green: a review of the clinical and experimental studies relating to safety [J]. Eye (Lond). 2009;23(3):504–18.
19. Gandorfer A, Messmer EM, Ulbig MW, et al. Indocyanine green selectively stains the internal limiting membrane [J]. Am J Ophthalmol. 2001;131(3):387–8.

Z. Zhang, U. Spandau, *Vitreoretinal Surgery*, https://doi.org/10.1007/978-3-032-25271-5

20. Okada Y, Nakamura S, Kubo E, et al. Analysis of changes in corneal shape and refraction following scleral buckling surgery [J]. Jpn J Ophthalmol. 2000;44(2):132–8.
21. Okamoto F, Yamane N, Okamoto C, et al. Changes in higher-order aberrations after scleral buckling surgery for rhegmatogenous retinal detachment [J]. Ophthalmology. 2008;115(7):1216–21.
22. Sato T, Kawasaki T, Okuyama M, et al. Refractive changes following scleral buckling surgery in juvenile retinal detachment [J]. Retina. 2003;23(5):629–35.
23. Lai MM, Lai JC, Lee WH, et al. Comparison of retrobulbar and sub-Tenon's capsule injection of local anesthetic in vitreoretinal surgery [J]. Ophthalmology. 2005;112(4):574–9.
24. Bergman L, Bäckmark I, Ones H, et al. Preoperative sub-Tenon's capsule injection of ropivacaine in conjunction with general anesthesia in retinal detachment surgery [J]. Ophthalmology. 2007;114(11):2055–60.
25. Errera MH, Liyanage SE, Moya R, et al. Primary scleral buckling for pediatric rhegmatogenous retinal detachment [J]. Retina. 2015;35(7):1441–9.
26. Lira RP, Takasaka I, Arieta CE, et al. Cryotherapy vs laser photocoagulation in scleral buckle surgery: a randomized clinical trial [J]. Arch Ophthalmol. 2010;128(12):1519–22.
27. Baino F. Scleral buckling biomaterials and implants for retinal detachment surgery [J]. Med Eng Phys. 2010;32(9):945–56.
28. Heimann H, Bartz-Schmidt KU, Bornfeld N, et al. Scleral buckling versus primary vitrectomy in rhegmatogenous retinal detachment: a prospective randomized multicenter clinical study [J]. Ophthalmology. 2007;114(12):2142–54.
29. Sigler EJ, Randolph JC, Calzada JI, et al. Pars plana vitrectomy with medium-term postoperative perfluoro-N-octane for recurrent inferior retinal detachment complicated by advanced proliferative vitreoretinopathy [J]. Retina. 2013;33(4):791–7.
30. Randolph JC, Diaz RI, Sigler EJ, et al. 25-gauge pars plana vitrectomy with medium-term postoperative perfluoro-n-octane for the repair of giant retinal tears [J]. Graefes Arch Clin Exp Ophthalmol. 2016;254(2):253–7.
31. Sigler EJ, Randolph JC, Calzada JI, et al. Anatomical and visual outcomes after two-port pars plana vitrectomy reoperation under silicone oil for epimacular membrane or recurrent retinal detachment [J]. Retina. 2014;34(10):1939–44.
32. Feng X, Li C, Zheng Q, et al. Risk of silicone oil as vitreous tamponade in pars plana vitrectomy: a systematic review and meta-analysis [J]. Retina. 2017;37(11):1989–2000.
33. Erakgun T, Egrilmez S. Surgical outcomes of transconjunctival sutureless 23-gauge vitrectomy with silicone oil injection [J]. Indian J Ophthalmol. 2009;57(2):105–9.
34. Rizzo S, Genovesi-Ebert F, Vento A, et al. Modified incision in 25-gauge vitrectomy in the creation of a tunneled airtight sclerotomy: an ultrabiomicroscopic study [J]. Graefes Arch Clin Exp Ophthalmol. 2007;245(9):1281–8.
35. Heimann H, Zou X, Jandeck C, et al. Primary vitrectomy for rhegmatogenous retinal detachment: an analysis of 512 cases [J]. Graefes Arch Clin Exp Ophthalmol. 2006;244(1):69–78.
36. Mendrinos E, Dang-Burgener NP, Stangos AN, et al. Primary vitrectomy without scleral buckling for pseudophakic rhegmatogenous retinal detachment [J]. Am J Ophthalmol. 2008;145(6):1063–70.
37. Minihan M, Tanner V, Williamson TH. Primary rhegmatogenous retinal detachment: 20 years of change [J]. Br J Ophthalmol. 2001;85(5):546–8.
38. Greenberg PB, Baumal CR. Laser therapy for rhegmatogenous retinal detachment [J]. Curr Opin Ophthalmol. 2001;12(3):171–4.
39. Qiang KT, Shunmugam M, Williamson TH. Characteristics of rhegmatogenous retinal detachments secondary to retinal dialyses [J]. Can J Ophthalmol. 2014;49(2):196–9.
40. Charteris DG, Sethi CS, Lewis GP, et al. Proliferative vitreoretinopathy-developments in adjunctive treatment and retinal pathology [J]. Eye (Lond). 2002;16(4):369–74.
41. Guidry C. The role of Müller cells in fibrocontractive retinal disorders [J]. Prog Retin Eye Res. 2005;24(1):75–86.
42. El GI, Powe DG, Orr G, et al. Apoptosis in proliferative vitreoretinopathy [J]. Invest Ophthalmol Vis Sci. 2004;45(5):1473–9.

43. Khan MA, Brady CJ, Kaiser RS. Clinical management of proliferative vitreoretinopathy: an update [J]. Retina. 2015;35(2):165–75.
44. Wong D, Van Meurs JC, Stappler T, et al. A pilot study on the use of a perfluorohexyloctane/silicone oil solution as a heavier than water internal tamponade agent [J]. Br J Ophthalmol. 2005;89(6):662–5.
45. Heimann H, Stappler T, Wong D. Heavy tamponade 1: a review of indications, use, and complications [J]. Eye (Lond). 2008;22(10):1342–59.
46. Hsu YJ, Hsieh YT, Yeh PT, et al. Combined tractional and rhegmatogenous retinal detachment in proliferative diabetic retinopathy in the anti-VEGF era [J]. J Ophthalmol. 2014;2014:917375.
47. Tao Y, Jiang YR, Li XX, et al. Long-term results of vitrectomy without endotamponade in proliferative diabetic retinopathy with tractional retinal detachment [J]. Retina. 2010;30(3):447–51.
48. Rahimy E, Pitcher JR, Gee CJ, et al. Diabetic tractional retinal detachment repair by vitreoretinal fellows in a county health system [J]. Retina. 2015;35(2):303–9.
49. Gandorfer A, Haritoglou C, Kampik A. Toxicity of indocyanine green in vitreoretinal surgery [J]. Dev Ophthalmol. 2008;42:69–81.
50. Taniuchi S, Hirakata A, Itoh Y, et al. Vitrectomy with or without internal limiting membrane peeling for each stage of myopic traction maculopathy [J]. Retina. 2013;33(10):2018–25.
51. Gass CA, Haritoglou C, Messmer EM, et al. Peripheral visual field defects after macular hole surgery: a complication with decreasing incidence [J]. Br J Ophthalmol. 2001;85(5):549–51.
52. Imai H, Ohta K. Microperimetric determination of retinal sensitivity in areas of dissociated optic nerve fiber layer following internal limiting membrane peeling [J]. Jpn J Ophthalmol. 2010;54(5):435–40.
53. Lin KL, Hirose T, Kroll AJ, et al. Prospects for treatment of pediatric vitreoretinal diseases with vascular endothelial growth factor inhibition [J]. Semin Ophthalmol. 2009;24(2):70–6.
54. Yu H, Li T, Luo Y, et al. Long-term outcomes of vitrectomy for progressive X-linked retinoschisis [J]. Am J Ophthalmol. 2012;154(2):394–402.
55. Trese MT. Enzymatic-assisted vitrectomy [J]. Eye (Lond). 2002;16(4):365–8.
56. Sharma T, Gopal L, Shanmugam MP, et al. Retinal detachment in Marfan syndrome: clinical characteristics and surgical outcome [J]. Retina. 2002;22(4):423–8.
57. Kreissig I. Minimal surgery for retinal detachment. Thieme; 2000. ISBN 3131110619.
58. Heimann H, Bartz-Schmidt KU, et al. Scleral buckling versus primary vitrectomy in rhegmatogenous retinal detachment: a prospective randomized multicenter clinical study. Ophthalmology. 2007;114(12):2142–54.

GPSR Compliance

The European Union's (EU) General Product Safety Regulation (GPSR) is a set of rules that requires consumer products to be safe and our obligations to ensure this.

If you have any concerns about our products, you can contact us on ProductSafety@springernature.com

In case Publisher is established outside the EU, the EU authorized representative is:

Springer Nature Customer Service Center GmbH
Europaplatz 3
69115 Heidelberg, Germany

Batch number: 10726133

Printed by Printforce, the Netherlands